Dentist's Guide to Medical Conditions and Complications

Dentist's Guide to Medical Conditions and Complications

Kanchan M. Ganda, M.D.

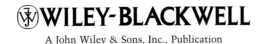
A John Wiley & Sons, Inc., Publication

Edition first published 2008
© 2008 Wiley-Blackwell

Blackwell Munksgaard, formerly an imprint of Blackwell Publishing was acquired by John Wiley & Sons in February 2007. Blackwell's publishing programme has been merged with Wiley's global Scientific, Technical, and Medical business to form Wiley-Blackwell.

Editorial Office
2121 State Avenue, Ames, Iowa 50014-8300, USA

For details of our global editorial offices, for customer services and for information about how to apply for permission to reuse the copyright material in this book please see our website at www.wiley.com/wiley-blackwell.

Disclaimer

Library of Congress Cataloguing-in-Publication Data

Ganda, Kanchan M.
   Dentist's guide to medical conditions and complications / by Kanchan M. Ganda.
      p. ; cm.
   Includes bibliographical references and index.
   ISBN 978-0-8138-0926-7 (alk. paper)
   1. Chronically ill—Dental care.   2. Sick—Dental care.   3. Oral manifestations of general diseases.   I. Title.
   [DNLM: 1. Stomatognathic Diseases—complications.   2. Dental Care—standards.   3. Medical History Taking.   4. Pharmaceutical Preparations,
Dental—administration & dosage.   5. Pharmaceutical Preparations,
Dental—contraindications.   6. Stomatognathic Diseases—diagnosis.   WU 140 G195d 2008]
   RK55.S53G36 2008
   617.6'026—dc22

                                                                    2008007433

A catalogue record for this book is available from the U.S. Library of Congress.

Set in 9.5 on 12 pt Palatino by SNP Best-set Typesetter Ltd., Hong Kong
Printed in Singapore by Markono Print Media Pte Ltd

2   2009

Dedication

This book is dedicated to all my students, past and present; to my late parents, Amrit Devi and Roop Krishan Dewan; and to my family for all their encouragement and loving support.

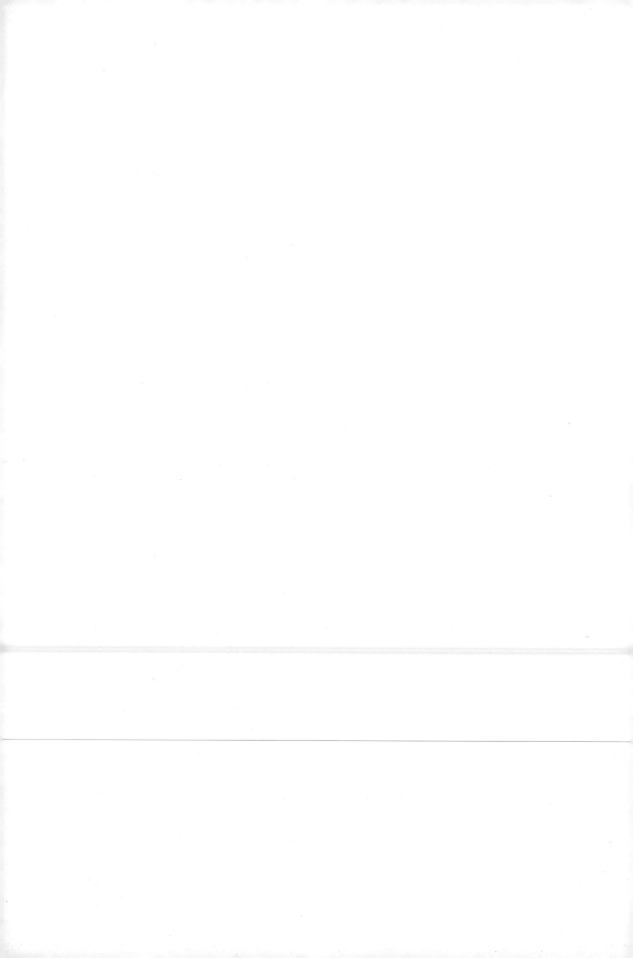

Contents

Acknowledgments

I wish to sincerely thank Dr. Bruce J. Baum, D.M.D., Ph.D., Chief, Gene Therapy and Therapeutics Branch, National Institute of Dental and Craniofacial Research, Bethesda, Maryland, who was instrumental in mentoring and motivating me to publish my work. Dr. Baum's vision for dentistry and the confidence that my work would make a difference is very humbling.

Thanks to my Dean at Tufts University School of Dental Medicine, Dr. Lonnie Norris, D.M.D, M.P.H., and our Dean of Curriculum, Dr. Nancy Arbree, D.D.S., M.S., for making a reality of my vision of integrating medicine into the dental curriculum and experiencing the outcome over the years. I was given the flexibility to create a medicine curriculum for our students and integrate this education through all the four years of dental curriculum. My sincere thanks to Dr. Noshir Mehta, D.M.D, M.S., Chair, Department of General Dentistry, Tufts University School of Dental Medicine, and to Dr. Catherine Hayes, D.M.D., D.M.Sc., Chair, Department of Public Health and Community Services, Tufts University School of Dental Medicine, for their support and critiquing of my work.

To all the past and present medicine course speakers and rotation directors, specialists in their respective fields of medicine, this unique dental education would have been incomplete without your active participation, dedication, and support. I wish to acknowledge and thank you all for your efforts and endless support.

I also would like to thank Patricia DiAngelis, Heidi S. Birnbaum, Lily Parsi, Amanda Jones, and Daniel M. Callahan for their unflagging support and help with the project.

I'd like to thank my son-in-law, Akshat Tewary, Esq., for his help with my book contract, my daughter Kiran for providing her not-so-computer-savvy mother with round-the-clock technical support, and my daughter Anjali and husband Om, both physicians, for the numerous discussions offering their insights about patient care.

Last but not least, I wish to thank all my students, who have been my constant source of inspiration. I could never have experienced the joy of teaching without their active participation and endurance in the learning of medicine!

Kanchan Ganda, M.D.

Introduction: Integration of Medicine in Dentistry

Dental care today holds many challenges for the dental practitioner. Patients live longer, often retaining their own dentition, have one or more medical conditions, and routinely take several medications.

Along with excellence in dentistry, the practicing dentist has the dual task of staying updated with the current concepts of medicine and pharmacology and should rightfully be called the "Physician of the Oral Cavity."

The integration of medicine in the dental curriculum has become a necessity, and this integration must begin with the freshman class for the students to gain maximum benefit and for the change to also gain credibility. The integration of medicine is best achieved when done in a case-based or problem-based format and correlated with the basic sciences, pharmacology, general pathology, oral pathology, and dentistry. There needs to be a true commitment and *constant* reenforcement of the integration in *all* the didactic and clinical courses.

The integration of medicine, pharmacology, and medically compromised patient care is best achieved when done in a pyramidal process, through the four years of dental education.

The foundation should instill a basic knowledge of:

1. Standard and medically compromised patient history taking and physical examination
2. Symptoms and signs of highest-priority illnesses along with the common laboratory tests evaluating those disease states
3. Anesthetics, analgesics, and antibiotics used in dentistry
4. Prescription writing

"Normal" patient assessment, when stressed in the first year, prepares students to better understand the changes prompted by disease states during the second year of their education, when didactic and clinical knowledge of highest-priority illnesses, associated diagnostic laboratory tests, and the vast pharmacopia used for the care of those diseases is added on. Case-based scenarios should be used to solidify this information.

The progressive learning up to the end of the second year prepares the student to "care" for the patient "on paper". With the start of the clinical years, the student is prepared to apply this knowledge toward "actual" patient care during the third and fourth years of education.

During the third year the student should participate in medical and surgical clinical rotations in a hospitalized setting and complete a Hospital Clerkship Program where the student is exposed to head-and-neck cancer care, emergency medicine, critical care, anesthesia, hematology, oncology, transplants, cardiothoracic surgery, etc. This will widen the student's knowledge, broaden clinical perception, and further enhance the link between medicine and dentistry.

During the clinical years, the students should complete faculty-reviewed medical consults for *all* their medically compromised patients, *prior* to dentistry. This patient-by-patient health status review will help correctly translate their didactic patient-care knowledge in the clinical setting.

The text is a compilation of materials needed for the integration of medicine in dentistry. It is a book all dental students *and* dental practitioners will appreciate both as a read and chairside.

The text provides information on epidemiology; physiology; pathophysiology; laboratory tests evaluation; associated pharmacology; dental alerts; and suggested deviations in the use of anesthetics, analgesics, and antibiotics for each disease state discussed.

The student will greatly benefit from the sections detailing history taking and physical examination; clinical and applied pharmacology of dental anesthetics, analgesics, and antibiotics; stress management; and management of medical emergencies in the dental setting.

Dentist's Guide to Medical Conditions and Complications

Patient Assessment

Routine History-Taking and Physical Examination

GENERAL OVERVIEW

Patient Interview Introduction

The primary job of the dental student starting clinical work is to learn to conduct a patient workup thoroughly and efficiently. The heart of every patient workup is a set pattern in sequential order of data collection and analysis.

Patient Workup Sequential Pattern

The sequential pattern of patient workup consists of the following:

1. History and physical examination
2. Laboratory data collection and analysis
3. Diagnostic and therapeutic plan formulation

The first step, the patient interview or the history, is probably the single most important task in the diagnostic patient workup because of its importance in diagnosis and in the development of a good doctor-patient relationship. The provider should have a professional manner that will put the patient at ease. During the interview, always listen carefully to the patient. Use interrogation sparingly or later, to aid a communicating patient or to restrict the rare patient who has a tendency to ramble!

Patient Interview Practical Points

Keep your appearance neat and clean. This will help gain your patient's trust. Always introduce yourself when meeting a patient and refer to the patient as "Mr. John Doe" or "Miss Jane Doe." Do not use first names during the initial encounter. Exchange a few brief pleasantries because this will help both you and the patient feel comfortable and at ease with each other.

Always have a friendly and sincere interest in your patient's problem(s). Always be courteous, respectful, and confidential and show a continued interest while you are with the patient.

Physical Examination Practical Points

Prior to the start of the physical examination let the patient know that you are going to take the pulse and blood pressure and examine the head and neck area. This explanation will enable the patient to understand that you will be "touching" him or her. Your attentive and respectful ways will enhance a good doctor-patient relationship.

The physical examination is an art that is learned by constant repetition. There are many styles and methods for conducting the general examination, and every clinician will ultimately choose one examination sequence to go by. Most clinicians, however, prefer the head-to-foot order. When examining any area of the body, it is usually best to follow an orderly sequence of inspection, palpation, percussion, and auscultation. This sequential routine ensures thoroughness.

The physical examination should always be conducted and assessed in the context of the patient's dental and medical history. The range of "normal" varies from patient to patient.

The student needs to become familiar with the use of the stethoscope and the blood pressure cuff. Fumbling with your equipment or the technique during patient examination will cause you embarrassment. The student also needs to practice the head and neck exam techniques often on friends or family to get a good sense of the normal.

History-Taking and Physical Examination Broad Conclusions

After the history and physical examination is completed, you should, in most cases, be able to answer the following questions:

- The disease states that exist in the patient and whether the patient's problems are acute or chronic
- The organ systems that may be involved
- The differential diagnosis of the patient's problems
- The laboratory tests that will be needed for the evaluation of the disease states
- Confirmation or exclusion of a diagnosis and/or whether to follow the course of a disease state

HISTORY-TAKING DETAILS

The purpose of medical history and physical examination is to collect information from the patient, examine the patient, and understand the patient's problems. The traditional history-taking has several parts, each with a specific purpose. In order to achieve maximum success, the medical history must be accurate, concise, and systematic.

Following is a standard outline in sequential order of the different components of history-taking. The introductory materials in the health history consist of collecting the following information from the patient.

Data Collection

The following information is obtained in all patients to gain a basic understanding of the patient:

Date of the visit: _____   Record Number: _____

Name:
_____ (last)   _____ (first)   _____ (middle)
Home address: _____   Home phone: _____
Business Address: _____   Business phone: _____

Occupation: _____   Date of birth: _____

Sex: M/F/Transgender _____
Marital status: S/M/D/W _____
Height: _____
Weight: _____
Referred by: _____

Chief Complaint

The chief complaint states in the patient's own words the reason for the visit, e.g., "I have a toothache" or "I need a root canal."

Present History

Present history lists, in clear chronological order, the details of the problem or problems for which the patient is seeking care. You will determine by interrogation the timeline of the following:

1. When did the patient's problem(s) begin?
2. Where did the problem(s) begin?
3. What kinds of symptoms did the patient experience?
4. Has the patient had any treatment for the problem(s)?
5. Has the treatment had any effect on the patient's condition?
6. Has the patient's lifestyle been affected by the problem(s)?

Past History

The past history gives you an insight about the health status of the patient until now. Check with the patient for the presence or absence of diseases by eliciting the **symptoms and signs** associated with the disease states. It is best to access the disease states with the patient in **alphabetical** order to ensure you address each disease state and not miss anything. Check by interrogation the following disease states:

Anemia

Determine the presence or absence of the nutritional, congenital, and acquired or chronic disease-associated anemias.

Bleeding Disorders

Determine the presence or absence of the congenital and acquired types of bleeding disorders.

Cardiorespiratory Disorders

Determine whether the patient has a history of angina, myocardial infarction, transient ischemic attacks (TIAs), cerebrovascular attacks (CVAs/strokes), hypertension, rheumatic heart disease, asthma, tuberculosis, bronchitis, sinusitis, and chronic obstructive pulmonary disease (COPD).

Drugs/Medications

Determine the patient's current medications. Check for prescribed, herbal, and over-the-counter (OTC) medications. Determine whether the patient is currently on corticosteroids or has been on them, by mouth or by injection, for 2 weeks or longer within the past 2 years. Check whether the patient has known allergies to any drugs, such as NSAIDS, aspirin, codeine, morphine, penicillin, sulpha antimicrobials, bisulfites, metabisulfites, or local anesthetics.

Endocrine Disorders

Check for diabetes, hyperthyroidism, hypothyroidism, parathyroid disorders, and adrenal disorders (Addison's disease or Cushing's syndrome).

Fits or Faints

Check for the presence of different kinds of seizures: grand mal epilepsy, petit mal epilepsy, temporal lobe or psychomotor epilepsy, or localized motor seizures.

Gastrointestinal Disorders

Check for oral ulcerations, esophagitis, gastritis, peptic ulcerations, Crohn's disease, celiac disease, ulcerative colitis, diverticulitis, polyps, and hemorrhoids.

Hospital Admissions

Determine the cause or causes for admission and whether the patient had any history of accidents or injuries. Determine whether the patient was given any anesthesia, either local or general. Determine whether there were any complications during the hospital admission due to the anesthesia or due to the medical/surgical condition for which the patient was admitted. Determine whether the patient was given any blood transfusion during hospitalization.

Immunological Diseases

Check for lupus, Sjögrens syndrome, rheumatoid arthritis, and polyarthritis nodosa.

Infectious Diseases

Check for infectious diseases of childhood: measles, mumps, chicken pox, streptococcus pharyngitis, rheumatic fever, scarlet fever. Also check for infectious diseases of adulthood: sexually transmitted diseases (STDs), hepatitis, HIV infection, and infectious mononucleosis.

Jaundice or Liver Disease

If the patient is jaundiced or has had jaundice, determine the cause. Is it due to viral hepatitis, alcoholic hepatitis, or gallstones? Determine whether there is any history of gallbladder dysfunction. Check whether there is any indication of improper liver function.

Kidney Disorders

Determine whether there is any indication of kidney dysfunction, renal stones, urinary tract infections, renal disease, renal failure, or renal transplant.

Likelihood of Pregnancy

Determine the date of the patient's last menstrual period (LMP) and whether the patient is pregnant. Always let the patient know that prior to dental radiographs, you need to know whether the patient is pregnant. You need to also know the pregnancy status as there are certain anesthetics, analgesics, and antibiotics that are contraindicated during pregnancy.

Musculoskeletal Disorders

Check for osteoporosis and other causes of impaired bone metabolism, Paget's disease, osteoarthritis, rheumatoid arthritis, psoriatic arthritis, gout, muscular dystrophy, polymyositis, and myasthenia gravis.

Neurological Disorders

Check for cranial nerve disorders, headaches, facial pains, migraine, multiple sclerosis, motor neuron disease, transient ischemic attacks (TIAs), or cerebrovascular accidents (CVAs) associated neurological deficits, Parkinson's disease, and peripheral neuropathies.

Obstetric and Gynecological Disorders

Check for conditions or diseases that can lead to bleeding or anemia. Also check for any tumors needing chemotherapy or radiotherapy.

Psychiatric Disease

Check for personality disorders, neuroses, anxiety, phobias, hysteria, psychoses, schizophrenia, and posttraumatic stress disorder (PTSD).

Radiation Therapy

Check for any radiation to the head and neck region and the rads or Gy of radiation received.

Skin Disorders

Lichen planus, phemphigus, herpes simplex, herpes zoster, eczema, unhealed skin lesions, and urticaria (itching of the skin) are conditions that should be checked for.

Tetanus

Determine the patient's immunization status for tetanus, hepatitis, influenza, and pneumonia.

Violence

Check for domestic violence and elder or child abuse.

Wound

Determine the patient's wound-healing capacity.

Personal History

In this part of the history, we try to get an insight into the patient's lifestyle, occupation, and habits. In the lifestyle component an attempt is made to understand what constitutes a typical day for the patient. What does the patient do for recreation, relaxation, etc.? What is the patient's job like? Are there any job-related toxic exposures? Is there any history of alcohol, coffee, or tea intake? How much of these does the patient consume? Is there any history of diarrhea or vomiting?

Is there any history of smoking cigarettes or using "recreational" drugs such as marijuana, cocaine, or amphetamines? Has the patient ever used intravenous (IV) drugs or swapped needles? Has the patient been exposed to any infectious diseases or sexually transmitted diseases (STDs)? Does the patient use any herbal medications or over-the-counter medications?

Does the patient use diet pills, birth control pills, laxatives, analgesics (aspirin, acetaminophen, NSAIDS, and other pain medications), or cough/cold medications?

Family History

Once the patient's medical history is completed, it is important to assess the health of the immediate family members. Determine whether certain common diseases run in the family or if a familial disease pattern exists. Determine the age and health of the patient's parents, siblings, and children. If any member is deceased, the age and cause of death is established.

Diseases with a strong hereditary component or tendency for familial clustering are sought. These diseases are coronary artery disease (CAD), heart disease, diabetes mellitus (DM), hypertension (Htn), stroke (CVA), asthma, allergies, arthritis, anemia, cancer, kidney disease, or psychiatric illness.

Review of Systems (ROS) Overview and Components

ROS is a final methodical inquiry prior to physical examination. All organ systems not already discussed during the interview are systematically reviewed here. It provides a thorough search for further, as yet unestablished, disease processes in the patient. If the patient has failed to mention certain symptoms, the process of ROS helps remind the patient. Also, if you have unknowingly omitted questioning the patient about certain aspects of his or her health, now is the time to include those.

Review of Systems Assessment Components

Constitutional

Determine whether there is any history of recent weight change, anorexia (loss of appetite), weakness, fatigue, fever, chills, insomnia, irritability, or night sweats.

Skin

Is there any history of allergic skin rashes, itching of the skin, unhealed lesions (probably due to diabetes, poor diet, steroids, or HIV/AIDS, etc.)? Is the rash acute or chronic? Is the rash unilateral or bilateral? Does the patient have any history of bruising or bleeding?

Head

Is there any history of headaches or loss of consciousness (LOC). LOC may be due to cardiovascular, neurologic, or metabolic causes, or due to anxiety.

Is there any history of seizures? Are the seizures generalized (with or without loss of consciousness) or focal? Are there any motor movements? Is there any history of head injury?

Eyes

Check for acuity of vision, history of glaucoma (can cause eye pain), redness, irritation, halos (seeing a white ring around a light source), blurred vision. Is there any irritation of the eyes or excessive tearing? These symptoms could be allergy-associated.

Ears

Check for recent change in hearing, ear pain, discharge, vertigo (dizziness) or ringing in the ears (tinnitus).

Lymph Glands

Check for lymph glandular enlargement in the neck or elsewhere. Are the nodes tender or painless? When did the patient first notice any changes in the nodes? Are the nodes freely mobile or are they anchored to the underlying tissues?

Respiratory System

Ask if there is any history of frequent sinus infections, postnasal drip, nosebleeds, sore throat, shortness of breath (SOB) on exertion or at rest. SOB can be due to respiratory, cardiac or metabolic diseases.

Check for wheezing (may be due to asthma, allergies, etc.); hemoptysis or blood in the sputum (may be due to dental causes or due to lung causes: bronchitis, tuberculosis). Check if the cough with expectoration is blood-tinged or is there frank blood in the sputum. Is there any history of bronchitis, asthma, pneumonia or emphysema?

Cardiovascular System

Is there any history of chest pain or discomfort or palpitations? Have the palpitations been associated with syncope (loss of consciousness)? Is there any history of either hypertension or hypotension? Does the patient experience any paroxysmal nocturnal dyspnea (shortness of breath experienced in the middle of the night)? Is there any shortness of breath (SOB) with exercise or exertion?

Is there any history of orthopnea (shortness of breath when lying flat in bed)? Does the patient use more than one pillow to sleep? Has this always been the case, or has the patient recently started using more pillows?

Is there any history of edema of the legs, face, etc? Does the patient experience any history of leg pains or cramps? Are the cramps relieved by rest? If yes, this is suggestive of intermittent claudication. If the cramping or leg pains are unremitting it is more likely to be muscular in origin.

Is there any history of murmur(s), rheumatic fever, varicose veins? Is there any history of hypercholerolemia, gout or excessive smoking that can lead to or worsen heart disease?

Gastrointestinal System

Check for a history of bleeding gums, oral ulcers, or sores. Is there any history of dysphagia? Can the patient point out and describe where the difficulty swallowing exists? Is there any history of heartburn, indigestion, bloating, belching or flatulence? Is there any history of nausea? Is it related to food? Determine the following:

- **Vomiting:** Is there any associated weight loss? Are there psychosocial factors, or medications causing it?
- **Hematemesis (vomiting blood):** Ask for associated ulcer history, food intolerance, abdominal pain or discomfort.
- **Jaundice:** Is the jaundice due to a viral cause or gallstones?

Is there a history of diarrhea/constipation or is there any change in color of stools?

Genitourinary System

Is there a history of polyuria (excessive urination) due to diabetes, renal disease or an unknown cause? Is it a recent change? Is there any history of nocturia (getting up at night to go to the bathroom)? Is this a recent change? Is there any history of dysuria (painful urination)? If dysuria is because of urinary tract infection (UTI), frequency and urgency will also be experienced. STDs will also be associated with similar symptoms. Always check to see if treatment for STD was completed. Check for renal stones, pain in the loins, frequent UTIs.

Menstrual History

Determine the date of the last menstrual period. Never forget to paraphrase this question, as discussed before. Check for any history of menorrhagia (heavy periods). Check whether the patient uses birth control or oral contraceptive pills. Let the patient know that oral antibiotics decrease the potency of oral contraceptives and the patient has to use extra barrier protection till the end of the next cycle. Additionally when prescribing an antibiotic, enter a case note in the record stating that the patient has been so informed.

Musculoskeletal System

Check for a history of joint pains and what joints are affected. Is the pain acute or chronic, unilateral or bilateral, and is it in the morning or evening? Are there any systemic symptoms? Is there a history of rheumatoid arthritis, osteoarthritis or gout?

Endocrine System

Check for symptoms associated with diabetes: polyuria (excessive urination), polydypsia (excessive thirst), polyphagia (excessive hunger) or weight change; thyroid: heat/cold intolerance, increased/decreased heart rate or goiter and adrenals: weight change, easy bruising, hypertension, etc?

Nervous System

Check for a history of stroke, cerebrovascular accident/stroke (CVA) or transient ischemic attack (TIA). Check for a history of muscle weakness, involuntary movements due to tremors, seizures or anxiety. Check for history of sensory loss of any kind, anesthesia (no sensation), parasthesias (altered sensation commonly experienced as pins and needles) or hyperesthesias (increased sensations). Check if there is any change in memory, especially a recent change.

History-Taking Conclusion

It is important at this point to collect the relevant data or all positive findings about the patient and then construct a logical framework of the case. You are now able to decide which organ or body area is affected and where to focus on during physical examination.

PHYSICAL EXAMINATION DETAILED DISCUSSION

Structure and Overview

The history serves to focus on and provides emphasis to the physical examination, in the sequence of patient workup. The patient is examined from head to toe, thus ensuring thoroughness and screening for abnormalities. Any specific physical findings suggested because of the history findings are sought.

PHYSICAL EXAMINATION ASSESSMENT COMPONENTS

The following are components of the physical examination in sequential order.

General Appearance

Note the patient's mental status, ability to interact, speech pattern, neatness, etc.

Vital Signs: Pulse, Respiration Rate, BP, Height, and Weight

Pulse

Note the rate, rhythm, volume, and regularity of the pulse. Count the pulse rate/minute. If the pulse rhythm is irregular, determine whether the irregular rhythm is regular or irregular. An irregularity, >5 beats/min, is pathological and should prompt a consult with the patient's M.D. Normal pulse: 65–85 beats/min.

Respiration Rate

Note the breathing pattern and the respiratory rate (RR)/min **while taking** the pulse, so the patient is unaware and anxiety does not alter the breathing. Normal RR: 12–16/min.

Blood Pressure (BP) Overview

Take the blood pressure in both arms during the patient's first visit. Always obtain two blood pressure readings during the patient's first visit. If the blood pressure is high, take two more readings at the next visit. An average of 3–4 readings will determine the mean blood pressure for the patient.

Always ensure that the patient has rested sufficiently in the chair prior to monitoring the BP. Certain physiological states can erroneously raise the blood pressure. Stress, caffeine, heavy meal consumption, improper positioning of the arm, or improper cuff size can all alter the BP readings. Normal BP reading: <120/80 mmHg.

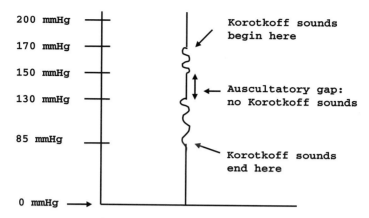

Figure 1.1. Blood pressure recording auscultatory gap.

Blood Pressure (BP) Recording

For a seated patient, place the patient's arm on the armchair and place the arms to the sides for a patient lying down. Fasten the cuff snugly over the arm such that the lower border of the cuff is about 1/4–1/2 inch above the elbow crease and the rubber tubes are over the brachial artery. The cuff should be at the cardiac level.

Place your fingers on the radial pulse and as you gradually raise the pressure to 200 mmHg, make a mental note of the reading where you lose the pulse. Continue to keep your fingers on the pulse and lower the pressure from 200 mmHg to 0 mmHg, making a mental note of the pressure where the pulse returns. The pressure where the radial pulse disappears and then reappears is the **same** and is the patient's **rough systolic pressure**. Next place your stethoscope on the brachial artery and raise the pressure to 30–40 mm above the rough systolic pressure. Now gradually lower the pressure and listen for the "tapping" of the Korotkoff sounds. The pressure where the Korotkoff sounds begin is the **true systolic pressure**, and the pressure where the tapping sounds disappear, is the **true diastolic pressure**. Always raise the pressure to 200 mmHg initially to overcome the **auscultatory gap** that may be present in an occasional hypertensive patient. As shown in Figure 1.1, the "tapping" sounds begin at the true **elevated** systolic pressure, disappear temporarily, reappear, and then disappear finally at the true diastolic pressure. If you **do not** raise the pressure to 200 mmHg, the reappearance of the tapping sounds can erroneously be thought of as the **start** of the tapping sounds.

Height and Weight

The height and weight of the patient is needed for the calculation of the basal metabolic index (BMI), the medication dosage prescribed during routine care or during a medical emergency, and the radiation dose for dental radiographs.

Examination of the Skin

Note the skin color, temperature, and turgor and look for skin lesions such as petechaie and bruises.

Examination of the Head

Note the quality of the hair. Is it coarse and dry or thin and sparse? Note the facial symmetry and look for any facial edema, butterfly rash, etc.

Examination of the Ears

Otitis Externa

Otitis externa is external ear infection or inflammation. Do the **ear tug test** by gently pulling on the earlobe. The test is positive, indicating infection in that ear, if the patient experiences pain with the pinna tug.

Otitis Media

Otitis media is middle ear infection or inflammation and is associated with mastoid tenderness. Gently press the mastoid tip with your thumb. The test is positive indicating otitis media in that ear, if the patient experiences pain on slight pressure.

Examination of the Eyes

Xanthelesma

Look for xanthelesma, which is a swelling near the medial end of the eyes. It can be benign or can be suggestive of hypercholesterolemia. Look for pallor, redness, and yellowing of the sclera by pulling down on the lower eyelid.

Exophthalmus

Exophthalmus or protrusion of the eyeballs can be familial or due to Grave's disease. The lid lag test is **positive** with Grave's disease and **negative** with familial cases.

The Lid Lag Test

Sit in front of the patient and hold the patient's head with your left hand. Now have the patient follow your moving right index finger as it moves from above the face to below the face. The upper eyelid does **not** roll over the eyeball with a positive lid lag test showing the white sclera.

Enophthalmus

Enophthalmus or sinking in of the eyeballs can be due to acute starvation, anorexia nervosa, or loss of body mass due to an underlying carcinoma.

Extraocular Movements

Sit in front of the patient and, holding the patient's head with your left hand, test for the extraocular movements. Have the patient follow your right index finger and test the patient's ability to look up, down, sideways (both right and left), and diagonally. The superior oblique muscle is innervated by cranial nerve (CN) IV, the lateral rectus muscle is supplied by CN VI, and the rest of the muscles are innervated by CN III, as shown in Figure 1.2.

The Light Reflex

To test for the light reflex, maintain the extraocular movements test position and have the patient look straight ahead. Bring a flashlight from the right side and shine it onto

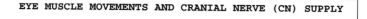

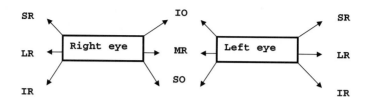

Figure 1.2. Extraocular muscle movements and associated cranial nerve innervations.

the right eye. Bridge the patient's nose with your hand to keep the light from spreading to the other eye. Observe the pupillary constriction in the right eye and also look for a simultaneous constriction in the left eye. The pupillary constriction in the right eye is the **direct** light reflex and the pupillary constriction in the left eye is the **indirect** or the **consensual** light reflex. Follow the same steps using the light, now from the left side. The afferent nerve for the light reflex is cranial nerve (CN) II and the efferent nerve is CN III.

Visual Fields

Maintain the same position as with the light reflex and have the patient look straight ahead. The patient should not move the head or eyes or gaze during the test. With your arms outstretched, gradually bring your wriggling fingers inward and have the patient inform at what point in the visual field he/she is able to see your fingers. Test the fields at points above, below, diagonally, and to the sides of the head, in a cross and x pattern.

Examination of the Nose and Sinuses

Check for sinus tenderness by tapping lightly over the ethmoid, maxillary, and frontal sinuses. Transient flexion of the neck toward the chest can bring out the pain associated with sinusitis.

Examination of the Mouth and Throat

Examine the teeth, gums, mucous membranes, tongue, oropharynx, and roof of the mouth. Gingival hypertrophy, when seen, can be due to puberty, pregnancy, leukemia, and drugs, phenytoin (Dilantin), an antiseizure drug; niphedipine (Procardia), a calcium channel blocker/high blood pressure medication; cyclosporine (Sandimmune), an anti-rejection drug for organ transplant).

Examination of the Neck: Lymph Glands, Thyroid, Trachea

Lymph Glands

Inspect the head and neck region for any lumps or bumps due to lymph node enlargement. Next, proceed with palpation of the lymph nodes. Stand behind or to the side of the patient and feel/palpate the lymph nodes in the neck with the pulp of your fingers. You may do this one side at a time or both sides at the same time.

Tonsillar nodes: Tonsillar nodes are the only nodes that should be palpated **one side at a time**. Simultaneous palpation of both sides can massage the carotid sinus causing bradycardia (slowing of the pulse). This could cause a problem, particularly in the elderly patient.

Normally, you are unable to feel any nodes. If you do feel some nodes, they should be soft, pea-sized, nontender, and freely mobile. These could be leftover nodes from a past infection. Tender nodes indicate a current infection and this should trigger assessment of disease-associated symptoms and signs.

Nontender, nonmobile, small, or enlarged nodes with irregular margins are highly suspicious for benign or cancerous tumors.

The preauricular, postauricular, and occipital nodes drain only the superficial tissues. The submental, submandibular, and tonsillar nodes drain superficial and deep tissues.

Bimanual palpation: Bimanual palpation of the floor of the mouth should always be done if the submental and submandibular nodes are enlarged. Using gloved hands, support the floor of the mouth firmly with your left palm under the chin. Place the fingers of your right hand inside the mouth and feel with pressure, the floor and sides of the mouth for any enlargements or swellings. Note the shape, size, mobility, and tenderness status of the swelling, when present.

Cervical Nodes

The cervical nodes that collect drainage from the above-mentioned nodes are anterior cervical, posterior cervical, and deep cervical. Firmly gripping the sternocleidomastoid (SCM) muscle, palpate the neck along the anterior border for the anterior cervical nodes, and along the posterior border for the posterior cervical nodes. The deep cervicals lie **under** the muscle and cannot be palpated.

Nape of the Neck Nodes

The nodes in this area include the trapezius and supraclavicular nodes.

Trapezius Nodes

Stand in front of or behind the patient and palpate on both sides at the nape of the neck, just below the occipital nodes.

Supraclavicular Nodes

Stand in front of the patient and have the patient flex the neck toward the chest. As the patient takes a **deep breath**, use the pulp of your fingers to feel the area behind both the clavicles adjacent to the suprasternal notch. Deep breathing brings to the surface any enlarged nodes, when present. These nodes are enlarged with liquid tumors or solid tumors affecting the lungs, breast, or upper abdomen. Section XVIII, "Oncology," outlines the head and neck lymphatic drainage disease states.

See Table 51.1 to learn more about specific tissues drained by each of the head and neck lymph nodes. The table also outlines direct or indirect drainage into the deep cervical chains.

Thyroid Gland

Use the following techniques:

1. **Inspection:** Stand in front of the patient and ask the patient to hyperextend the neck and swallow. Note the free mobility of the thyroid gland in the neck.
2. **Palpation:** Palpate the thyroid gland by standing behind the patient. Place your palm on the patient's neck and check whether the gland feels warmer than the surrounding skin. Check whether the surface is smooth. Palpate each lobe separately, as stated next, to note the size and margins of the gland. Move the left gland toward the right, to feel the right margin of the gland. The margin if felt, should be soft and smooth. Repeat the process on the left side by moving the right gland toward the left.
3. **Auscultation:** Occasionally an arterial bruit may be heard over a highly vascular enlarged gland.

Trachea

The trachea is normally located in the **midline**. Deviation to the right or left may suggest tumor, pneumothorax, or lung collapse.

Examination of the Hands

Check the skin temperature, appearance, and color of the hands, nails, joints, palms, and palmar creases and look for any deformity if present. Compare the patient's palm color with the color of your own palms. White palmar creases indicate hemoglobin level that is less than 50% of normal. Palmar erythema is frequently seen in alcoholics. If the knuckle joints and the proximal interphalangeal joints are swollen and affected bilaterally, it is indicative of **rheumatoid arthritis**. If the distal interphalangeal joints are affected unilaterally, it is suggestive of **osteoarthritis**. Look for and note any changes in the nails.

Examination of the Nails

Clubbing or convexity of the nails can be associated with chronic cardiopulmonary diseases.

Spooning or koilonychia can be seen with iron deficiency anemia.

Splinter hemorrhage in the nails can be associated with subacute bacterial endocarditis (SBE).

Examination of the Back

Inspection

Look for any spinal deformity.

Palpation

The spine should be palpated along the entire length of the spinal column to elicit any areas of tenderness.

Movements

Ask the patient to bend forward, backward, and sideways to check for mobility of the spine. Patients with limitation in movements should be assisted in and out of the dental chair. Rheumatoid arthritis affects the mobility of the cervical spine and the temporo-mandibular joint (TMJ). Osteoarthritis affects the lumbosacral joint mobility.

Examination of the Lower Extremities

Inspection

Inspect for any skeletal or muscular deformity, varicose veins, joint deformity, and loss of hair on the toes, shin, and feet. Loss of hair occurs due to poor circulation.

Palpation

Palpate the joints for any tenderness or swelling. Also, with the back of your hands check for the relative warmth of the feet and toes and indirectly assess perfusion.

Examination of the Lungs or Pulmonary Examination

Inspection

Note the shape and symmetry of the chest. Barrel chest is seen with obstructive lung disease and with emphysema (hyperinflated lungs). Note the rate, rhythm, and regularity of respiration, if yet incomplete. Normal respiration rate for adults is 12–16 breaths/min. Resting shallow tachypnea (rapid shallow breathing) is seen with restrictive lung disease. Hyperpnea (rapid deep breathing) is commonly seen with anxiety, exertion, or metabolic acidosis. The rapid deep breathing as seen in metabolic acidosis is called *Kussmaul's respiration.*

Palpation

Strap the chest with your hands and note the equality of chest excursions on both sides simultaneously, with deep breaths. Test from the apex to the base of the lungs.

Palpation of the Apex of the Lungs

To palpate the apex of the lungs, place your palms on the patient's shoulders and press down firmly as the patient inhales deeply. Check whether the apex of both lungs rises up equally. In the adult patient, a collapsed apex is usually due to tuberculosis (TB).

Percussion

Compare percussion notes at the same intercostal levels over both lung fields. The normal percussion note is resonant. Dullness on percussion is caused by consolidation of the lungs, as in pneumonia, or due to fluid collection, as in pleural effusion. A hyperresonant note occurs with pneumothorax.

Auscultation

Auscultate the right and left lung fields, at the same intercostal level, for comparison of auscultatory findings. Note the quality of the breath sounds and determine whether any adventitious sounds like rales, ronchi, or wheezes are present. The vesicular breathing pattern as seen in Figure 1.3 is heard over normal lung parenchyma. In this pattern, the inspiration limb is longer than the expiration limb.

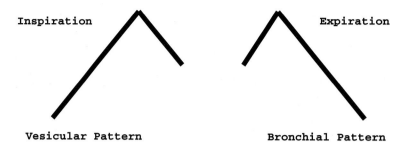

Inspiration   Expiration

Vesicular Pattern   Bronchial Pattern

Figure 1.3. Breathing patterns.

Bronchial Breath Sounds

The expiratory sound is higher pitched and louder than that heard with the vesicular breath sounds. Also, the expiratory component is equal to or greater than the inspiratory component (Figure 1.3). Bronchial breath sounds, when heard over the lung parenchyma, are **abnormal** and indicate underlying disease. Bronchial sounds heard over the **bifurcation** of the trachea, however, are **normal** in occurrence.

Adventitious Breath Sounds

Adventitious breath sounds heard on auscultation are:

- **Wheezes,** as with asthma, are whistling sounds caused by constriction of the bronchioles.
- **Rales and ronchi** are crackling sounds indicating presence of fluid in the lungs that can be due to bronchitis or congestive heart failure (CHF). Rales are coarse crackles and ronchi are soft crackles.

Examination of the Cardiovascular System

Inspection

Lay the patient at a 30–40° angle and note the jugular venous pulsation (JVP) in the neck. Normally, the JVP will be seen at or below the clavicle. If the JVP is seen in the neck, it is suggestive of decreased forward flow/cardiac output or increased backward flow. The apex beat, which is usually located in the fifth intercostal space medial to the midclavicular line, is also noted during inspection of the heart. Confirm the apex beat location with your palm, during palpation.

Palpation

Locate the carotid pulse with the tips of your fingers along the anterior border of the sternomastoid muscle in the middle of the neck, one carotid at a time. Once located, gently press down and establish the pulse rate/min. Never use your thumb to feel for pulsations because the thumb has its own pulsation. This can interfere with the patient's pulsation. Never palpate the carotid at the angle of the mandible because this will compress the carotid sinus and cause the pulse to slow down. This can become problematic in the elderly patient and may result in the patient experiencing dizziness or fainting. Note the pulse rate/minute of each carotid artery. Disparity of pulse rates between the two carotids will require you to auscultate for carotid bruits, as discussed below under "Auscultation."

Palpate the radial pulse at the wrist with the tips of your fingers, but never your thumb. Support the patient's hand in your hand and feel the radial pulse, which is located on the side of the thumb, with the fingers of your other hand. Let the pulse stabilize for a few seconds and then count the rate/minute. Determine the rhythm of the pulse. If there is a rhythm irregularity, assess whether it is regular (regularly irregular rhythm as in cardiac conduction defects) or irregular (irregularly irregular rhythm as in atrial flutter or atrial fibrillation). Palpate over the cardiac area with your palm to feel for the presence of any other pulses or thrills. A thrill is a purring sensation, felt on palpation. Thrills are caused by a loud heart murmur. Murmurs are sounds produced by turbulent blood flow or they can occur due to vibrating heart valves.

Percussion

Percussion of the heart is done to outline the right and left border of the heart.

Auscultation

There are two associated auscultation techniques:

1. **Carotid Artery Auscultation:** When there is disparity in rates between the two carotids, auscultate over the arteries as the patient **holds** the breath. Turbulence of blood flow in the partially obstructed carotid artery causes a swooshing sound or **bruit** over the carotid artery with the **lesser** pulsation. Holding the breath is important as a bruit, and breath sounds are similar sounding.
2. **Heart Sounds Auscultation:** As shown in Figure 1.4, the first heart sound or S_1 is caused by the **closure** of the **mitral** and the **tricuspid** valves, and the second heart sound or S_2 is caused by the **closure** of the **aortic** and the **pulmonic** valves. The phase between S_1 and S_2 is the **systolic** or **ventricle** contraction phase, and the phase between S_2 and S_1 is the **diastolic** or the **atrial** contraction phase. Auscultation must be done in the four cardiac areas, shown in Figure 1.5. The **aortic** area is located in the **second right** intercostal space, next to the sternum. The **pulmonic** area is located in the **second left** intercostal space, next to the sternum. The **tricuspid** area is located in the third and fourth intercostal spaces; along the left border of the sternum and the **mitral** area is located in the fifth intercostal space, medial to the midclavicular line. The **apex beat** is located in the mitral area.

Systolic murmurs, as shown in Figure 1.6, can be due to aortic stenosis (AS), pulmonary stenosis (PS), tricuspid incompetence (TI), or mitral incompetence/regurgitation (MI). Diastolic murmurs, as shown in Figure 1.7, can be caused by mitral stenosis (MS), tricuspid stenosis (TS), aortic incompetence (AI), or pulmonary incompetence (PI).

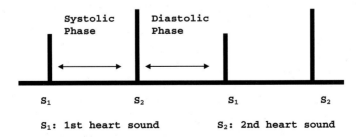

Figure 1.4. Heart sounds: Systolic and diastolic phases.

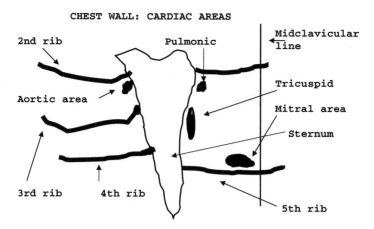

CHEST WALL: CARDIAC AREAS

Figure 1.5. Cardiac areas surface anatomy.

Examination of the Heart: The Systolic Phase

Systolic Murmurs: PS or AS or TI or MI

R. atrium	L. atrium
T	M
R. ventricle	L. ventricle
P	A

Blood flows through pulmonic (P) and aortic (A) valves

Figure 1.6. Systolic murmurs.

Examination of the Heart: The Diastolic Phase

Diastolic Murmurs: TS or MS or PI or AI

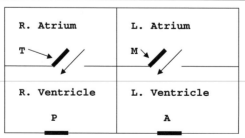

R. Atrium	L. Atrium
T	M
R. Ventricle	L. Ventricle
P	A

Blood flows through tricuspid (T) and mitral (M) valves

Figure 1.7. Diastolic murmurs.

Table 1.1. Cranial nerve (CN) examination

CN #	CN Name	Cranial Nerve (CN) Action
CN I	**Olfactory**	Causes the sense of smell.
CN II	**Optic**	Afferent nerve for vision.
CN III	**Oculomotor**	Causes all extraocular muscle movements (except those caused by lateral rectus and superior oblique muscles) and pupillary constriction.
CN IV	**Trochlear**	Innervates the superior oblique muscle to move the eye down and in.
CN V	**Trigeminal**	Sensory fibers to the face via the ophthalmic, maxillary, and mandibular divisions. Motor fibers to the muscles of mastication, the temporal and masseter muscles. **CN V Sensory Exam:** Have the patient **shut** the eyes. Touch the skin in the ophthalmic, maxillary, and mandibular areas with a cotton tip. Sense of touch is intact with optimal sensory function. **CN V Motor Exam:** Put your hands on either side of the patient's face and feel the equality of the masseter muscle tone as the patient clenches. Next place your hands on either side of the forehead to test the temporalis muscle tone as the patient clenches.
CN VI	**Abducens**	Innervates the lateral rectus muscle and moves the eye laterally.
CN VII	**Facial**	Motor nerve to most facial muscles and anterior tongue taste. Ask the patient to blow, whistle, and frown.
CN VIII	**Acoustic**	Responsible for hearing and balance.
CN IX	**Glossopharyngeal**	Sensory and motor to pharynx and posterior tongue plus responsible for taste.
CN X	**Vagus**	Motor to the palate, larynx, pharynx; sensory to pharynx and larynx. Test IX and X CNs together. Ask the patient to say a deep "aah." Use flashlight to see whether the palate rises equally on both sides.
CN XI	**Spinal Accessory**	Motor nerve to sternocleidomastoid and trapezius muscles. To test trapezius muscle, stand behind the patient and press down on both shoulders with your hands. Ask patient to shrug against pressure and note equality of tension on both sides. Sternocleidomastoid test: Place your palm on patient's **right** cheek and feel the tension in **left** sternomastoid as the patient tries to turn his face to the right against resistance. Next, test the right sternomastoid muscle.
CN XII	**Hypoglossal**	Motor to tongue. Ask patient to protrude the tongue. It should be in the midline and have no tremors. CN damage causes the tongue to deviate toward the **affected** side.

Examination of the Musculoskeletal System

Warm tender elbow joints with subcutaneous nodules are commonly seen with rheumatoid arthritis. Wrists swollen bilaterally are suggestive of rheumatoid arthritis. Palpable enlargement of bones in hands, also called *nodules,* is suggestive of osteoarthritis. If the large toe is affected, think of gout.

Examination of the Cranial Nerves

Review Table 1.1.

History and Physical Assessment of the Medically Compromised Dental Patient (MCP)

MCP HISTORY AND PHYSICAL (H&P) INTRODUCTION

A medically compromised patient is one who suffers from one or more diseases and is taking one or more medications for the care of those disease states. The management of the medically compromised dental patient is a multitiered process (discussed below) that requires detailed organized assessment of several aspects associated with the patient, and this process can sometimes take more than one dental visit. Every medically compromised patient should have a thorough assessment of the medical and dental histories during the first visit. The dentist needs to decide what laboratory tests to obtain from the patient's primary care physician (PCP) and/or the specialist(s). Evaluation of the tests will help determine the control status of the patient's disease states. The dentist also needs to assess the vital organ status; the patient's American Society of Anesthesiology (ASA) status; the need for stress management; the dental treatment plan; and the final anesthetics, analgesics, and antibiotics (AAAs) that can be safely used during dentistry.

It is important that all pertinent information collected prior to dentistry, be incorporated in the patient's record as a "medical consultation" case note. This note can be referenced any time during patient care and should be updated when there is a change in the health history or the list of medications.

MEASURES ESTABLISHED WITH THE COMPLETE HEALTH HISTORY

The complete health history will provide

- The date of the last physical examination
- The name, address, and telephone number of the primary care physician (PCP) and the specialists
- The disease state(s) being managed in the patient

The control status of disease state(s) is determined by assessment of appropriate laboratory test results, as with diabetes, or by following standard guidelines, as with blood pressure readings.

Diabetes Assessment Example

To assess diabetes, evaluate the fasting blood sugar (FBS), postprandial/postmeal blood sugar (PPBS) and the HbA₁C. The well-controlled patient will have FBS: <125 mg/dL; PPBS: <140 mg/dL; and HbA₁C: <7% (Normal: 4–6%).

Hypertension Assessment Example

To evaluate hypertension, assess the blood pressure (BP), and categorize the patient's BP readings as normal, high-normal, mild, moderate, or severe and determine the following:

- The presence of symptoms of an as yet undiagnosed condition
- Whether medical emergencies have occurred in past dental visits
- Whether the patient requires premedication (at a minimum, successive appointments should be scheduled 7 days apart when using the same premedication antibiotic)
- The prescribed, OTC, or herbal medications the patient is taking.

Always confirm whether the patient is compliant with the medications—never presume! Assess the drug-drug interactions (DDIs) between the drugs that the patient is taking and the anesthetics, analgesics, and antibiotics, (AAAs) used in the dental setting. A thorough assessment of all medications is necessary to prevent adverse reactions or drug-related emergencies during dental treatment. Evaluate every drug by assessing its mechanism of action; what condition (s) does it treat and what are the DDIs between the drug and the AAAs.

Digoxin and theophylline, as examples, are discussed below to demonstrate the way drugs should be assessed.

Lanoxin (Digoxin) Assessment

Digoxin, a cardiac glycoside is used to treat congestive heart failure (CHF) and atrial fibrillation (AF). AF is also called *supraventricular arrhythmia*.

Digoxin Mechanism of Action

Digoxin binds to and inhibits the magnesium and adenosine triphosphate (ATP) dependent Na⁺ and K⁺ ATP-ase, thereby increasing the influx of calcium ions in the cardiac smooth muscle. This increase in calcium ions enhances the myocardial contractility.

Digoxin and Local Anesthetics

Avoid local anesthetics with epinephrine in the presence of digoxin because epinephrine can be counterproductive (Table 2.1). It is safe to use 3% mepivacaine HCL (Carbocaine) or 4% prilocaine HCL (Citanest Plain) instead.

Digoxin and Analgesics

Avoid aspirin and NSAIDS with digoxin. Aspirin decreases digoxin absorption from the gut and displaces digoxin from the protein binding sites. NSAIDS increase serum digoxin levels by decreasing the renal clearance of digoxin. Use acetaminophen (Tylenol), oxycodone + acetaminophen (Percocet), hydrocodone + acetaminophen (Vicodin) or acetaminophen + 30 mg codeine (Tylenol #3) instead, depending on the needs of the patient and if no contraindications exist to the use of centrally acting pain medications.

Table 2.1. Digoxin and AAAs

Avoid with Digoxin	Use with Digoxin
ANESTHETICS	**ANESTHETICS**
All local anesthetics with epinephrine	a. 3% Mepivacaine (Carbocaine) b. 4% Prilocaine HCL without epinephrine (Citanest Plain)
ANALGESICS	**ANALGESICS**
a. Aspirin b. NSAIDS	a. Acetaminophen (Tylenol) b. Tylenol with Codeine (Tylenol #3) c. Tylenol with Hydrocodone (Vicodin) d. Tylenol with Oxycodone (Percocet)
ANTIBIOTICS	**ANTIBIOTICS**
a. Clarithromycin (Biaxin) b. Tetracyclines	a. All Penicillins b. All Cephalosporins c. Clindamycin d. Azythromycin

Digoxin and Antibiotics

Avoid macrolides, erythromycin, clarithromycin, and all tetracyclines with digoxin because these drugs increase serum digoxin levels. Use the penicillins, cephalosporins, clindamycin, or azithromycin (macrolide) instead.

Theophylline (Theo-Dur) Assessment

Theophylline is a xanthine-derivative bronchodilator that is used in the management of moderate to severe asthma. It has a very narrow "therapeutic index," which means that there is a very small difference between the therapeutic dose and the toxic dose.

Theophylline and Anesthetics

Thoephylline can become toxic in the presence of epinephrine. It is advised you use 3% mepivacaine HCL (Carbocaine) or 4% prilocaine HCL (Citanest Plain) instead.

Theophylline and Antibiotics

Avoid macrolides because theophylline can become toxic in the presence of macrolides erythromycin, azithromycin, or clarithromycin.

Note: Penicillin, aspirin, and NSAIDS can precipitate asthma attacks in some patients. Thus, always check whether the patient is allergic to or has had an adverse reaction with aspirin, codeine, morphine, local anesthetics, sulfa drugs, bisulfites, or penicillin. Avoid the use of those specific drugs.

Over-the-Counter (OTC) Drugs

Determine the specific OTC drugs the patient is taking and the frequency of intake. Check if the patient is consuming cough/cold medications, laxatives, diet pills, or herbals.

Morphine and Codeine Cross-Reactivity

Check whether the patient was given morphine for pain during past hospitalization. If there was no untoward reaction, this patient could be prescribed codeine during dentistry.

Corticosteroid History

Check whether there is a current or past history of steroid intake for 2 weeks or longer within the last 2 years. If the answer is yes, consult with the patient's physician to determine whether extra steroids are needed for major dental work.

Recreational Drugs

Check whether the patient is using any recreational drugs. Determine whether these drugs will affect the anesthetics, analgesics, and antibiotics (AAA's) or the patient's medications. Cocaine enhances the action of local anesthetics containing epinephrine. Alcohol enhances the utilization of local anesthetics, resulting in shorter duration of anesthesia. Alcohol also decreases the potency of antiseizure medications. The patient needs to be drug-free **for 24 hr**, and you should **defer** dental treatment in the **intoxicated** patient to avoid accidental needle sticks.

Oral Contraceptives (OCs)

Check whether the patient is on OCs. Have the patient take extra precautions until the end of the **next cycle** when prescribing **any oral** antibiotic with OCs. Oral antibiotics do not affect the systemic contraceptives, Norplant or Implanon. Norplant contains progestin. It is not as effective as originally thought, so it is now being phased out. Implanon is a new systemic contraceptive drug inserted under the skin of the upper arm; it contains the progestin etonogestrel and provides contraception for 3 years.

How Does the Patient Feel About Dentist Visits?

Presence of anxiety, phobia, or fear calls for stress management during dentistry.

MEASURES ESTABLISHED WITH THE PHYSICAL EXAMINATION

On completion of the medical history, the following are assessed on physical examination:

- Pulse
- Blood Pressure
- Respiration
- Height and weight
- Head and neck
- Status of the major systems
- Status of the vital organs

TREATMENT PLAN ASSESSMENT

Complete history and physical examination leads into the treatment plan, which determines the following:

Table 2.2. Medical consultation case note example

Dental Chief Complaint: "My mouth is a mess and I can only eat on one side."
Anticipated Dental Treatment: Full mouth extractions with immediate denture
Age: 59; **Gender:** F; **Ethnicity:** Hispanic; **Allergies:** None
Height: 5'2"; **Weight:** 155 lb; **Pulse:** 86/min; **BP:** 125/75 mmHg; **Respiration:** 14/min;
   ASA Status: II
List of Medical Conditions: Depression; social anxiety; Hepatitis C; anemia of chronic illness.
Patient has effectively been in a substance abuse program for 10 months. **Avoid** narcotics,
   sedatives, hypnotics, and alcoholic mouthwashes because she is a recovering addict.
Laboratory Tests Requested with Results Against Each Test:
- **LFTs** were "mildly abnormal" per physician.
- **CBC w/ WBC differential: WBC:** 6.2: Normal (N);
RBC: 4.26: Low (L); **Hgb:** 13.1: (L); **Hct:** 39.0: (L);
MCH: 30.8: (N); **MCV:** 91.6: (N); **RDW:** 14.1: (N);
Platelet count: 213: (N). **Assessment:** Mild anemia.
List of Medications (Prescribed, OTC, & Herbals) and DDIs:
Zoloft: 250 mg/day; Neurontin: 900 mg/day; Wellbutrin: 100 mg/day; Buspar: 60 mg/day;
   Triazadone: 150 mg HS; Centrum and Multivitamin.
Zoloft (Sertraline): SSRI antidepressant. Avoid sedatives, especially Benzodiazepenes. Zoloft
   causes bruxism.
- Anesthetics: Zoloft increases Lidocaine levels, avoid use
- Antibiotics: No Erythromycin or Clarithromycin
- Analgesics: No NSAIDS (risk of bleeding); no codeine, hydrocodone, oxycodone (levels
   decreased by Zoloft)
Neurontin (Gabapentin): Used for anxiety disorders. It has an additive effect with sedatives.
   Avoid barbiturates and opioid analgesics. It causes xerostomia and dry throat.
- Anesthetics; antibiotics: no contraindication (CI)
- Analgesics: No opioid analgesics
Wellbutrin (Bupropion): Dopamine reuptake inhibitor antidepressant. Causes abnormal taste
   and severe xerostomia
- Anesthetics: Use caution with epinephrine because Wellbutrin blocks the reuptake of
   Norepinephrine (NE)
- Antibiotics: No CI
- Analgesics: No opioid analgesics
Buspar (Buspirone): Non-Benzodiazepine anxiolytic. It causes xerostomia.
- Anesthetics; analgesics: No CI
- Antibiotics: Avoid CYP3A4 inhibitors drugs Doxycycline, Clarithromycin, and Azole antifungals
Trazadone: Serotonin reuptake inhibitor.
- Anesthetics: No CI
- Antibiotics: Avoid CYP3A4 inhibitor drugs
- Analgesics: No opioids, oxycodone, or hydrocodone
- **Centrum multivitamin:** No CIs with the AAAs
- **Need for Premedication:** No
Final List of Anesthetics Safe for Dentistry:
- 0.5% Bupivacaine (Marcaine); 4% Prilocaine HCL (Citanest Forte); 3% Mepivacaine HCL
   (Carbocaine): Maximum 2 carpules
Final List of Analgesics Safe for Dentistry:
- Regular or extra strength Tylenol
Final List of Antibiotics Safe for Dentistry:
- Penicillins, Cephalosporins, or Clindamycin

- The final list of AAAs that can be safely used
- Whether the patient needs shorter appointments (ASA-III/IV patients) or appointments 7 days apart
- Whether the patient needs to be given morning or afternoon appointments, dependent on when the patient eats. The patient needs to be on a full stomach to prevent hypoglycemia.

Never **presume** that the patient has eaten; always **ask** and know **how much** the patient has eaten! Morning appointments are needed for myasthenia gravis patients and for patients needing a steroid boost prior to dentistry. Whether the patient needs to bring his own medications to the dental office, especially if there is a history of asthma, angina, or hypoglycemia.Whether stress management is needed using oral or systemic sedation. See Chapter 10, "Oral and Parenteral Conscious Sedation for Dentistry; Assessment, Analysis, and Associated Dental Management," for details.

The Medical Consultation Case Note

The medical consultation case note for the medically compromised dental patient contains an assessment of all pertinent facts (medical status, laboratory tests, medications, and safe AAAs), associated with patient care and should be referenced for all appointments. See Table 2.2.

Pharmacology

Prescription Writing, DEA Schedules, and FDA Pregnancy Drug Categories

OVERVIEW

The goal of accurate prescription writing is to improve patient care and reduce errors. You need to have a good understanding about the specifics of prescription writing because this can help you, your patient, and the pharmacy expedite the dispensing and use of the appropriate medications.

You can legally prescribe only those drugs that are appropriate to your practice, and you should prescribe only for patients you see in your practice. Never prescribe for friends or family, as a "favor." Prescribe only those drugs with which you are familiar, and do not allow the patient to dictate what to prescribe!

Do not abbreviate details of the prescription. Write clear and complete instructions in ink and do not use "as directed."

Prescribe the correct quantity, e.g., 5–7 days' supply for most full-course antibiotic therapies or 2–3 days' supply for analgesics and/or sedatives. Maintain complete records of what you prescribe. Store all controlled substances appropriately and keep necessary records.

Communicate telephone orders directly and clearly to a pharmacist when telephoning prescriptions. Establish a rapport with a pharmacist and use him/her as an information source when in doubt. Establish a good rapport with the patient and explain how to use the prescribed medication. Instruct the patient to:

1. Read the label on the prescription container before taking the drug.
2. Store the drugs appropriately.
3. Use all the medication prescribed.
4. Discard any excess medications after 1 year.

You should know the patient's current Medical History, current list of medications and the current status of underlying disease states. You need to check the drug-drug interactions (DDIs) between the medications already in use by the patient and what you plan on prescribing, **before** you prescribe.

Always confirm and document any history of medication allergies and take that into consideration when writing a prescription.

Example: Severe allergy to penicillin prevents you from prescribing cephalexin (Keflex), a cephalosporin.

Prescribe doses that are both correct and measurable. Prescriptions should be written using the metric system: (gram, g; milligram, mg) and not the apothecary system: (grain; dram; ounce, oz). You need, however, to be familiar with the metric-to-apothecary or metric-to-household system conversions because an occasional patient may be on a medication using either the apothecary or household measurements.

Metric, Apothecary, Liquid Weight, and Household Measurement Systems

Metric-to-Apothecary Systems Dry-Weight Measurements
3.89 g = 1 dram
60 mg = 1 grain

Liquid Weight Measurements: Metric Versus Household Measurements
15 mL = 1 Tbsp
5 mL = 1 tsp
1 mL = 15–16 drops

Prescription Abbreviations

Listed are the commonly used abbreviations every provider should know:

qd or od: every day
bid: twice daily
tid: thrice daily
qid: 4 times daily
ac: before meals
pc: after meals
hs or qhs: at bedtime
disp: dispense
prn: as needed
po: by mouth (orally)
IV: intravenous
IM: intramuscular
stat: immediately
sq or sc: subcutaneous
sig or signa: directions for use
mcg or μg: micrograms

Prescription Writing Regulations

Each state's department of public health decides on the specifics of prescription writing and then publishes the regulations. It is important for you to be familiar with the prescription-writing requirements in your state. Some states require you to have a state prescribing number in addition to a DEA number. The state number does not get listed on the prescription form.

Drug Enforcement Agency (DEA) Number

You are required by law to register with the Drug Enforcement Agency (DEA) in Washington, to store, dispense, or prescribe drugs, and your prescription forms must contain a space for your DEA number. The DEA license is renewed every 2 years.

DEA Drug Schedules

The controlled substance act ranks drugs according to their potential for abuse and dependency into categories, called *schedules*. All states in the U.S. except Massachusetts have 5 schedules: Schedules I–V. Massachusetts has Schedules I–VI. The DEA number is required for all controlled substances. Many pharmacies additionally require the DEA number for any telephonically communicated prescription. Scheduled drugs are prescribed for the treatment of cough, diarrhea, mild anxiety, and pain, including postsurgical pain.

DEA Drug Schedule I

Drugs in this category have a significant abuse potential and there are no proven therapeutic indications to prescribe them.

Drugs included in this category: heroin and marijuana.

DEA Drug Schedule II

Drugs in this category have a high abuse potential and they can be associated with severe psychic or physical dependency. Narcotics, stimulants (amphetamines) and depressants belong to this category. **No refills** can be ordered for **Schedule II** drugs, and the prescription is invalid after **30 days**. Emergency telephone orders, when taken, need to immediately be followed by a written prescription from the provider. Prescription records have to be maintained at the pharmacy and at the provider's office.

Schedule II drugs used in dentistry: hydromorphone (Dilaudid), meperidine (Demerol), methadone, morphine, and oxycontin, or oxycodone + acetaminophen (Percocet).

DEA Drug Schedule III

Schedule III drugs have a lesser abuse potential than Schedule II drugs. This category includes compounds containing limited quantities of certain narcotic and non-narcotic drugs. Abuse of these drugs can lead to moderate or low physical dependence or high psychological dependence. Records need to be maintained, as in Schedule II, but a maximum of **five** refills can be prescribed in **6 months**.

Schedule III drugs used in dentistry: codeine + acetaminophen (Tylenol #1–4), and hydrocodone + acetaminophen (Vicodin).

DEA Drug Schedule IV

The abuse potential for Schedule IV drugs is less than that with the Schedule III drugs. Abuse is associated with limited physical or psychological dependency. Records need to be maintained, as in Schedule III, and a maximum of **five** refills can be prescribed in **6 months**.

Schedule IV drugs used in dentistry: diazepam (Valium), flurazepam (Dalmane), midazolam (Versed), pentobarbital, dextropropoxyphene (Darvon), and pentazocine (Talwin-NX).

DEA Drug Schedule V

The abuse potential for Schedule V drugs is less than that with the Schedule IV drugs. Schedule V drugs include preparations containing limited amounts of certain narcotics and stimulant drugs, for antitussive (cough), antidiarrheal, and analgesic purposes. Laws and regulations vary by state for drugs in this category. Records need to be maintained, as in Schedule IV, and a maximum of **five** refills can be prescribed in **6 months**.

   Schedule V drugs: cough preparations with <200 mg codeine/mL or per 100 g (Robitussin AC), and phenergan with codeine.

DEA Drug Schedule VI

This category is only in Massachusetts and all preparations known as "legend" drugs are included in this category. *Legend* refers to the FDA-required statement: *"Caution— Federal Law Prohibits Dispensing Without a Prescription."* Records need to be maintained, as in Schedule V, and a maximum of **five** refills can be prescribed in **6 months**.

   Schedule VI drugs: tolbutamide (Orinase), ibuprofen (Motrin), and idomethacin (Indocin).

Pregnancy Drugs Categories A–X

The Food and Drug Agency (FDA) classifies drugs into five categories according to their level of safety for the fetus during pregnancy. Categories **A and B** drugs are considered **safe** during pregnancy. Prior to writing a prescription for a pregnant patient, always know the FDA category for the drug.

Category A

Category A drugs have been used in pregnant women and are proven safe throughout the pregnancy.

Category B

A drug is classified as category B if animal studies have shown no risk to the fetus but pregnant women have not been tested. Alternatively, animal studies may have shown risk but studies in pregnant women have shown no risk to the fetus in any trimester.

Category C

A drug is classified as a category C drug if animal studies have shown an adverse effect and pregnant women have not been tested. Alternatively, no studies in pregnant women or animals have been conducted.

Category D

A drug is classified as category D if studies in pregnant women have shown risk to the fetus. The drug, however, may be used in a life-threatening situation if safer drugs are ineffective.

Category X

Drugs in this category have shown positive fetal risk.
   Example: isotretinoin (Accutane)

ELEMENTS OF PRESCRIPTION WRITING

The following sections describe elements of a prescription (Figure 3.1).

Patient Specificity

The prescription should be written **only** for the patient **you** are treating.

Date

The date on which you write the prescription is important because the pharmacy will not honor an undated prescription. As discussed earlier, Schedule II prescriptions are invalid after 30 days and all others are invalid after 6 months. The date therefore is required for this guideline to be implemented.

```
            Dental Clinic Prescription Form

Doctor's Name: John Brown D.M.D

Doctor's Address: One Main Street

                  Boston, MA 02111

Doctor's Telephone #: 617-555-1212

Prescription Date: 01/14/08

Patient's Name: Ms. Jane Doe

Patient's Address: One Center St

                   Apt # 1

                   Boston, MA 02111

Rx: Amoxicillin (Amoxil), 500 mg/tablets,

    for oral infection

Disp: 15 tablets

Sig: Take 1 capsule PO tid for 5 days

Refill: 0 (zero)

□: No Substitution

◪: Label

Practitioner's Signature: Jb

Practitioner's Name Printed: John Brown, D.M.D
```

Figure 3.1. Prescription form for Amoxicillin (Amoxyl).

Patient's Name and Address

Print the patient's name and address very clearly.

Drug Name

Confirm through proper drug reference that the **correct** drug is prescribed for the patient's problem and clearly print the name of the drug.

Example: **Amoxicillin (Amoxil)**—generic name (trade name)

Write both the generic and trade name of the drug, to avoid confusion at the pharmacy. Many drugs have similar-sounding names, such as lanoxin (digoxin), a cardiac glycoside, versus levoxyl (Levothyroxine), a thyroid hormone! The common antibiotics used in dentistry are all available in generic form and the pharmacist is mandated by law to dispense this form, unless otherwise indicated by you, the provider, in the "no substitution" box.

No Substitution Box

If you do not want to dispense the generic form of the drug, write the trade name of the drug you want to prescribe and check off the No Substitution box. This confirms for the pharmacists that you want to prescribe only that drug.

Example: Amoxil 500 mg with the **No Substitution box checked off** indicates that the pharmacist cannot dispense the generic version of amoxicillin.

Drug Strength

You must clearly list the right drug strength per tablet/capsule/ml.

Example: Amoxicillin, **500 mg/tablet**

Drug Dose

You must clearly indicate the correct dosage schedule and number of times in the day you want the patient to take the drug.

Example: Amoxicillin, 500 mg **tid/three times/day**. You avoid confusion by additionally spelling it out as "three times/day." This can be important, especially when prescribing for patients that get easily confused or don't recall abbreviations well.

Route of Administration

Indicate the correct route of administration.

Example: Amoxicillin 500 mg **PO (oral)** tid

Duration of the Prescription

Indicate on the prescription the correct duration for which the drug is prescribed.

Example: Amoxicillin (Amoxil), 500 mg tid × **5 days (for 5 days)**

Total Amount of Drug Dispensed

Indicate the total number of tablets you plan to dispense.

Example: **Dispense 15 Amoxicillin tablets**.

Total Number of Refills

Points to consider prior to writing refills are drug safety, drug regulations, managed care guidelines, and convenience.

Drug Safety

This should be considered for drugs with high abuse potential.

Example: Oxycodone + Acetaminophen (Percocet). **No refills**.

Drug Regulations

Some states implement a maximum length of time that certain specific medications can be prescribed (30/60 days). A new prescription is needed in such cases if the drug is to be continued. You need to check with the local state board to know the specifics for your state.

Managed Care Guidelines

Insurance plans often dictate the maximum amount of drug dispensed at one given time, for the patient to obtain insurance drug coverage.

Convenience

If a patient is getting treated for a stable underlying disease state, a practitioner could write a prescription for 90 days. This option is commonly used by a medical practitioner and not a dentist because medications for dentistry are usually dispensed short-term. If you plan on giving refills, you must write that in the section specified for refills. In the dental setting antibiotics for premedication prophylaxis often need refills, especially if the patient is to be seen for months at a stretch for several procedures. Determine how much the patient will need and indicate that on the refill line. Do not overprescribe. Write the numerical value and spell it out, to avoid confusion. If you plan on giving no refills, spell that out too.

Example: 0 (zero) refills; 2 (two) refills

The patient's name, date, drug, dose, units, quantity, route, frequency, refills, signature, and the "No Substitution" check-off are required by Massachusetts prescription regulations.

Label Box Check-Off and Drug Indication

By law, any specific information about the drug or drug indication that needs to be on the dispensing label is provided by the practitioner in the prescription. The practitioner needs to check off the Label box when this is desired.

Drug Indication helps the patient and the pharmacy know the reason for which the drug is dispensed.

Example: Amoxicillin (Amoxil) 500 mg/tablet **for oral infection**

Local Anesthetics Commonly Used in Dentistry: Assessment, Analysis, and Associated Dental Management Guidelines

LOCAL ANESTHETIC CLASSIFICATION AND PHARMACOTHERAPEUTICS

There are two distinct types of local anesthetics: amides and esters. Amides are subdivided into amides with epinephrine and amides without epinephrine (Table 4.1).

Classification of Amides with Epinephrine

- 2% lidocaine with 1:100,000 epinephrine (Xylocaine)
- 4% prilocaine HCL with 1:200,000 epinephrine (Citanest Forte)
- 0.5% bupivacaine with 1:200,000 epinephrine (Marcaine)
- 4% septocaine with 1:100,000 and 1:200,000 epinephrine (Articaine)

Amide with Levonordefrin (NeoCobefrin)

- 2% mepivacaine HCL (Carbocaine) with 1:20,000 levonordefrin (NeoCobefrin), a sympathomimetic amine

Classification of Amides Without Epinephrine

- 3% mepivacaine HCL (Carbocaine)
- 4% prilocaine HCL (Citanest Plain)

Classification of Ester Local Anesthetics

- Injectable propoxycaine and procaine (Ravocaine)
- Topical benzocaine

Metabolism of Local Anesthetics

All amide local anesthetics are metabolized in the liver. 4% prilocaine HCL (Citanest) additionally is metabolized in the kidney and plasma. Ester local anesthetics are metabolized in the plasma by plasma cholinesterase, and plasma cholinesterase is **synthesized** in the liver. So there is no real advantage using ester local anesthetics over the amides in a cirrhotic patient. Benzocaine as a topical anesthetic is the only ester used today in dentistry.

Table 4.1. Summary: Local anesthetics (LAs)

LAs: Generic/Trade Name	LAs: Facts, Advice, or Alerts
AMIDE LA WITH EPINEPHRINE **Amide Local Anesthetic Alerts**	Use **only 2 carpules** of any LA in compromised patients. **Avoid LAs with epinephrine and epinephrine cords with:** Hyperthyroidism; severe coronary artery disease; MAO and Tricyclic antidepressants; Prophylthiouracil (PTU); Lanoxin (Digoxin); Theophylline; bisulfite allergy; G6PD anemia and serum creatinine >2 mg/dL or CrCl <50/min. Use 5–10% Aluminum chloride (Hemodent) cords when needed.
2% Lidocaine (Xylocaine) with 1:l00,000 Epinephrine: Pregnancy Category: B	**Concentration/carpule:** 36 mg **Lasts:** 60 min **Recommended Dose:** 3.0 mg/lb **Healthy adult:** Max. 11.5 carpules
4% Prilocaine HCL (Citanest Forte) with 1:200,000 Epinephrine: Pregnancy Category: B	**Concentration/carpule:** 72 mg **Lasts:** 2 h **Recommended Dose:** 2.7 mg/lb **Healthy adult:** Max. 5 carpules **Avoid with:** Congenital methemoglobinemia; ASA III/IV status hypoxic states; moderate to severe anemia/kidney disease, and multiple sclerosis
0.5% Bupivacaine (Marcaine) with 1:200,000 Epinephrine: Pregnancy Category: C	**Concentration/carpule:** 9 mg **Lasts:** 90 min or longer **Recommended Dose:** 0.6 mg/lb **Healthy adult:** Max. 9 carpules
4% Septocaine (Articaine) with 1:100,000/1:200,000 Epinephrine: Pregnancy category: C	**Concentration/carpule:** 72 mg **Lasts:** 45–75 min **Recommended Dose:** 3.2 mg/lb **Healthy adult:** Max. 6 carpules Has 1.5 times Lidocaine potency. Action occurs within 1–3 min. **Avoid use in all conditions listed under Citanest Forte.**
AMIDE WITH LEVONORDEFRIN **2% Mepivacaine (Carbocaine) with 1:20,000 Levonordefrin (NeoCobefrin):** Pregnancy Category: C	**Infiltration/block anesthesia** **Dose:** 36 mg/carpule **Healthy adult:** Max. 5 carpules **Avoid with:** Hyperthyroidism, severe coronary disease, MAO-Is, bisulfite allergy, G6PD anemia
AMIDES WITHOUT EPINEPHRINE **3% Mepivacaine HCL (Carbocaine):** Pregnancy Category: C	**Concentration/carpule:** 54 mg **Lasts:** 20 min **Recommended Dose:** 3.0 mg/lb **Healthy adult:** Max. 7.5 carpules Safe with G6PD anemia.

Table 4.1. *Continued*

LAs: Generic/Trade Name	LAs: Facts, Advice, or Alerts
4% Prilocaine HCL (Citanest Plain): Pregnancy category: B Safe to use in the hypertensive pregnant patient	**Concentration/carpule:** 72 mg **Lasts:** 30 min **Recommended Dose:** 2.7 mg/lb. **Healthy adult:** Max. 5 cartridges **Avoid in all conditions listed under Citanest Forte.**
ESTER ANESTHETICS	
Propoxycaine and Procaine (Ravocaine): Pregnancy Category: C	**Concentration/carpule:** 43.2 mg **Lasts:** 30–40 min. **Healthy adult:** Max. 9 cartridges **Not available;** highly allergenic
Topical Benzocaine: Pregnancy Category: C	**Avoid in all states listed under Citanest Forte.**

Factors Affecting Onset and Duration of Local Anesthetics

The onset and duration of action depends on multiple factors:

1. **Tissue pH:** With infection, the pH of the tissue decreases, becoming more acidic. An acidic pH is responsible for the delayed effectiveness or ineffectiveness of the local anesthetic.
2. **Lipid solubility:** The greater the lipid solubility of the local anesthetic, the more rapid is the onset of action.
3. **Local anesthetic concentration formulation:** The high-concentration local anesthetics prilocaine (Citanest) and septocaine (Articaine) require fewer injections compared to the low-concentration local anesthetics such as lidocaine. Low-concentration preparations are preferred for use in the pediatric population and 0.5% bupivacaine (Marcaine) should be avoided in children.
4. **Presence of a vasoconstrictor:** By themselves, local anesthetics cause vasodilation, diffuse very rapidly, and last for a shorter duration of time. Presence of a vasoconstrictor improves the duration and depth of anesthesia, thus decreasing the need for more anesthetic use per visit. There are two types of vasoconstrictors used in dentistry: epinephrine and levonordefrin.
   a. **Epinephrine:** Epinephrine is the most common vasoconstrictor added in 1:50,000, 1:100,000 or 1:200,000 concentrations in various local anesthetics. Epinephrine causes vasoconstriction by stimulating the α_1 receptors in the mucus membranes. Epinephrine also affects the β_1 receptors in the heart and the β_2 receptors in the skeletal muscles. Stimulation of the β_1 receptors causes **tachycardia and an increased systolic blood pressure (SBP)**. Stimulation of the β_2 receptors causes vasodilation and a **decreased diastolic blood pressure (DBP)**. The reflex tachycardia triggered by epinephrine becomes an issue in patients with significant cardiovascular disease and should thus be avoided.
   b. **Levonordefrin (NeoCobefrin):** Levonordefrin (NeoCobefrin) is a sympathomimetic amine that acts as a vasoconstrictor, producing less cardiac and CNS stimulation than epinephrine. It has a fast onset of action, providing effective

anesthesia and has very few side effects. Levonordefrin increases the systolic and diastolic BP but it causes a reflex **bradycardia** (decreased heart rate). Reflex bradycardia is a beneficial side effect in patients with mild to moderate cardio-vascular heart disease. The potency of 1:20,000 Levonordefrin is equivalent to the potency of 1:100,000 epinephrine.

5. **Infiltration versus block anesthesia:** Infiltration anesthesia is more rapid in onset compared to block anesthesia, but it is shorter lasting than block anesthesia.

Local Anesthetics and Cross-Reactivity

True allergy to the amides is very rare. Allergy to one amide does not contraindicate the use of the other amides. A patient may occasionally be allergic to the antioxidant metasulfite or bisulfite preservative in the local anesthetic. The preservative preserves the potency of the epinephrine. Switching to an amide without epinephrine is an appro-priate option in such situations.There is definite cross-reactivity among the ester local anesthetics. Each ester has a common breakdown allergenic compound, paraaminoben-zoic acid, which causes a hypersensitivity reaction.

Local Anesthetic Adjuncts

Epinephrine containing retraction cords have 8% racemic epinephrine, and they are used to provide adequate bloodless fields during dentistry. Retraction cords mechani-cally displace gingival tissue causing tissue contraction and hemostasis. The higher the concentration of epinephrine in the cords, the greater is the chance for the epinephrine to be systemically absorbed. Epinephrine containing cords should be **avoided** in the presence of hyperthyroidism, severe coronary artery disease, MAO-Is for depression, bisulfite allergy, G6PD anemia, and kidney disease associated with serum creatinine >2 mg/dL or CrCl < 50/min. It is best to use aluminum chloride (a potent astringent) containing cords when epinephrine containing cords are contraindicated. 5–10% alumi-num chloride (Hemodent) gingival retraction cords are available for use and are con-sidered very safe when used in the medically compromised dental patient.

AMIDE AND ESTER LOCAL ANESTHETICS DETAILED DISCUSSION

Amide Local Anesthetics

2% Lidocaine (Xylocaine) with 1:100,000 Epinephrine

- Pregnancy category: **Category B**
- Concentration per carpule: 36 mg lidocaine
- Duration of action: 60 min
- Recommended dose for 2% lidocaine (Xylocaine): 3.0 mg/lb
- Maximum number of carpules for a healthy 140 lb adult: 11.5

4% Prilocaine HCL (Citanest Forte) with 1:200,000 Epinephrine

- Pregnancy category: **Category B**
- Concentration per carpule: 72 mg prilocaine
- Duration of action: 2 hr
- Recommended dose for 4% prilocaine (Citanest Forte): 2.7 mg/lb
- Maximum number of carpules for a healthy 140 lb adult: 5

0.5% Bupivacaine (Marcaine) with 1:200,000 Epinephrine
- Pregnancy category: **Category C**
- Concentration per carpule: 9 mg bupivacaine
- Duration of action: 90 min or longer
- Recommended dose for 0.5% bupivacaine (Marcaine): 0.6 mg/lb
- Maximum number of cartridges in a healthy 140 lb adult: 9

4% Septocaine (Articaine) with 1:100,000/1:200,000 Epinephrine
- Pregnancy category: **Category C**
- Concentration per carpule: 72 mg septocaine
- Duration of action: Depending on the epinephrine concentration, the effects last for 45–75 min.
- Recommended dose for septocaine (Articaine) 3.2 mg/lb
- Maximum number of cartridges in a healthy 140 lb adult: 6

Articaine is 1.5 times **more potent** than lidocaine and has an onset of action within **1–3 min** of injection. Articaine **should not** be given to patients with disease states associated with hypoxia and patients with a history of allergy to metasulfites or bisulfites.

2% Mepivacaine (Carbocaine) with 1:20,000 Levonordefrin (NeoCobefrin)
- Pregnancy category: **Category C**
- Concentration per carpule: 36 mg mepivacaine HCL/carpule
- Duration of action: 60 min
- Average amount per visit for a healthy adult: 5 carpules
- Average amount per visit for a medically compromised patient: 2

It is available in the U.S. for **infiltration and block** anesthesia. The anesthetic contains bisulfites to prevent the oxidation of levonordefrin. Avoid use in patients with demonstrated bisulfite allergy and patients with G6PD anemia. Also avoid in patients with a history of hyperthyroidism or severe coronary artery disease and in patients on MAO inhibitors, to prevent a rise in the blood pressure. Systemic injection of the anesthetic can cause bradycardia, decreased cardiac output, anxiety, restlessness, confusion, and seizures. Always aspirate prior to injecting the anesthetic.

3% Mepivacaine HCL (Carbocaine)
- Pregnancy category: **Category C**
- Concentration per carpule: 54 mg mepivacaine
- Duration of action: 20 min
- Recommended dose for 3% mepivacaine (Carbocaine): 3.0 mg/lb
- Maximum number of cartridges in a healthy 140 lb adult: 7.5

4% Prilocaine HCL (Citanest Plain)
- Pregnancy category: **Category B** local anesthetic
- Concentration per carpule: 72 mg prilocaine
- Duration of action: 30 min
- Recommended dose for 4% prilocaine (Citanest Plain): 2.7 mg/lb
- Maximum number of cartridges in a healthy 140 lb adult: 5

4% prilocaine HCL (Citanest Plain) **should be** the local anesthetic of choice for a **hypertensive** pregnant patient.

Ester Local Anesthetics

Propoxycaine and Procaine (Ravocaine)

These anesthetics are not currently available.

- Ravocaine pregnancy category: **Category C**
- Concentration per carpule: 43.2 mg
- Duration of action: 30–40 min
- Maximum number of cartridges in a healthy 140 lb adult: 9

Topical Benzocaine

- Pregnancy category: **Category C**

Benzocaine use is contraindicated in the pregnant patient, patients allergic to esters, and patients with congenital methemoglobinemia.

LOCAL ANESTHETIC DENTAL ALERTS AND SUGGESTED DENTAL GUIDELINES

The following are dental alerts and guidelines for local anesthetics:

1. Use no more than 2 carpules of local anesthetic per visit in any medically compromised patient. You thus avoid excessive use of local anesthetics and associated emergencies.
2. Avoid amides with epinephrine in patients presenting with a history of sulfite or bisulfite allergy. Both early and late IgE-mediated reactions can occur with the sulfites. The patient can experience bronchospasm, rhinitis, conjunctivitis, urticaria, or anaphylactic shock.
3. There is no cross-reactivity between the sulpha antimicrobials, sulphur, and the metasulfites or bisulfites. Patients presenting with allergy to the sulpha antimicrobials or sulphur **can be given** epinephrine-containing local anesthetics.
4. A true IgE-mediated reaction to local anesthetics is **rare**. Often the reaction is due to hyperventilation, vasovagal reaction, numbness of the pharynx from extravasated local anesthetic, or an inadvertent intravascular injection of epinephrine. It is suggested you inject a 0.2 mL subcutaneous (SC) local anesthetic challenge and look for a reaction in someone who has never had a local anesthetic or thinks there could be local anesthetic–associated allergy. It is safe to proceed with the local anesthetic if there is no reaction within 5 min of the injection.
5. Toxicity of the amide local anesthetics can occur with significant liver disease, but liver disease **does not** increase the duration of action of the amides. Dental treatment in a cirrhotic patient must therefore be **simplified** and completed over **multiple** appointments. Treat one area of the oral cavity at a time, rather than working on different areas of the mouth per appointment, to minimize the total amount of anesthetic used.
6. 2% lidocaine (Xylocaine), 4% prilocaine HCL with 1:200,000 epinephrine (Citanest Forte), or 4% prilocaine HCL (Citanest Plain) are **category B** drugs that are **safe** during pregnancy.

7. 0.5% bupivacaine (Marcaine), 4% septocaine with 1:100,000 and 1:200,000 epinephrine (Articaine), 3% mepivacaine HCL (Carbocaine) and 2% mepivacaine (Carbocaine) with 1:20,000 levonordefrin (NeoCobefrin) are **Category C** drugs that **should not be used** during pregnancy.

8. Old age does not contraindicate the use of local anesthetics. However, use caution with the total number of carpules and epinephrine or levonordefrin used in elderly patients with compromised liver function or coronary artery disease.

9. Excessive accumulation of prilocaine, septocaine, and benzocaine associated metabolites can cause methemoglobinemia. They should be avoided in patients presenting with congenital methemoglobinemia. Methemoglobinemia causes cyanosis, which **does not** respond to 100% oxygen.

10. Prilocaine and septocaine have been implicated in causing lingual nerve associated parasthesias and prolonged anesthesia after dental use, and it can last for 8 weeks or longer.

11. Local anesthetics are **not** associated with malignant hyperthermia and are **safe** to use. Inhaled general anesthetics and succinylcholine should be avoided in patients who are genetically predisposed to the condition.

12. Avoid local anesthetics containing epinephrine in patients with a history of hyperthyroidism, patients with severe cardiac and pulmonary disease, and patients on MAO-I (monoamineoxidase inhibitors), tricyclic antidepressants, propylthiouracil (PTU), lanoxin (digoxin) or theophylline.

13. All local anesthetics when used in excess will cause restlessness, anxiety, confusion, tremors, dizziness, and seizures.

LOCAL ANESTHETIC COMPLICATIONS

Local anesthetics can cause two types of complications:

- Localized
- Generalized: local anesthetic and/or epinephrine overdose

Localized Complications

Localized complications at the site of the injection are:

1. **Pain on injection:** Pain is caused by a dull needle or by rapid injection of the local anesthetic. Use sharp needles, topical anesthesia, and inject slowly to avoid pain on injection.

2. **Burning on injection:** Rapid injections, pH of the local anesthetic, and "warmed" local anesthetic are the main causes. Burning rapidly disappears as the local anesthetic takes effect if the pH is the cause. Rapid injection or an overly "warmed" local anesthetic may cause trismus, edema, or paresthesia. Always store local anesthetics at room temperature in a clean container without alcohol or other sterilizing agents.

3. **Persistent anesthesia or paresthesia:** Anesthesia can persist for days, weeks, or months. Trauma to any nerve or bleeding around a nerve can cause paresthesia. The patient experiences an electric shock sensation throughout the distribution of the nerve. 4% prilocaine (Citanest) and 4% septocaine (Articaine) are often associated with paresthesia when compared with other local anesthetics, and they should be avoided in patients with multiple sclerosis (MS). Most paresthesias resolve within

8 weeks without treatment, though severe damage can be permanent. Reassure the patient and provide frequent follow-up visits to reassess the condition. A highly symptomatic or anxious patient can be given 2 mg/5 mg diazepam (Valium) at bedtime.

4. **Trismus:** Prolonged spasm of the jaw muscles is associated with a locked jaw and trismus can become chronic and a problem to manage. The most common etiology is trauma to the muscles or blood vessels in the infratemporal fossa. Low-grade infection following local anesthesia injection can also cause trismus. Symptoms usually develop 1–6 days posttreatment. To prevent the occurrence of trismus decrease multiple needle penetrations in an area and do not inject excessive volumes of the anesthetic solution into a restricted area. The patient can be treated with heat therapy, warm saline rinse, analgesics, and, if necessary, diazepam (Valium). Give 10 mg diazepam, bid until the patient is able to tolerate the trismus or has recovered.

5. **Hematoma:** Nicking of an artery or a vein during injection can release blood into the extravascular spaces causing a painful bruise or swelling that persists for 7–14 days. Treatment consists of applying direct pressure at the site of bleeding for about 2 min followed by **icing** the area on the **first** day. Prescribe analgesics and advise the patient to use heat application when needed **after** the first day to avoid vasodilation and worsening of symptoms.

6. **Infection:** Injecting local anesthetic into an area of infection does not produce optimal anesthetic effect. If, however, the local anesthetic is injected under pressure, bacteria from the local site may be forced into the adjacent tissue. The patient is best treated with antibiotics, heat, analgesics, and benzodiazepines.

7. **Facial nerve paralysis:** Facial palsy can occur when the local anesthetic is introduced into the deep lobe of the parotid gland. Within seconds, the patient will sense a weakening of muscles on the affected side. Treatment: Reassure the patient. The situation will last for a few hours without residual effects. Apply an eye patch to the affected eye after removing the contact lens, when present. Reschedule and follow up.

Generalized Complications

Generalized reactions to local anesthetics can manifest as a local anesthetic overdose or epinephrine overdose reaction. Please refer to Chapter 9, "Management of Medical Emergencies in the Dental Setting: Assessment, Analysis, and Associated Dental Management Guidelines," for a detailed discussion of this topic.

Analgesics Commonly Used in Dentistry: Assessment, Analysis, and Associated Dental Management Guidelines

OVERVIEW

Analgesics are a very important adjunct in dentistry to assure quick recovery from pain. It is best to prescribe analgesics for no more than 2–3 days, and patients experiencing pain beyond 2–3 days should be reassessed before any additional analgesics are prescribed. Having a tight hold on the amount of analgesics you dispense keeps drug addicts away from your practice!

To assure selection of a "safe" analgesic for the compromised patient, the dentist needs to address multiple factors, such as the following:

- The patient's current medical status
- The patient's vital organs status, which includes the status of the liver and the kidneys
- Assessment of other medications the patient is on and associated drug-drug interactions
- Assessment of the appropriate analgesic dose and whether the patient should be dispensed a peripheral or centrally acting analgesic or a combination of both.

ANALGESICS CLASSIFICATION

Analgesics are classified according to their site of action:

I. **Peripherally acting analgesics:** Acetaminophen (Tylenol), aspirin, nonsteroidal antiinflamatory drugs (NSAIDS), and COX-2 inhibitors belong to this category of analgesics.
II. **Centrally acting opioid analgesics:** Codeine, morphine, hydromorphone (Dilaudid), oral transmucosal fentanyl citrate (OTFC), oxycodone, hydrocodone, propoxyphene, meperidine (Demerol) and centrally acting non-narcotic opioid analgesic, tramadol (Ultram) belong to this category.

PERIPHERALLY ACTING ANALGESICS

Acetaminophen (Tylenol)

Acetaminophen Pharmacology

Acetaminophen or Paracetamol, a pregnancy category B drug, is also known by its chemical name N-acetyl-p-aminophenol (APAP). The half-life of Tylenol is 2–4 hr and the therapeutic dose is 4 g/day. More than 90% of the acetaminophen dose is metabolized by the liver to sulfate and glucuronide conjugates, which are water soluble and eliminated in the urine. Conversion to sulfate is the primary pathway until the age of 10–12 years. Glucuronidation is the primary pathway in adolescents and adults. Only 2% of an acetaminophen dose is inactivated by glutathione and then excreted by the kidneys.

Tylenol Toxicity

Tylenol is the most common overdosed medication. Alcohol, liver disease, starvation, and protein malnutrition **decrease** glutathione levels and **increase** the chances of Tylenol toxicity. Hepatotoxicity due to Tylenol is most pronounced in the **fasting** patient and patients taking drugs primarily metabolized by the liver.

CYP3A4-induced Tylenol hepatotoxicity occurs from the formation of the reactive and toxic metabolite N-acetyl-benzoquinoneimine (NAPQI). Typically, glutathione binds to NAPQI and excretes NAPQI as nontoxic mercapturate conjugates. When glutathione stores are diminished, NAPQI binds to the liver cells causing hepatic necrosis. Alcohol consumption with Tylenol increases NAPQI production, so alcoholics **can overdose** with a therapeutic dose. Acetaminophen use is absolutely contraindicated *with* **alcohol** *and* in the presence of **alcohol-associated liver disease.**

Tylenol toxicity–induced acute liver failure can cause impaired hepatic synthetic function, the extent of which can be judged by monitoring the PT/INR (Table 5.1). The PT/INR is **increased** when the acutely injured liver is unable to produce clotting factors. The Tylenol toxicity prognosis is good when the PT/INR is **normal** in the presence of

Table 5.1. Summary: Acute acetaminophen (Tylenol) toxicity–associated liver function test (LFT) changes

LFT Marker	Marker Status
Total Protein	Normal
Albumin (A)	Normal
Globulin (G)	Normal
A:G ratio	Normal
ALT/SGPT	>10,000 IU/L; rapidly normal on recovery
AST/SGOT	Increased, but less than ALT
ALT:AST ratio	ALT>AST
GGT	Normal
Alkaline Phosphatase (AP)	Increased
PT/INR	Acutely prolonged with liver failure
Total Bilirubin	Normal
Direct-B	Normal
Indirect-B	Normal

increased ALT and AST. Renal failure, encephalopathy, and cerebral edema can additionally occur with Tylenol toxicity–associated acute liver failure. Immediate liver transplant is the only treatment in such cases.

Tylenol Toxicity Symptoms and Signs

Tylenol toxicity can present with an irregular pulse, nausea, vomiting, diarrhea, sweating, abdominal pain, seizures, and coma.

Tylenol Toxicity Laboratory Test Assessment

Tylenol toxicity causes an acute rise in the ALT and AST to >10,000 U/L within 24 hr after ingestion or within 8–16 hr in very severe cases, and peak levels occur at 48–72 hr.

As discussed earlier, the PT/INR, serum creatinine, and blood urea nitrogen (BUN) levels must also be assessed.

Tylenol Toxicity Treatment

The first step in management of Tylenol toxicity is gastrointestinal decontamination with activated charcoal. *N*-acetylcysteine (NAC) given PO (oral) or IV (intravenous) is the antidote and most patients recover if NAC is given within 8 hr of ingestion of the toxic dose. Glutathione levels are replaced by the sulfhydryl compounds from NAC causing reversal of the toxicity.

N-acetylcysteine (NAC) dose: Initial dose: 140 mg/kg, followed by 70 mg/kg every 4 hr × 17 doses, after the initial dose.

Tylenol Dosing

1. **Normal Tylenol Dose:** 325–650 mg q4–6h OR 1,000 mg 3–4 times/day. Do not exceed 4 g/day and avoid alcohol.
2. **Tylenol Dose with Kidney Disease:** Tylenol dose must be adjusted in renal failure because metabolites can otherwise accumulate. Use the following guidelines for dosing with kidney disease:
   a. **CrCl >50 mL/min or serum creatinine <2.0 mg/dL: Dose normally.** Give 325–650 mg **q4–6h** *or* 1,000 mg, 3–4 times/day.
   b. **CrCl 10–50 mL/min or serum creatinine >2.0 mg/dL to predialysis:** Prescribe 325–650 mg **q6h** only.
   c. **CrCl <10 mL/min or the renal failure/dialysis patient:** Prescribe 325–650 mg **q8h** only.
3. **Tylenol Dose with Liver Disease:** Use Tylenol with caution in the presence of hepatic impairment. Cases of hepatotoxicity at daily acetaminophen dosages <4 g/day have been reported. Limited, low-dose therapy is usually well tolerated with hepatic disease or cirrhosis. Avoid **chronic** use in hepatic impairment. The maximum daily dose of acetaminophen should be no more than **2 g/day** in patients with cirrhosis or chronic active hepatitis. Use the following guideline for dosing with liver disease:
   a. **Chronic inactive hepatitis:** Give Tylenol 325–650 mg **q6h**.
   b. **Chronic active hepatitis or cirrhosis:** Give Tylenol 325–650 mg **q8h**.

Nonsteroidal Antiinflammatory Drugs (NSAIDS)

NSAIDS Overview and Classification

Cyclo-oxygenase-1 (COX-1) is expressed in most normal tissues producing protective prostaglandins, which help maintain the gastric mucosa, normal renal function and platelet aggregation. NSAIDS work by **inhibiting** prostaglandin synthetase or cyclo-oxygenase (COX). Dependent on their action on cyclo-oxygenase (COX), NSAIDS are subdivided into nonselective and highly selective COX-1 and COX-2 inhibitors. Salicylates, aspirin and the traditional NSAIDS, indomethacin, ibuprofen, naproxen, ketoprofen and ketorolac belong to the class of the nonselective COX-1 inhibitors. Aspirin and the traditional NSAIDS, inhibit the vasodilator prostaglandins. Celecoxib and Valdecoxib belong to the class of highly selective COX-2 inhibitors.

NSAIDS and Vital Organs

NSAIDS are metabolized by the liver via conjugative and oxidation pathways and patients with liver disease should specifically **avoid** Aspirin and Ibuprofen. Some NSAIDS are more hepatotoxic than others. Patients with liver cirrhosis are at **increased risk of kidney damage** due to NSAIDS. NSAIDS should therefore be avoided in patients with cirrhosis.

NSAIDS and Pregnancy

NSAIDS are contraindicated during pregnancy for the following reasons:

- NSAIDS can alter the renal cortical function in the mother and decrease the fetal renal output. In the first trimester NSAIDS use is associated with an increased tendency towards miscarriages. In the third trimester, NSAIDS can increase the risk of closure of the fetal ductus arteriosus (FDA) or patent ductus arteriosus (PDA), resulting in fetal death.

NSAIDS Adverse Side Effects

NSAIDS can cause gastric irritability, platelet dysfunction, renal insufficiency and hepatotoxicity. The gastric irritability by NSAIDS is mediated in two ways, direct and indirect. Directly, the acidic molecules in the NSAIDS irritate the mucosa, and indirectly, NSAIDS inhibit COX-1. The combined effect causes a significant reduction of protective prostaglandins.

NSAIDS **temporarily** affect platelet cohesiveness and the platelets regain their cohesiveness once the NSAIDS have cleared the system. NSAIDS can usually be stopped 24 hr prior major surgery, after consulting with the patient's M.D. NSAIDS-associated renal damage is due to selective inhibition of the vasodilator prostaglandins, resulting in unapposed action of vasoconstrictor prostaglandins and consequent reduction in renal blood flow. Short-term, low dose NSAIDS use does not cause this side effect. The risk of renal toxicity with NSAIDS increases with old age and when used in the presence of renal disease, diuretics, cirrhosis and other nephrotoxic drugs.

Aspirin and NSAIDS can cause rhinosinusitis, polyps and asthma in patients allergic to these medications, by blocking the cyclo-oxygenase-1 enzyme, which triggers an overproduction of leukotrienes. Leukotrienes in turn cause bronchoconstriction.

Aspirin

Aspirin Facts

Aspirin is a pregnancy category C drug that becomes a category D drug in the third trimester of pregnancy. Aspirin has an analgesic efficacy equivalent to 5–10 mg, IM Morphine. The lowest effective aspirin dose should be used. Aspirin has to be used for several days to maximize effect and achieve optimal plasma levels. Aspirin has analgesic, antiinflammatory and antipyretic activity. The antipyretic activity is central in action.

Aspirin Metabolization

Aspirin is mainly metabolized in the liver and excreted through the kidneys. Patients with a creatinine clearance <50 mL/min or with serum creatinine >2 mg/dl should be given aspirin **q6h** only. **Avoid** Aspirin use in patients with **severe liver disease** and in patients on dialysis, with a CrCl <10 mL/min.

Aspirin Alert

Aspirin when taken daily, permanently affects platelet cohesiveness for the entire life span of the platelets, which is 10–14 days. Aspirin-associated platelet effect, affects **primary homeostasis** causing a prolonged Bleeding Time (BT). Aspirin does not affect the platelet count, PT/INR or the APTT.

The patient's physician must always be contacted prior to any major dental procedure to determine **if and when** the aspirin can be stopped. Consultation with the M.D. is absolutely necessary as it is the M.D. who clearly knows the patient's risk for thrombosis. In most cases, the adult or baby aspirin is usually stopped 7 days prior to the major surgical procedure but in the presence of high daily doses of aspirin for arthritis care, aspirin may have to be stopped for 10 days. Aspirin should be restarted **1–2 days** after the procedure, to ensure good primary hemostasis. Tylenol may be substituted in the interim period for pain control.

Aspirin Dose

Aspirin is available as an 81 mg tablet (baby aspirin) and a 325 mg tablet (adult aspirin). **Dose:** 325–650 mg q4–6h PRN, maximum dose: 4 g/day. Reduce the dose in the elderly and avoid in patients with **hypoalbuminemia and a CrCl <10 mL/min** (this is the patient on dialysis).

Ibuprofen and Naproxen

Ibuprofen and Naproxen Facts

NSAIDS have an analgesic efficacy equivalent to 5–10 mg, IM Morphine and the lowest effective NSAID dose should be used. NSAIDS have to be used for several days to maximize effect and achieve optimal plasma levels. Ibuprofen and Naproxen are pregnancy category C drugs that become category D drugs in the third trimester of pregnancy.

Ibuprofen and Naproxen Actions

They have analgesic, antiinflammatory and antipyretic activity. The antipyretic activity is central in action.

Ibuprofen and Naproxen Metabolization

They are mainly metabolized in the liver and excreted through the kidneys. NSAIDS use must be avoided in patients with any form of kidney or liver disease. The clearance of Naproxen is decreased in chronic hepatitis.

Ibuprofen and Naproxen Dose

1. **Ibuprofen (Motrin) Dose:** 200–400 mg PO q4–6h PRN; maximum dose: 1,200 mg/day
2. **Naproxen (Naprosyn) Dose:** 250–500 mg PO q8–12h PRN; maximum dose: 1,500 mg/day

COX-2 Inhibitors

COX-2 Inhibitors Facts

COX-2 production is induced by inflammation and is associated with pain. COX-2 inhibition has analgesic, antiinflammatory and antipyretic activity. The analgesic activity is similar to that of the COX-1 inhibitors. The COX-2 inhibitors are effective for acute and chronic pain associated with rheumatoid and osteoarthritis. Unlike the COX-1 inhibitors, they do not affect platelets and the gastric mucosa. COX-2 inhibitors are pregnancy category C drugs that become category D drugs in the third trimester of pregnancy. Celecoxib has a sulfa tail that can cause a reaction and it is avoided in patients with **Sulfonamide** antimicrobial allergy.

COX-2 Metabolization

COX-2 drugs are metabolized in the liver and excreted through the kidneys. They have renal effects similar to the COX-1 inhibitors. COX-2 inhibitors should be avoided in the elderly and in patients with renal, hepatic or cardiac impairment.

Celecoxib Dose

Celecoxib, 100–200 mg q12h PRN

CENTRALLY ACTING OPIOID ANALGESICS

The opioid analgesics have morphinelike effects and they act by interacting with the opioid receptors. All opioids need a prescription and many of them cannot be prescribed with a refill.

Opioids Classification

Opioids commonly used in dentistry are codeine; morphine; hydromorphone (Dilaudid); oral transmucosal fentanyl citrate (OTFC); oxycodone; oxycodone + acetaminophen (Percocet); hydrocodone + acetaminophen (Vicodin/Lortab); hydromorphone (Dilaudid); propoxyphene (Darvon); propoxyphene + acetaminophen (Darvocet N); meperidine (Demerol); and tramadol (Ultram), which is a non-narcotic opioid.

Opioid Metabolism and the Liver

Essentials for the proper processing of drugs metabolized by the liver are adequate liver function, optimal albumin levels, and good blood flow to the liver. Metabolism is also dependent on whether the drug is a high- or low-extraction drug. High-extraction drugs are efficiently removed from the bloodstream by the liver. Liver disease is thus associated with a decrease in clearance and increase in plasma concentration and elimination half-life of drugs metabolized by the liver. The liver is the major site for biotransformation of the opioids and most of them are metabolized by oxidation. Hepatic metabolism converts drugs into products that are less potent than the original drug, and these products are eventually more easily excreted. Some products, however, may be more potent than the original drug. The metabolism of opioids is impaired in liver and kidney disease. Liver failure is associated with **decreased oxidation** of opioids and **decreased clearance**, particularly affecting meperidine, propoxyphene, pentazocine, and tramadol. **Lower the dose and prolong the interval** if an opioid has to be used in a patient with liver disease. Use caution with codeine, morphine and oxycodone because their active metabolites are cleared through the kidneys. Avoid meperidine, propoxyphene, pentazocine, and tramadol with liver or kidney disease. Hydromorphone or fentanyl are recommended for use in liver or kidney failure.

Narcotic Side Effects

Narcotic side effects are nausea, vomiting, lightheadedness, dizziness, dry mouth, mental sluggishness, difficulty urinating, and constipation.

Opioid Alerts and Facts Significant for Dentistry

The following are alerts and facts significant for dentistry:

1. Oral narcotics should be prescribed for only 2–3 days and further pain management should be continued with non-narcotic pain medications.
2. Chronic narcotic use accelerates the liver enzymes causing faster drug metabolization and consequent need for larger and more frequent doses. Physical dependence and tolerance can thus occur with long-term use.
3. Opioids increase alcohol effects and should not be combined.
4. Avoid opioid analgesic use just prior to birth (last 2–4 weeks of pregnancy), because this can cause serious breathing problems in the newborn.
5. Limit use in the lactating patient as opioids pass through the breast milk.
6. Opioid use should be restricted in patients with a history of seizures, severe asthma, COPD, severe emphysema, uncontrolled hypothyroidism, Addison's disease, gallstones, diverticulitis, enlarged prostate, urinary retention problems, drug abuse, and recovering addicts.
7. Do not prescribe narcotic analgesics to patients on antipsychotics, CNS depressants, or TCAs because this can cause narcotic analgesic toxicity.
8. Morphine, codeine, and meperidine are nonspecific histamine liberators that bind to a specific receptor on the mast cells causing histamine release. Patients with severe symptoms can be given an opioid pain medication with a non-sedating antihistamine or a nonopioid pain medication such as tromethamine (Toradol).
9. Do not combine opioid analgesics with sedating antihistamines, CNS depressants; tricyclic antidepressants (TCAs), muscle relaxants, or warfarin (Coumadin).
10. Do not combine Demerol with monoamine oxidase (MAO) inhibitors; do not combine Darvocet N or Darvon with antiseizure medications; do not combine morphine with zidovudin (AZT).

Codeine

Codeine Facts

Codeine is similar to morphine but is milder and causes more constipation. Codeine activity depends on its conversion to morphine by the CYP2D6 enzyme. Codeine is metabolized in the liver and excreted through the kidneys. With liver failure, codeine conversion is impaired and its analgesic activity is compromised. The active metabolites accumulate in renal failure, and there are reports of serious adverse effects in renal failure patients. **Dose adjustments** are recommended in patients with **hepatic and renal** insufficiency.

   Codeine pregnancy category: Category **A**.

Codeine Caution

A patient allergic to morphine will be allergic to codeine due to cross-reactivity.

Codeine Preparations

Codeine is typically used in combination with acetaminophen as:

Tylenol #1: 7.5 mg codeine +300 mg acetaminophen (APAP)
Tylenol #2: 15 mg codeine +300 mg APAP
Tylenol #3: 30 mg codeine +300 mg APAP: Most prescribed
Tylenol #4: 60 mg codeine +300 mg APAP

Codeine Dosing

1. **Normal Dose:** The usual dose is 30–60 mg/1–2 tablets q4–6h, maximum 12 tablets/24 hr. Do not exceed 4 g/day of acetaminophen.
2. **Dose with Kidney Disease:**
    a. **CrCl >50 mL/min or serum creatinine <2.0 mg/dL:** Dose normally, use 30–60 mg codeine. Dispense 1–2 Tylenol #3 q4h PRN.
    b. **CrCl 10–50 mL/min or serum creatinine >2.0 mg/dL to predialysis:** Decrease codeine dose by 50%, use 15–30 mg codeine. Dispense 1–2 Tylenol #2 q6h PRN.
    c. **CrCl <10 mL/min or in the Renal Failure/Dialysis Patient:** Decrease the codeine dose by 75% and use 7.5–15 mg codeine. Dispense 1–2 Tylenol #1 q8h PRN.
3. **Dose with Liver Disease:**
    a. **Mild or chronic inactive hepatitis:** Dose normally, give 30–60 mg codeine. Give 1–2 Tylenol #3 **q4h** PRN.
    b. **Moderate-severe or active hepatitis:** Dispense 50% dose, give 15–30 mg codeine. Give 1–2 Tylenol #2 **q6h** PRN.
    c. **Cirrhosis:** Reduce dose by 75%, give 7.5–15 mg codeine. Give 1–2 Tylenol #1 **q8h** PRN.

Morphine

Morphine Facts

Morphine is metabolized mainly in the liver by glucuronidation and some metabolism occurs in the kidney and the gastrointestinal tract. Morphine clearance is decreased in liver failure. Renal failure is associated with an accumulation of morphine metabolites. Morphine can thus cause hepatotoxicity and nephrotoxicity.

Morphine Use

Morphine is used in the management of moderate to severe pain. Avoid use in the elderly and in patients with severe pulmonary disease.

Morphine pregnancy category: Category **C**.

Morphine Dose

1. **Normal Oral Morphine:** 10–20 mg q3–4h
2. **Normal IV Morphine:** 2 mg q2–3h

Morphine is a high-extraction drug and its bioavailability increases in patients with advanced liver disease or cirrhosis. The dosing interval of morphine should be increased by 1.5–2 times the regular dosing interval if you *have* to use it in a patient with liver disease. Ideally, morphine should **not** be used in the presence of liver and kidney disease.

Hydromorphone (Dilaudid)

Hydromorphone Facts

Hydromorphone is metabolized in the liver and excreted in the urine. Hydromorphone is used in the management of moderate to severe pain.

Hydromorphone pregnancy category: Category **C/D** at term.

Hydromorphone Caution

Dilaudid tablets contain metabisulfite, and the drug should not be used in patients with a history of allergy to sulfites or history of G6PD anemia. Avoid in elderly patients and in patients with severe pulmonary disease. Hydromorphone **can be used** in kidney or liver failure.

Hydromorphone Dose

Dilaudid is available as a 2, 4, or 8 mg tablet. The following are the usual doses:

1. **Oral Hydromorphone:** 2–4 mg q4h
2. **IV Hydromorphone:** 1.5 mg q4h

Oral Transmucosal Fentanyl Citrate (OTFC)

Oral Transmucosal Fentanyl Citrate (OTFC) Facts

OTFC is used for breakthrough pain in cancer patients who are already on opioids. It is 100 times more potent than morphine. 25–50% absorption is transmucosal and the rest is via slow gastrointestinal absorption. OFTC becomes effective in 5–10 min and the effect lasts for 1–3.5 hr. Fentanyl metabolism is **unaffected** with liver disease.

Fentanyl citrate pregnancy category: Category **C/D**.

Fentanyl Citrate Side Effects

Fentanyl causes dizziness, nausea, and drowsiness.

Fentanyl Citrate (OTFC) Dose

Start with 1 200 µg lozenge and use it over 15 min, holding it between the gums and the cheek and moving it from one side to the other side. Do not place it on the tongue because this will slow the absorption of OTFC. Wait 15 min and use a second 200 µg lozenge if the pain does not immediately subside. Do not use more than 2 lozenges at a given time.

Oxycodone: Oxycodone + Acetaminophen: Percocet

Percocet Facts

Oxycodone is typically combined with acetaminophen (Percocet) or aspirin (Percodan). Percocet is the only preparation advised for dentistry and not Percodan, because Percodan can trigger aspirin-induced platelet dysfunction bleeding. Percocet is used for mild, moderate, or severe pain.

Oxycodone is metabolized in the liver and excreted through the kidneys. It is converted to its active form in the liver by the CYP2D6 enzyme. Percocet action lasts for 4–6 hr. Prescribe with **caution** and careful monitoring in **renal failure** patients, and use with **caution** in the presence of **hepatic impairment**; in the elderly; and in the presence of **severe** liver, kidney, and pulmonary disease. **Limited, low-dose** therapy is usually well tolerated in hepatic disease or cirrhosis. However, cases of hepatotoxicity at daily acetaminophen dosages <4 g/day have been reported. Avoid chronic use in the presence of hepatic impairment.

Percocet DEA Schedule

Percocet is a Schedule II drug that requires a written prescription, which must be filled in 30 days. No refills are allowed for Percocet.

Percocet pregnancy category: Percocet is a category B drug when used short-term and in smaller doses. However, when Percocet is used for a prolonged period at term or in high doses, it can become a category D drug causing breathing difficulty and even death in the newborn.

Percocet Preparations

Percocet is available in the following strengths:

2.5 mg oxycodone + 325 mg acetaminophen (APAP): 2.5/325
5 mg oxycodone + 325 mg APAP (original tablet): 5/325
7.5 mg oxycodone + 325 mg APAP: 7.5/325
7.5 mg oxycodone + 500 mg APAP: 7.5/500
10 mg oxycodone + 650 mg APAP: 10/650

Percocet Dosing

1. **Normal Percocet Dose:oxycodone + APAP (Percocet):** 2.5–5 mg oxycodone **q4–6h**
   In the healthy adult depending on the pain intensity: Dispense one 2.5/325 or 5/325 Percocet tablet **q4–6h** PRN. It is better to dispense one 5/325 tablet instead of two 2.5/325 tablets for severe pain so that the total Tylenol intake can be kept down.
2. **Percocet Dose with Kidney Disease:**
   a. **Predialysis: 1,** 2.5/325 tablet **q6h** PRN
   b. **Dialysis: 1,** 2.5/325 tablet **q8h** PRN
3. **Percocet Dose Schedule with Liver Disease:**
   a. **Hepatitis: 1,** 2.5/325 tablet **q6h** PRN
   b. **Cirrhosis: 1,** 2.5/325 tablet **q8h** PRN

Hydrocodone: Hydrocodone + Acetaminophen (Vicodin)

Vicodin Facts

Vicodin is metabolized in the liver and excreted in the urine. Administer with **caution** and careful monitoring in patients with **renal failure** and use with **caution** in the presence of **hepatic impairment**. Limited, low-dose therapy is usually well tolerated in hepatic disease or cirrhosis. However, cases of hepatotoxicity at daily acetaminophen dosages <4 g/day have been reported. Avoid chronic use in the presence of hepatic impairment.

Vicodin or Lortab is used for the management of moderate to severe pain, and it is a Schedule III drug.

Vicodin Pregnancy Category: Category **B**; Category **C/D** at term.

Vicodin Preparations

1. **Each Vicodin tablet contains:** 5 mg hydrocodone +500 mg acetaminophen (APAP)
2. **Vicodin ES contains:** 7.5 mg hydrocodone +500 mg APAP
3. **Vicoprofin contains:** 7.5 mg hydrocodone +200 mg ibuprofen. Vicoprofin is particularly useful in the presence of pain and inflammation.

Vicodin Dosing

1. **Normal Dose:** 5–10 mg hydrocodone: Give **1–2** tablets **q6h** PRN.
2. **Vicodin Dose with Kidney Disease:**
   a. **Predialysis:** Vicodin, **1** tab **q6h** PRN
   b. **Dialysis:** Vicodin, **1** tab **q8h** PRN
3. **Vicodin Dose with Liver Disease:**
   a. **Hepatitis:** Vicodin, **1** tab **q6h** PRN
   b. **Cirrhosis:** Vicodin, **1** tab **q8h** PRN

Dextropropoxyphene (Darvon)

Darvon Facts

Darvon levels increase in patients with chronic liver disease or cirrhosis, resulting in hepatotoxicity. Propoxyphene's metabolite norpropoxyphene also accumulates with kidney disease, causing sedation and confusion. A**void** Darvon or Darvocet in patients with liver and kidney disease.

Darvon Pregnancy Category: Category **C**.

Darvon Preparations

1. **Darvocet N:** 50 mg propoxyphene +325 mg acetaminophen. **Dose:** 1–2 tablets q4h PRN, maximum 600 mg propoxyphene napsylate/day
2. **Darvocet N 100:** 100 mg propoxyphene +650 mg acetaminophen

Darvon Dose

1 tablet q4h, maximum 600 mg propoxyphene napsylate/day

Meperidine (Demerol)

Meperidine Facts

Meperidine is metabolized in the liver and excreted through the kidneys. It is a high-extraction drug and its bioavailability increases in patients with advanced liver disease or cirrhosis. Its metabolite normeperidine accumulates with kidney disease causing CNS toxicity. Thus meperidine should **not** be used in patients with liver disease or kidney disease. Meperidine should only be used for the management of moderate to severe *acute* pain. It should not be used for *chronic* pain. Avoid meperidine in the pregnant patient and patients taking MAO inhibitors.

 Meperidine Pregnancy Category: Category **C/D**.

Meperidine Dose

Oral: 50 mg q3–4h PRN

Tramadol (Ultram)

Tramadol Facts

Tramadol, a category **C** drug is an atypical centrally acting non-narcotic opioid analgesic that is **not** considered a controlled substance. It therefore can be obtained with a regular prescription. On ingestion, the CYP2D6 enzyme in the liver converts tramadol to its active form, O-desmethyl-tramadol. Inactive metabolites of this product are excreted by the kidney. Avoid in the presence of severe liver or kidney disease, with seizure medications, TCAs, or SSRIs.

Tramadol Preparation

Ultracet: 37.5 mg tramadol + 325 mg APAP

Tramadol Dose

50–100 mg Ultram PO q4–6h PRN

ANALGESIC PRESCRIPTIONS FOR MILD, MODERATE, OR SEVERE PAIN

1. **Mild pain analgesic prescriptions:**
    a. **Aspirin:** 325 mg/tab; Rx: 2 tabs q6h PRN (not advised)
    b. **Ibuprofen:** 200 mg/tab; Rx: 2 tabs q6h PRN
    c. **Naproxen (Aleve):** 200 mg/tab; Rx: 1 tab q8h PRN
    d. **Acetaminophen (Tylenol):** 325 mg/tab or 500 mg/tab; Rx: 2 tabs q6h PRN
    e. **Ketoprofen (Orudis):** 500 mg/tab; Rx: 1 tab q 8–12 hr PRN
    f. **Ibuprofen (Motrin):** 800 mg/tab; Rx: 1 tab q8h PRN
     Avoid using aspirin for pain relief because aspirin permanently affects the cohesiveness of the platelets, causing excessive postoperative bleeding.
2. **Moderate pain analgesic prescriptions:**
    a. **Codeine and acetaminophen (Tylenol #3):** 30 mg codeine and 300 mg acetaminophen/tab. Rx: 1 tab q6h PRN
    b. **Hydrocodone and acetaminophen (Vicodin):** 5 mg hydrocodone and 500 mg acetaminophen/tab Rx: 1 tab q6h PRN. Vicodin is preferred over Percocet because it is less addicting than Percocet.

Table 5.2. Analgesics summary

Analgesic	Analgesic Doses: All Used PRN
Acetaminophen (Tylenol): Pregnancy Category B Strengths available: 325/500 mg/tablet	Normal Dose: 325–650 mg q4–6 h/ 1000 mg 3–4 times (x)/day. Avoid alcohol use. Normal Maximum Dose: 4 g/day Liver Disease Dose: <2 g/day Chronic inactive hepatitis: 325–650 mg **q6h** Chronic active Hepatitis or Cirrhosis: 325–650 mg **q8h** Kidney Disease Dosages: i. S. Creatinine (Cr) <2.0 mg/dL: Give normal dose ii. S. Cr >2.0 mg/dL to Predialysis: 325–650 mg **q6h** iii. Dialysis: 325–650 mg **q8h**
Aspirin: Pregnancy Category: C; Category D in 3rd trimester Strengths available: 81 mg/325 mg/tablet	Normal Dose: 325–650 mg q4–6 h Maximum Dose: 4 g/day. Reduce dose in the elderly. Kidney Disease Dose: S. Cr >2 mg/dL to Predialysis: Dose aspirin q6h only Avoid with cirrhosis and in patients on dialysis. Avoid aspirin use in dentistry.
Ibuprofen (Motrin): Pregnancy Category: B; Category D in 3rd trimester Strengths available: 200/400/800 mg/tablet	Normal Dose: 200–400 mg q4–6 h Maximum Dose: 1200 mg/day Avoid with liver and kidney disease.
Naproxen (Naprosyn): Pregnancy Category: B; Category D in 3rd trimester Strengths available: 250/500 mg/tablet	Normal Dose: 250–500 mg PO q8–12 h Maximum Dose: 1500 mg/day Avoid with liver and kidney disease.
Celecoxib (Celebrex): Pregnancy Category: B; Category D in 3rd trimester Strengths available: 100/200 mg/tablet	Normal Dose: 100–200 mg q12h Avoid with liver or kidney disease.
Codeine: Pregnancy Category: A Strengths available: Tylenol #1: 7.5 mg Codeine + 300 mg Acetaminophen (APAP) Tylenol #2: 15 mg Codeine + 300 mg APAP Tylenol #3: Most prescribed strength 30 mg Codeine + 300 mg APAP Tylenol #4: 60 mg Codeine + 300 mg APAP	Normal Dose: 30–60 mg/1–2 tabs q4–6 h. Maximum 12 tabs/24 h and <4 g/day of Tylenol Kidney Disease Dosages: i. S. Cr. <2.0 mg/dL: Normal Dose ii. S. Cr. >2.0 mg/dL to Predialysis: 1–2 Tylenol #2 **q6h** iii. Dialysis: 1–2 Tylenol #1 q8h Liver Disease Dosages: i. Mild or chronic inactive Hepatitis: Dose normally: 1–2 Tylenol #3 q4h ii. Moderate-severe or active Hepatitis: 1–2 Tylenol #2 **q6h** iii. Cirrhosis: 1–2 Tylenol #1 **q8h**

Table 5.2. *Continued*

Analgesic	Analgesic Doses: All Used PRN
Morphine: Pregnancy Category: C Strength: 10 mg/tablet	Normal Dose: Oral: 10–20 mg q3–4 h IV: 2 mg q2–3 h Avoid with liver or kidney disease.
Hydromorphone (Dilaudid): Pregnancy category: C; Category D at term	Normal Dose: Oral: 2–4 mg q4h IV: 1.5 mg q4h Liver/Kidney Disease: Can be used in liver or kidney failure.
Oral Transmucosal Fentanyl Citrate (OTFC): Pregnancy Category: C Category D in late term	Normal Dose: Suck on 1, 200 µg lozenge over 15 min. Use another 200 µg lozenge after 15 min if pain persists.
Oxycodone + APAP (Percocet): Pregnancy Category: B Category D in late term Strengths available: **2.5/325:** 2.5 mg Oxycodone + 325 mg Acetaminophen (APAP) **5/325:** 5 mg Oxycodone + 325 mg APAP (original tablet) **7.5/325:** 7.5 mg Oxycodone + 325 mg APAP **7.5/500:** 7.5 mg Oxycodone + 500 mg APAP **10/650:** 10 mg Oxycodone + 650 mg APAP	Normal Dose: One 2.5/325 or 5/325 Percocet tablet **q4–6 h** Kidney Disease Dosages: i. Predialysis: One 2.5/325 tab **q6h** ii. Dialysis: One 2.5/325 tab **q8h** Liver Disease Dosages: i. Hepatitis: One 2.5/325 tab **q6h** ii. Cirrhosis: One 2.5/325 tab **q8h**
Hydrocodone + Acetaminophen (Vicodin): Pregnancy Category B; Category C/D at term Strengths available: **Each Vicodin tablet contains:** 5 mg Hydrocodone + 500 mg Acetaminophen (APAP) **Vicodin ES:** 7.5 mg Hydrocodone + 500 mg APAP **Vicoprofin:** 7.5 mg Hydrocodone + 200 mg Ibuprofen	Normal Dose: 1–2 tablets **q6h** Kidney Disease Dosages: i. Predialysis: 1 tab **q6h** ii. Dialysis: 1 tab **q8h** Liver Disease Dosages: i. Hepatitis: 1 tab **q6h** ii. Cirrhosis: 1 tab **q8h**
Dextropropoxyphene + Acetaminophen (Darvocet N or Darvocet N 100): Pregnancy Category: C Strengths available: **Darvocet N:** 50 mg Propoxyphene + 325 mg Acetaminophen **Darvocet N 100:** 100 mg Propoxyphene + 650 mg Acetaminophen	Darvocet N Dose: 1–2 tablets q4h; maximum 600 mg Propoxyphene Napsylate/day Darvocet N 100 Dose: 1 tablet q4h; maximum 600 mg Propoxyphene Napsylate/day **Avoid** with kidney/liver disease.

Table 5.2.   *Continued*

Analgesic	Analgesic Doses: All Used PRN
Meperidine (Demerol): Pregnancy Category: C; Category D in late term Strength: 50 mg/tablet	Normal Dose: 50 mg q3–4 h **Avoid** in kidney/liver disease.
Tramadol (Ultram): Pregnancy Category: C Strength available: **Ultracet 37.5/325:** 37.5 mg Tramadol + 325 mg APAP	Normal Dose: 50–100 mg PO q4–6 h **Avoid** in severe liver and kidney disease.
Aspirin NSAIDS Extra-strength Tylenol Meperidine (Demerol) Propoxyphene (Darvon) Pentazocine Tramadol (Ultram)	**Avoid all** these analgesics in the presence of kidney or liver disease.
Regular-strength Tylenol Dose modified Codeine with Tylenol; Oxycodone or Hydrocodone with Tylenol Hydromorphone (Dilaudid) or Fentanyl	These analgesics **can be used** with kidney or liver disease.

    c. **Oxycodone and aspirin (Percodan):** 4.88 mg oxycodone and 325 mg aspirin/tab Rx: 1 tab q6h PRN. Percodan is not recommended because it contains aspirin.

    d. **Oxycodone and acetaminophen (Percocet):** 5 mg oxycodone and 325 mg acetaminophen/tab Rx: 1 tab q6h PRN

    e. **Meperidine (Demerol):** 50 mg/tab Rx: 1 tab q6h PRN

    f. **Propoxyphene (Darvocet-N100):** propoxyphene 100 mg plus 650 mg acetaminophen/tab Rx: 1 tab q4h PRN

3. **Non-narcotic and narcotic analgesic prescriptions for severe pain:**

    a. **Non-narcotic preparation: pentazocine lactate (Talwin):** Dose: 30 mg SC, IM or IV, q4h PRN

    b. **Narcotic preparations:**

        i. **Codeine sulphate dose:** 15–60 mg SC or IM q4h

        ii. **Meperidine HCL (Demerol):** Dose: 50–150 mg SC/IM q4h PRN

        iii. **Morphine sulphate:** Dose: 5–20 mg SC/IM q4h

ANALGESICS SUMMARY

Review Table 5.2.

Odontogenic Infections and Antibiotics Commonly Used in Dentistry: Assessment, Analysis, and Associated Dental Management Guidelines

ODONTOGENIC INFECTION OVERVIEW AND MANAGEMENT FACTS

Odontogenic infections when present are typically treated with incision and drainage (I&D) of an abscess, when possible; antibiotics; pain and fever relief with appropriate analgesics; and removal of the source of infection once the patient is stabilized, e.g., extraction of an infected tooth.

FACTORS ASSESSED PRIOR TO ANTIBIOTIC USE

The following factors should be considered, assessed, or evaluated prior to prescribing antibiotics:

- Infection presentation: localized or generalized
- The specific organisms involved
- The duration for which the patient has been symptomatic
- Specific antibiotic facts: half-life, therapeutic window, spectrum of activity, mechanism of action of the antibiotic, the bactericidal or bacteriostatic status of the antibiotic, location(s) where the antibiotic is metabolized and cleared, the appropriate dosage and duration of antibiotic use, the drug-drug interactions (DDIs) between the patient's medications and the antibiotic prescribed, antibiotic side effects, and immune system status of the patient
- Mechanisms to maintain the intestinal bacterial flora during the antibiotic intake
- Water or fluid consumption with the antibiotic intake
- Antibiotic prescription in the presence of oral contraceptives
- Antibiotic use during breast-feeding

ODONTOGENIC INFECTIONS: ORGANISMS AND DURATION OF INFECTION

Odontogenic infections usually have a mixed aerobic and anaerobic flora. Early infections or infections symptomatic for less than 3 days are predominantly aerobic, and gram-positive streptococcus viridans or alpha-hemolytic streptococcus is the predominant bacteria. It responds extremely well to penicillin, clindamycin, or cephalosporins. Penicillin VK is the first drug of choice for **early** infections. Clindamycin or cephalexin (Keflex), are alternate first-choice drugs for an early infection in a penicillin-allergic patient. As the infection matures the patient's defenses take over and the flora becomes mostly anaerobic. Anaerobes are therefore associated with late infections or infections symptomatic for more than 3 days. **Staphylococcus aureus** predominates in **late** infections, but occasional isolates in early oral infections can also show staphylococcus aureus. Patients with staphylococcus aureus infection respond extremely well to clindamycin and poorly to penicillin. Clindamycin is the treatment of choice for **late** odontogenic infections. Clindamycin additionally has **replaced** erythromycin as the drug of choice for patients allergic to penicillin. Periodontal infections are often polymicrobial, and anaerobic bacteria predominate. Peri-implant disease is mostly plaque-induced, and bacteria when isolated are similar to those associated with periodontal infection. An aerobic flora comprising streptococcus viridans or alpha-hemolytic streptococcus is most commonly associated with dental caries. Dental pulp involvement is associated with a more anaerobic flora. Gram-negative bacilli are more likely to be associated with periapical infections.

Odontogenic Infection and Associated Antibiotic Protocol

Infection symptomatic for fewer than 3 days:

- Start with Pen VK/clindamycin (penicillin-allergic patient).
- Switch to clindamycin (first choice), azythromycin, clarithromycin, or penicillin VK and metronidazole if there is no response in 24–48 hr.

Infection symptomatic for more than 3 days:

- Start with clindamycin (first choice).
- Azythromycin, clarithromycin, or Pen VK and metronidazole are alternate drugs if clindamycin cannot be used.

Periodontal Infections

- Amoxicillin, clindamycin, metronidazole, doxycycline, and tetracycline are antibiotics commonly used for treatment of periodontal infections.

Odontogenic Infection Types

Odontogenic infections can be localized or generalized. Localized infections can present as a dry socket causing pain, swelling, and redness or as an abscess/localized pus-forming process that can cause fever, malaise, mild prostration, and localized lymphadenopathy.

Generalized/spreading infections can spread into anatomic sites causing cellulites and septicemia. The patient presents with rapidly progressing fever, chills, malaise, tachycardia, diffuse swelling at the site of infection, moderate to severe prostration, and lymphadenopathy. Always assess the mental status and patient interactiveness. A spreading infection is associated with a noninteractive status. Also assess the respiratory status in the presence of a generalized infection. Ludwig's angina compromising the sublingual and submandibular spaces should be considered if the patient is experiencing breathing difficulty. Swelling around the eyes or a generalized swelling of the face is localized cellulites that have the potential for spreading.

Table 6.1. Antibiotics summary

Antibiotic	Antibiotic Doses: Normal/Modified
Penicillin VK: Category B Strength: 250/500 mg/tab	1. **Normal Dose:** 250–500 mg PO q6h/qid Renal dose determined using serum creatinine (S.Cr) or creatinine clearance (CrCl). 2. **S.Cr. <2.0 mg/dL or CrCl >50 mL/min:** Dispense normal dose. 3. **S.Cr 2.0 mg/dL to Predialysis or CrCl 10–50 mL/min:** 250–500 mg q8–12 h 4. **Dialysis:** 250–500 q12–16 h
Penicillin G: Category B Strength: 1.2 MU/injection	1. **Normal Dose:** 1.2 million units Penicillin G, IM q12h 2. **Patient with both Liver and Kidney Disease:** Use half the normal dose.

Amoxicillin (Amoxyl):
Category B
Strengths:
  250/500/875 mg/capsule
	1. **Normal Dose:**
	  i. 250–500 mg PO q8h or 500–875 mg PO q12h × 5–7 days
	  ii. 3 g or 6, 500 mg capsules twice in 8 h (1-day treatment [Rx] for severe acute infection)
	2. **Premedication:** 2 g PO 1 h prior to Rx
	3. **Kidney Disease:**
	  i. **CrCl >30 mL/min or a S.Cr <3.3 mg/dL:** Dispense the normal dose.
	  ii. **CrCl 10–30 mL/min or S.Cr >3.3 mg/dL to Predialysis:** Prolong the interval and avoid the 875 mg tablet: Give 250–500 mg PO q12h.
	  iii. **CrCl <10 mL/min or Dialysis:** Prolong the interval and give 250–500 mg PO q24h **after** dialysis.
	4. **Liver Disease:** Use normal dose.
	5. **Liver and Kidney Disease:** Use renal dose guidelines.

Augmentin: Category B Strength: 250/500 mg/capsule	1. **Normal Dose:** 250/500 mg q8h 2. **Kidney Disease:** Decrease dose by 50% with kidney disease.
Ampicillin: Category B Strength: 250/500 mg/capsule	1. **Normal Dose:** 250–500 mg q6h for 5–7 days 2. **Premedication Dose:** 2.0 g IV/IM 30 min prior to procedure
Dicloxacillin: Category B Strength: 250/500 mg/capsule	1. **Normal Dose:** 250–500 mg qid × 5–7 days 2. **Kidney Disease:** Use 50% of normal dose.

Cephalexin (Keflex): Strength: 250/500 mg/capsule
Cefadroxil (Duricef): Strength 250/500 mg/capsule
Cefazolin (Ancef): Injection
Ceftriaxone (Rocephin): Injection
All Cephalosporins are Category B
	1. **Cephalexin (Keflex):**
	  i. **Normal Dose:** 250–1000 mg q6h/qid × 5–7 days, maximum 4.0 g/day
	  ii. **Kidney Disease Dose:** q12h or q24h
	2. **Cefadroxil (Duricef):** Normal Dose: 1–2 g/day in 2 divided doses × 5–7 days
	3. **Premedication Prophylaxis with Cephalexin or Cefadroxil:** 2 g PO 1 h prior to procedure
	4. **Cefazolin (Ancef):** 1 g IV/IM 30 min prior to procedure
	5. **Ceftriaxone (Rocephin):** 1.0 g IV/IM 30 min prior to the procedure
	6. **Kidney and Liver Disease:** All Cephalosporins can be used with **50%** dose reduction.

Table 6.1. *Continued*

Antibiotic	Antibiotic Doses: Normal/Modified

Clindamycin (Cleocin):
Category B
Strengths: 150/300 mg/tablet
Note: 150/300 mg PO is a static dose;
150/300 mg IV/IM is a cidal dose;
600 mg PO or IV/IM is a cidal dose
	1. **Normal Dose:** 150–450 mg q6–8 h/qid PO × 5–7 days. Best to prescribe the lower dose, 150 mg tid or q8h to minimize adverse side effects.
	2. **Refractory Cases of Periodontal Infection**: 600 mg/day × 7 days
	3. **Premedication Prophylaxis:**
	  i. 600 mg PO 1 h prior to treatment
	  ii. 600 mg, IV 30 min before procedure
	4. **Hepatitis:** No dose change.
	5. **Cirrhosis:** Decrease dose by 50%.
	6. **Kidney Disease:** No dose change with kidney disease or renal failure.
	7. **Kidney and Liver Disease:** Can be used with a 50% dose reduction.

Azithromycin (Zithromax/Z-pak): Category B Strength: 250/500 mg/capsule	**Azithromycin:** 1. **Azithromycin Normal 5-day Dose:** 250 mg bid or 500 mg HS on day one, then 250 mg/day for the next 4 days 2. **Azithromycin Normal 3-day Dose:** 500 mg/day × 3 days 3. **Azithromycin and Kidney Disease:** No dose change. 4. **Azithromycin and Liver Disease:** Avoid.
Clarithromycin (Biaxin): Category C Strength: 250/500 mg/capsule	**Clarithromycin:** 1. **Clarithromycin Normal Dose:** 250 or 500 mg bid for 5–7 days 2. **Clarithromycin and Kidney Disease:** Avoid. 3. **Clarithromycin and Liver Disease:** Can be used if kidney status is normal. **Premedication Prophylaxis with both:** Azithromycin or Clarithromycin, 500 mg PO 1 h prior to procedure
Metronidazole (Flagyl): Category B Strength: 250/500 mg/capsule	1. **Normal Dose:** 250 mg q6h or 500 mg q8h × 5–7 days. Best to give lower dose (250 mg) instead of the 500 mg dose, to minimize dry mouth and metallic taste. 2. **Alternate Rx for Bacterial Infection:** 7.5 mg/kg BW (max. 1 g), q6h × 7 days 3. **"Poor Man's Augmentin":** 250 mg Pen VK/ Amoxicillin + Metronidazole 250 mg q6h or 500 mg q8h × 5–7 days 4. **Initial/1st recurrence of mild or moderate Pseudomembranous Colitis:** 500 mg q8h × 10–14 days. Repeat one more cycle if infection persists. 5. **Kidney Failure/Dialysis:** 500 mg PO q12h, given after dialysis 6. **Mild Liver Disease:** Normal dose **Moderate/severe disease:** Use 50% dose reduction. 7. **Liver and Kidney Disease:** 250 mg q12h

Table 6.1.   *Continued*

Antibiotic	Antibiotic Doses: Normal/Modified
Tetracycline HCL: Category D Strength: 250/500 mg per capsule	**Tetracycline HCL:** 1. **Tetracycline HCL Normal Dose:** 250 mg qid PO on empty stomach × 5–7 days 2. **Tetracycline and Liver/Kidney Disease:** Avoid with liver or kidney disease or both liver and kidney disease.
Doxycycline (Vibramycin): Category D Strength: 50/100 mg per capsule	**Doxycycline:** 1. **Doxycycline, 100 mg/capsule Normal Dose:** 200 mg PO 2 h prior to bed on day one; 100 mg, also 2 h prior to bed/day for days 2–10 2. **Doxycycline, 50 mg/capsule Normal Dose:** 100 mg PO 2 h prior to bed, on day one; 50 mg, also 2 h prior to bed/day for days 2–10 3. **Doxycycline with Liver/Kidney Disease:** Normal dose. 4. **Kidney and Liver Disease:** Normal dose.

Vancomycin (Vancocin):
Category C
Oral Vancomycin:
    125/250 mg per pulvule
IV Vancomycin:
    500 mg/1 g vial
	1. **Vancomycin HCl pulvules for 2nd recurrence or severe Pseudomembranous Colitis:** 125 mg qid × 10–14 days
	2. **Vancomycin for Systemic Infections:** 7.5 mg/kg BW or 500 mg–1 g IV q6–12 h
	    Kidney Disease: Avoid.
	    Liver Disease: No dose change.

Symptoms, Signs, Patient Immunity, and Vital Organ Status

Oral infections cause pain, fever, malaise, minimal to significant swelling, and erythema. If the infection is localized and the patient's immunity is adequate, an incision-drainage (I&D) and pain medications are all that is needed. Avoid antibiotic use in the **absence** of fever and facial swelling. This practice will **reduce** future antimicrobial resistance. Antibiotics are definitely needed to treat an infection when adequate drainage cannot be achieved, the patient is significantly symptomatic, the infection is spreading and/or compromising the airways, or the patient is immune compromised. The antibiotic selected should match the organisms that need to be targeted. The practitioner must focus on the patient's immunity and the patient's vital organ status or functioning capacity when prescribing an antibiotic. For example, use antibiotics that clear through the kidney if the patient has hepatitis or cirrhosis.

The response to infection(s) largely depends on the patient's medical status and his/her ability to ward off or fight the infection. Diabetes, chemotherapy, radiotherapy, neutropenia, status postsplenectomy, chronic steroid use, systemic lupus erythematosus (SLE), HIV/AIDS, compromised hepatic/renal status, leukemia, or severe anemias are some of the disease states where the patient may respond poorly to an infection. These systemic conditions must be **simultaneously** brought under control with the help of the patient's physician, along with the management of the odontogenic infection.

ANTIBIOTIC PHARMACOTHERAPEUTIC CONSIDERATIONS AND FACTS FOR ODONTOGENIC INFECTIONS

Antibiotics and Dose Selection Criteria

The patient's weight should always be taken into consideration when making a decision on what antibiotic dose to prescribe. Opportunistic infections, particularly yeast over-growth in female patients and intestinal bacterial flora washout can occur with larger antibiotic doses or when antibiotics are prescribed for longer duration than necessary. It is suggested you use 140 lb as a cutoff, when selecting the antibiotic dose. As an example, prescribe 250 mg Pen VK qid for a patient under 140 lb and 500 mg qid for a patient over 140 lb.

Occasionally, a patient can be prescribed a **loading dose** of the antibiotic to achieve an effective dose in the bloodstream quickly. This becomes particularly important when treating the patient who has significant infection and/or inflammation.

Minimum Inhibitory Concentration (MIC)

The minimum inhibitory concentration (MIC) is the smallest concentration of an anti-microbial needed to stop bacterial growth. The MIC needs to be maintained for a period of time to completely eradicate the bacterial infection and this, in turn, correlates with the duration for which an antibiotic is prescribed. Most antibiotics in the dental setting are prescribed for 5–7 days. The rule of thumb typically is to have the patient take the antibiotics for an additional 5 days following improvement of the initial symptoms and signs. Infections that are mild to moderately symptomatic should be treated for 5 days, to prevent future antibiotic resistance.

Antibiotic Half-Life

The half-life of a drug determines the dosage length or time period for which the drug is prescribed. Penicillin has a shorter half-life when compared to Amoxicillin or azithro-mycin (Zithromax). Penicillin is prescribed qid (4 times/day) or q6h (every 6 hr), as opposed to amoxicillin, which is prescribed tid (3 times per day) or q8h (every 8 hr). Azithromycin (Zithromax) is taken once a day for 3/5 days. The effect of azithromycin (Zithromax) lasts for about 7 days.

Therapeutic Window

For any drug to be effective there is a desired therapeutic concentration range at which the drug needs to be maintained. Above this range the drug becomes toxic and below this range the drug is not effective.

Antibiotic Spectrum of Activity

Any given antibiotic is effective against certain specific types of bacteria only. This is the criteria used to classify an antibiotic's spectrum of activity: narrow, extended, or wide. Penicillin is an example of a narrow-spectrum antibiotic, amoxicillin is an example of an extended-spectrum antibiotic, and tetracycline is an example of a broad-spectrum antibiotic. It is best to target early infections (infection symptomatic for less than 3 days), with narrow-spectrum antibiotics and late infections (infection symptomatic for more than 3 days) with broader-spectrum antibiotics. This strategy will prevent secondary infections and antibiotic resistance. Incorporating the antibiotic spectrum of activity information, penicillin, cephalexin (Keflex), or cephadroxyl (Duricef) are very effective for **recent** onset dental infections or infections that have been symptomatic for **less** than 3 days. Clindamycin, azithromycin (Zithromax) or Clarithromycin (Biaxin) are very effective for **late** infections or infections that have caused symptoms for **more** than 3 days.

Bactericidal and Bacteriostatic Activity

Bactericidal drugs kill the bacteria by inhibiting the bacterial cell wall synthesis. Bacteriostatic antibiotics are protein synthesis inhibitors that prevent bacterial growth, and thus allow the patient's immune system ultimately to eradicate the bacteria. Cidal and static antibiotics should never be prescribed together because the cidal drugs require active bacterial growth and the static drugs stop bacterial growth. A cidal drug is made **less** effective in the presence of a static drug.

On occasion you may encounter an oral infection in a patient on a long-term, daily, single-dose antibiotic, e.g., tetracycline or minocycline (bacteriostatic drugs) for acne management. You will need to prescribe either a bacteriostatic or bactericidal antibiotic from **another** antibiotic family to treat this infection. The static antibiotic could be taken **along** with the tetracycline/minocycline, but a **6-hr interval** would have to be maintained between the static tetracycline/minocycline and the cidal antibiotic you plan on using for the infection.

Protein Synthesis Inhibitors

Bacteria have ribosomal subunits 30S and 50S. Specific bacteriostatic antibiotics selectively target these subunits. Tetracycline targets the 30S subunit; erythromycin and clindamycin target the 50S subunit.

Antibiotic Resistance Mechanism

Bacterial resistance to the penicillins occurs through the production of beta-lactamase, which has the ability to break the beta-lactam ring structure of penicillin. This prevents penicillin from reaching its binding sites. Penicillin is ineffective against gram-negative infections because it cannot penetrate the multilayer gram-negative bacterial cell wall. Beta-lactamase stable antibiotics, augmentin (Amoxicillin + clavulanic acid), and clindamycin are antibiotics that work against the beta-lactamase–producing bacteria. Clavulanic acid has the beta-lactam ring that acts as a decoy for the enzyme. The enzyme destroys this ring, thus letting amoxicillin target the bacteria.

Antibiotic Drug-Drug Interactions (DDIs)

The DDI could be with dietary items, as with tetracycline and metal cations. When tetracycline is taken with milk of magnesia, Tums, or Mylanta, it gets precipitated out in the gastrointestinal tract. The antibiotic does not get absorbed and never reaches the bacteria.

Antibiotics and Allergy

Always ask the patients about allergies to antibiotics. Determine whether the reaction was mild, moderate, or severe. Clindamycin is the antibiotic of choice for a patient allergic to penicillin VK or any other member of the penicillin family. The penicillins and the cephalosporins share a common chemical structure; consequently, patients presenting with severe or anaphylactoid-type allergy to the penicillins can have a 5–15% cross-reactivity with the cephalosporins. Clindamycin, azithromycin (Zithromax), or clarithromycin (Biaxin) are alternate drugs that can be prescribed instead.

Antibiotics and Intestinal Bacterial Flora

Any antibiotic when used in large doses or for prolonged periods has the potential to eradicate the intestinal bacterial flora, cause diarrhea, clostridium difficile overgrowth, and pseudomembranous colitis. It is suggested that you always recommend the use of probiotics or acidophilus-containing yogurt with the antibiotic because this will maintain the bacterial flora and minimize or prevent this very untoward side effect.

Antibiotics and Water/Fluid Consumption

Always have the patient drink 6–8 glasses of water when taking an antibiotic. This will help flush the kidneys and prevent adverse effects due to poor antibiotic clearance. Always remember that dehydration impairs the renal clearance of drugs.

Oral Antibiotics and Oral Contraceptives

Routinely, oral contraceptives are absorbed into the bloodstream and delivered to the liver. They are inactivated in the liver and delivered back to the gut where the intestinal bacteria reactivate the birth-control pill, thus rendering it effective. If bacteria in the gut are insufficient in number to reactivate the pill, the pill remains inactive and is excreted without providing adequate contraceptive effect. Oral contraceptives thus are rendered less effective when taken with **oral** antibiotics that wash out the bacterial flora. You must warn your patient to use external contraception when taking oral antibiotics. Systemic contraceptives etonogestrel (Implanon) and levonorgestrel (Norplant) implants are not affected with oral antibiotic use.

Antibiotics and Breast-Feeding

Minimize the use of antibiotics with breast-feeding because of the risk of altering the baby's intestinal flora. Excessive or inappropriate use of antibiotics may promote growth of resistant pathogens. When antibiotic use is absolutely needed, have the patient take the antibiotic **after** the feed.

ANTIBIOTICS USED IN DENTISTRY

Classification

Dentistry antibiotics are classified as the following:

1. **Penicillins:** penicillin VK, amoxicillin, amoxicillin + clavulanic acid (Augmentin), ampicillin, and dicloxacillin.
2. **Cephalosporins:** cephalexin (Keflex), cephadroxyl (Duricef), cephazolin (Ancef), and ceftriaxone (Rocephin).
3. **Lincomycin group antibiotic:** clindamycin
4. **Macrolides:** erythromycin (older macrolide) and the newer macrolides, azithromycin (Zithromax), and clarithromycin (Biaxin)

5. **Metronidazole (Flagyl)**
6. **Tetracy clines:** tetracycline HCL, doxycycline (Vibramycin)
7. **Vancomycin**

PENICILLINS

Overview

Penicillins are beta-lactam bactericidal antibiotics that cause death of the bacteria by inhibiting the cell wall synthesis. They cross the placenta and are distributed in the breast milk. This is an important point to remember especially when prescribing any one of the penicillins to a lactating mother. All penicillins primarily have a **renal** elimination. Penicillins can cause an allergic reaction in some patients. Allergy toward one member of the penicillin family indicates allergy toward all other members of the family. Allergies are more common with parenterally administered penicillins, and less common with the orally administered penicillins. When planning on using any of the penicillins in the renal-compromised patient, you need to reduce the **dose or increase** the dosing **interval**. It is therefore suggested that you use a drug like clindamycin instead. Clindamycin can be safely used in a renal-compromised patient even in the presence of dialysis or end-stage renal disease (ESRD). Alternatively, you can use the full dose of azithromycin to treat an infection in a renal-compromised patient because azithromycin is metabolized in the liver. All oral penicillins should be taken **1 hr prior** to eating **or 1 hr after eating**, to prevent binding of the penicillins to food and avoid acid inactivation.

Penicillin VK

Penicillin VK Spectrum of Activity

Penicillin VK is a narrow-spectrum bactericidal antibiotic that targets gram-positive aerobic cocci and the major pathogens of mixed anaerobic infections. It is effective against some, but **not all**, staphylococci. Pen VK has a large therapeutic window and minimal drug interactions, if any. Being a narrow-spectrum antibiotic, Pen VK causes minimum disturbance to the intestinal flora. Pen VK is an ideal antibiotic for treating infections that have been symptomatic for less than 3 days.

Penicillin VK: Drug Uptake and Clearance

After oral ingestion peak serum levels occur within 1 hr and almost the entire drug is excreted unchanged through the kidneys. The dose must be adjusted in renal failure.

    Penicillin VK Pregnancy Risk Factor: B.

Penicillin VK Prescription for Adults and Children Above Age 12

1. **Rx: Pen VK:** 250 mg or 500 mg/tab
   Disp: 20 or 28 tablets
   Sig: 250 mg or 500 mg q6h/qid ×5–7 days
2. **Pen VK with Kidney Disease:**
   a. **In the presence of serum creatinine <2.0 mg/dL or the CrCl is >50 mL/min:** Pen VK is dosed normally at 250–500 mg PO **q6h**.

    b. **In the presence of CrCl 10–50 mL/min or serum creatinine between 2.0 mg/dL to Predialysis:** Pen VK is dosed at 250–500 mg **q8–12h.**

    c. **In the Dialysis Patient:** Pen VK is dosed at 250–500 **q12–16h.**

3. **Pen VK with Liver Disease:** No dose alteration is needed.

Penicillin G

Penicillin G Facts

Penicillin G is mainly excreted through the kidneys when the renal status is normal. If the renal status is compromised, the liver becomes the major route of excretion via bile. Penicillin G **can be prescribed** for treatment of infection with a 50% dose reduction in a patient with a compromised liver **and** kidney status.

    Penicillin G Pregnancy Risk Factor: B.

Penicillin G Dose

1.2 MU (million units) penicillin G, IM q12h

Amoxicillin

Amoxicillin Spectrum of Activity

Amoxicillin is an extended-spectrum penicillin. It is **less** effective against gram-positive cocci compared to Pen VK and has a **similar** coverage to penicillin against anaerobic bacteria. It does provide coverage against gram-negative enteric bacteria, but oral infections in the immune-competent patient do not require this coverage.

Amoxicillin Drug Uptake

Amoxicillin is **better absorbed** from the gut and has **more stable** blood concentrations over time, compared to penicillin. Amoxicillin is metabolized in the liver and excreted through the kidneys and the dose must be adjusted in the renal-compromised patient.

Amoxicillin Use

Amoxicillin is *the* antibiotic recommended by the American Heart Association (AHA) for the prevention of subacute bacterial endocarditis (SBE) in patients not allergic to the penicillins. Amoxicillin can be prescribed for infections symptomatic for less than 3 days, but because it is an extended-spectrum antibiotic, it is suggested that you prescribe Pen VK instead. This conscious effort to prescribe a narrow-spectrum antibiotic will prevent antibiotic resistance in the future. Amoxicillin should be considered first, however, when treating oral infections in an immune-compromised patient, because gram-negative enteric bacteria may be present at the infection site.

    Amoxicillin Pregnancy Risk Factor: B.

Amoxicillin Prescriptions

Amoxicillin is prescribed tid (three times per day) or q8h (every 8 hr) because it has a longer half-life compared to Pen VK. Amoxicillin can be prescribed in the following ways:

1. **Rx: Amoxicillin** 250, 500, or 875 mg/capsule
    Disp: Variable
    Sig: 250/500 mg q8h or 500–875 mg PO q12h ×5–7 days

Note: The 875 mg tablet should not be used in patients with CrCl <30 mL/min or the patient with a serum creatinine >3.3 mg/dL.

2. A high-dose 1-day short-course of amoxicillin can be used for treatment of a **very symptomatic acute** dento-alveolar abscess. The 1-day course has been found to be as effective as the conventional 5-day, 250 mg qid course of penicillin VK.
   Rx: Amoxicillin 500 mg/capsule
   Disp: 12 capsules
   Sig: 3 g (6, 500 mg capsules) amoxicillin twice, in 8 hr

3. **Amoxicillin for Premedication Prophylaxis:**
   Rx: Amoxicillin 2 g PO 1 hr prior to procedure

4. **Amoxicillin Dose Guidelines with Kidney Disease:**
   a. **Cr Cl >30 mL/min or a serum creatinine <3.3 mg/dL:** Dispense the normal dose of amoxicillin, 250–500 mg PO **q8h.**
   b. **Cr Cl 10–30 mL/min or a serum creatinine >3.3 mg/dL to Predialysis:** Prolong the interval and avoid using the 875 mg tablet. Rx: 250–500 mg PO **q12h.**
   c. **Cr Cl <10 mL/min or Dialysis**: Prolong the interval: **Rx:** 250–500 mg PO **q24h.** The dose during hemodialysis is the same as that given for CrCl <10 mL/min and the dose must be given **after** completion of dialysis on the days of dialysis.

5. **Amoxicillin Dose with Liver Disease:**
   The dose of amoxicillin does not need to be adjusted in the presence of liver failure.

   Amoxicillin can be used in a patient with **both** kidney and liver disease with dose adjustments according to the renal guidelines.

Amoxicillin-Clavulanic Acid (Augmentin)

Augmentin Spectrum of Activity

The beta-lactamase (penicillinase) inhibitor potassium clavulanate extends amoxicillin's spectrum of activity to include beta-lactamase–producing strains of staphylococcus aureus, haemophilus influenzae, and many strains of enteric gram-negative bacilli. This combination is useful for the oral treatment of bite wounds, otitis media, sinusitis, some lower respiratory infections, and urinary tract infections.

Amoxicillin-Clavulanic Acid (Augmentin) Adverse Effects

Augmentin can very easily wash out the intestinal bacterial flora, causing a higher incidence of diarrhea and other gastrointestinal symptoms compared to amoxicillin alone. Augmentin can thus increase the effectiveness of warfarin (Coumadin). It is suggested that you minimize the use of Augmentin because of its side effects and cost.
   Augmentin Pregnancy Risk Factor: B.

Amoxicillin-Clavulanic Acid (Augmentin) Prescription

Each Augmentin capsule contains 125 mg clavulanic acid and 250/500/875 mg amoxicillin

1. **Rx: Augmentin** 250 mg or 500 mg/tablet
   Disp: 15 or 21 tablets
   Sig: 250/500 mg q8h for 5–7 days

2. **Amoxicillin-Clavulanic Acid (Augmentin) and Kidney Disease:**
   Decrease the dose by at least 50% in renal-compromised patients.

Ampicillin

Ampicillin Spectrum of Activity and Overview

Ampicillin is a semisynthetic penicillin and, like amoxicillin, it is classified as an extended-spectrum antibiotic. It is as effective as penicillin G in pneumococcal, streptococcal, and meningococcal infections.

Ampicillin is also active against many strains of salmonella, shigella, proteus mirabilis, and escherichia coli along with most strains of haemophilus influenzae. Some strains of H. influenzae, however, are now resistant to ampicillin, and the drug is not effective for the treatment of infections caused by penicillinase-producing staphylococci. It is very effective against pseudomonas.

Ampicillin Adverse Effects

Rashes are more frequent with ampicillin than with the other penicillins.

Ampicillin Drug Uptake

Ampicillin does concentrate in the bile, but the major excretion occurs through the kidneys. Use caution in the presence of liver disease.
  Pregnancy Risk Factor: B.

Ampicillin Prescriptions

1. **Rx: Ampicillin** 250 mg or 500 mg/capsule
    Disp: 20 or 28 capsules
    Sig: 250–500 mg q6h for 5–7 days
2. For premedication prophylaxis in patients unable to take oral preparations
    Rx: Ampicillin 2.0 g, IV/IM 30 min prior to procedure
3. **Ampicillin and Kidney Disease:** The dosage of ampicillin should be **decreased** by at least 50% in the renal-compromised patient.

Dicloxacillin

Dicloxacillin is a beta-lactamase–resistant semisynthetic penicillin that is effective against penicillinase-producing staphylococcus infection.

Dicloxacillin Drug Alert

Dicloxacillin increases the effectiveness of anticoagulants.

Dicloxacillin Prescriptions

1. **Normal Dose:** 250–500 mg qid × 5–7 days
2. **Dicloxacillin and Kidney Disease:** As with all penicillins, use dicloxacillin with caution in the renal-compromised patient and decrease the dose by at least 50%.

CEPHALOSPORINS

Cephalosporins Spectrum of Activity and Overview

Cephalosporins, like the penicillins, contain a beta-lactam chemical structure and are cell wall synthesis inhibitors. They are completely cleared through the renal system.

The cephalosporins are subgrouped into first-, second-, and third-generation drugs, and each generation has a broader-spectrum of activity than the one before.

The first-generation cephalosporins have very good bone penetration and increased activity against staphylococcus aureus. They are an excellent choice for joint prosthesis prophylaxis. Cephalosporins should **not** be prescribed to patients with an anaphylactoid reaction toward penicillins because there is a 5–15% cross-reactivity with the cephalosporins.

The first-generation cephalosporins, dispensed in oral dose form are cephalexin (Keflex) and cephadroxyl (Duricef). Cephazolin (Ancef) is also a first-generation **injectable** drug, recommended by the AHA for premedication prophylaxis in penicillin-allergic patients unable to take oral medications. As of April 2007, AHA has added a third-generation cephalosporin, ceftriaxone (Rocephin) to its list of injectable premedication antibiotics, for penicillin-allergic patients unable to take oral medications.

Cephalosporins Adverse Effects

Cephalosporins and the other broader-spectrum antibiotics can wash out the intestinal bacterial flora, decrease Vitamin K absorption, and cause increased bleeding, particularly in patients on warfarin (Coumadin).

Cephalosporins Drug Use

The first-generation drugs are excellent at treating **early** oral infections because they kill aerobic gram-positive streptococci and staphylococci bacteria very effectively, but they are **not** effective against many anaerobes. This accounts for the first-generation cephalosporins **not** being effective for **late** infections. The first-generation cephalosporins are considered a good second alternative to clindamycin for treatment of oral infections in **nonanaphylactoid**, penicillin-allergic patients.

Cephalosporins Pregnancy Risk Factor: B.

Cephalosporins Prescriptions

1. **Rx: Cephalexin (Keflex), 250 or 500 mg/capsule**
    Disp: Variable
    Dose: 250–1,000 mg PO q6h/qid × 5–7 days, maximum 4.0 g/day
      The renal dosing of Keflex should be q12h or q24h, in the presence of kidney disease.
2. **Rx: Cephadroxyl (Duricef), 250 or 500 mg/capsule**
    Disp: Variable
    Dose: 1–2 g/day PO in two divided doses × 5–7 days
3. **For Premedication Prophylaxis:**
    a. **Cephalexin or cephadroxyl,** 2 g PO, 1 hr prior to procedure
    b. **Cephazolin (Ancef)** 1 g, IV/IM 30 min prior procedure
    c. **Ceftriaxone (Rocephin)** 1.0 g IV/IM, 30 min prior to the procedure
4. **Cephalosporins and Kidney Disease:** Almost all of the cephalosporins used for management of odontogenic infections are excreted unchanged by the kidneys. Reduce the dose of cephalosporins by 50% in a renal-compromised patient. Cephalosporins can be used in a patient with **both** kidney and liver disease but with a 50% dose reduction.

LINCOSAMIDE GROUP ANTIBIOTIC, CLINDAMYCIN

Clindamycin Spectrum of Activity and Overview

Clindamycin is a broad-spectrum antibiotic that is very effective against aerobic, anaerobic, and beta-lactamase–producing bacteria. It is a protein synthesis inhibitor that targets the 50S ribosomal subunit. Clindamycin also has a stimulatory effect on the host immune system. At **low** doses for treatment of infections, clindamycin is bacteriostatic in action. At **high** doses, as with the AHA-recommended antibiotic prophylaxis, it is bactericidal in action.

Clindamycin Drug Uptake

Peak clindamycin levels are attained in about 1 hr after oral ingestion. Clindamycin attains high levels in the saliva, gingival tissue, and bone. The half-life of clindamycin is 2–3 hr. Clindamycin is **partially** metabolized in the liver and intestinal mucosa. The metabolites are excreted through the kidneys, feces, and bile.

Clindamycin Adverse Effects

Pseudomembranous colitis due to clostridium difficile overgrowth after the first few pills or even months after taking a full course of clindamycin has often been cause for concern for a very long time. Recent literature however **downplays** this side effect and states that clindamycin **does not** cause the pseudomembranous colitis, when used appropriately in an outpatient setting. The literature further states that not just clindamycin but **any** antibiotic that washes out the intestinal bacterial flora can cause pseudomembranous colitis.

In the presence of antibiotic-induced colitis, the offending antibiotic should be stopped and metronidazole (Flagyl) or vancomycin pulvules (oral vancomycin) prescribed, to treat the clostridium difficile–associated infection.

Clindamycin Drug Uses

In the early stages of oral infections the bacterial population is more aerobic, and in the late stages it switches from aerobic to anaerobic. This is the reason why clindamycin is *the* drug of choice for treatment of oral infections symptomatic for more than 3 days. Clindamycin 600 mg PO (oral) is the drug of choice for joint prosthesis prophylaxis, in penicillin-allergic patients.

Clindamycin Pregnancy Risk Factor: B.

Clindamycin Prescriptions

1. **Rx: Clindamycin**, 150 or 300 mg/tablet
    Disp: Variable
    Dose: 150–450 mg q6–8h/qid PO ×5–7 days
    Note: At this dose, clindamycin is static in action. It is best to prescribe the lower dose of clindamycin, **150 mg, tid or q8h** because this **minimizes** the adverse side effects. Clindamycin serum levels are known to exceed the MIC for bacterial growth for at least 6 hr after consumption of the recommended dose.
2. **Refractory Cases of Periodontal Infection**: These patients are best treated with 600 mg/day of **clindamycin** ×7 days.

3. **Premedication Prophylaxis:**
   a. **Clindamycin:** 600 mg PO, 1 hr prior to treatment. This is a cidal dose.
   b. **Clindamycin** 600 mg, IV 30 min prior to procedure. This is a cidal dose.
4. **Clindamycin and Liver Disease:**
   a. **Hepatitis:** The full dose of clindamycin can be used in the presence of nonacute, nonfulminant hepatitis.
   b. **Cirrhosis:** Decrease clindamycin dose **by 50%** in patients with liver cirrhosis.
5. **Clindamycin and Kidney Disease:** No dose change is needed in the presence of kidney disease or renal failure.

Clindamycin can be used with a 50% dose reduction in a patient with **both** kidney and liver disease.

MACROLIDES

Macrolides Overview and Spectrum of Activity

Macrolides are considered narrow-spectrum antibiotics that are effective against many gram-positive and gram-negative aerobic and anaerobic bacteria.

Erythromycin and azithromycin are metabolized in the liver and excreted mainly through the feces and bile. Some minimal excretion also occurs through the kidneys. The metabolism of clarithromycin is partly hepatic, where it is metabolized by the CYP3A4 enzyme and part of the metabolism occurs by conversion to 14 OH clarithromycin, an active metabolite. Clarithromycin is primarily excreted through the kidneys.

Clarithromycin and azithromycin can be given with food and do not cause the gastrointestinal upset associated with erythromycin.

Erythromycin and clarithromycin suppress the cytochrome P4503A4 enzyme in the liver and gut. The 3A4 enzyme metabolizes many useful therapeutic drugs and is also involved in the conversion of some prodrugs into active functional metabolites. With suppression of the 3A4 enzyme the nonmetabolized drugs accumulate in the liver and become toxic while the prodrugs are rendered ineffective.

Azithromycin is the **safest** of all the three macrolides. It **does not** affect the P4503A4 enzyme. Azithromycin has, rarely, been associated with allergic reactions, including angioedema, anaphylaxis, and dermatologic reactions, such as Stevens-Johnson syndrome and toxic epidermal necrolysis.

Erythromycin is no longer used in the dental setting. Bacterial resistance, severe gastrointestinal upsets, and cytochrome P4503A4 enzyme–associated DDIs were all cause for the loss in popularity of erythromycin. Erythromycin additionally can aggravate the weakness experienced by patients with myasthenia gravis.

Azithromycin and clarithromycin are recommended as alternates for SBE prophylaxis by the AHA, in the penicillin-allergic patient. Both of these drugs are also used in the management of odontogenic infections symptomatic for more than 3 days, in the penicillin-allergic patient. Since clarithromycin is associated with several DDIs, it is suggested that you use azithromycin instead.

Drugs Interacting with Erythromycin and Clarithromycin

Drugs interacting with erythromycin and clarithromycin are theophylline, oral anticoagulants, lanoxin (Digoxin), methylprednisolone, phenytoin sodium (Dilantin), carbamazepine (Tegretol), cyclosporine (Sandimmune), and ergot alkaloids.

Erythromycin and Azithromycin Pregnancy Risk Factor: B.
Clarithromycin Pregnancy Risk Factor: C.

Macrolides Prescriptions

1. **Rx:** 5-day supply: **Azithromycin** 250 mg/capsule
    Disp: 6 capsules
    Sig: 250 mg bid or 500 mg hs on the first day, and then 250 mg/day for the next 4 days
2. **Rx:** 3-day supply: **Azithromycin** 500 mg/capsule
    Disp: 3 capsules
    Sig: 500 mg/day × 3 days
3. **Azithromycin and Kidney Disease:** Use full dose azithromycin in the renal-compromised patient.
4. **Azithromycin and Liver Disease:** Specific guidelines for azithromycin dosing in presence of liver disease have not been established, so it is best to **avoid** azithromycin in patients with liver disease.
5. **Rx: Clarithromycin** 250 or 500 mg/cap
    Disp: Variable
    Sig: 250 or 500 mg bid for 5–7 days
6. **Clarithromycin and Kidney Disease:** It is best to **avoid** clarithromycin use in the renal-compromised patient, but, if needed, use the following guidelines:
    a. CrCl 30–60 mL/min or a serum creatinine <3.3 mg/dL: Decrease the dose by 50%: **Give 250 mg q12h.**
    b. CrCl <30 mL/min or a serum creatinine >3.3 mg/dL to predialysis: Decrease the dose by 75%: **Give 125 mg q12h.**
    c. In presence of CrCl <10 mL/min or dialysis: Dose clarithromycin at **125 mg q24h.**
7. **Clarithromycin and Liver Disease:** No clarithromycin dose adjustment is needed in the liver compromised patient **as long as** the renal function is normal.
8. **Macrolides for Premedication Prophylaxis:**
    Give azithromycin or clarithromycin, 500 mg PO 1 hr prior to the procedure.

METRONIDAZOLE (FLAGYL)

Metronidazole (Flagyl) Spectrum of Activity and Overview

Metronidazole kills bacteria by interfering with their ability to make new DNA. Metronidazole is used for treatment of trichomoniasis, amebiasis, giardiasis, Gardnerella vaginitis, and anaerobic bacterial infections only. The anaerobic organisms have the ability to metabolize metronidazole to its active form within the anaerobic cells. Metronidazole is metabolized in the liver and excreted through the kidneys and feces. Bacterial resistance to metronidazole is very rare.

Metronidazole (Flagyl) and Pen VK/amoxicillin are often dispensed when the patient's infection does not respond to penicillin alone in the treatment of a mixed aerobic and anaerobic bacterial infection. This combination is called the "poor man's augmentin." Metronidazole is also available for intravenous administration, in the treatment of anaerobic bacterial infections.

Metronidazole is the first drug of choice for the treatment of an initial bout or first recurrence of mild or moderate clostridium difficile infection (CDI)–associated pseudomembranous colitis.

Metronidazole Adverse Effects

Frequent: Nausea, headache, dry mouth, and metallic taste
Occasional: Vomiting, diarrhea, insomnia, and weakness stomatitis, vertigo, paresthesia, rash, urethral burning, and phlebitis at the injection site
Rare: Seizures, encephalopathy, ataxia, leukopenia, and pancreatitis

Metronidazole and Drug-Drug Interactions (DDIs)

Metronidazole interferes with the metabolism of alcohol with a consequent buildup of acetaldehydes, resulting in vomiting and extreme nausea. This disulfiram or Antabuse-type reaction occurs when metronidazole is combined with alcohol. The patient should not consume alcohol when taking metronidazole and must continue to avoid alcohol for an additional 48 hr after the last dose.

Metronidazole increases the effect of anticoagulants. There is decreased effect of metronidazole with Antabuse pentobarbital. There is possible increased toxicity with cimetidine. Metronidazole inhibits the excretion of lithium leading to lithium toxicity and consequent renal damage.

Metronidazole (Flagyl) Pregnancy Risk Factor: B.

Metronidazole (Flagyl) Prescriptions

For treatment of anaerobic infection or in combination with 250 mg Pen VK or 250 mg amoxicillin:

1. **Rx: Metronidazole (Flagyl),** 250 or 500 mg/tab
   Disp: Variable
   Sig: 250 mg q6h or 500 mg q8h × 5–7 days
   It is best to dispense the **lower dose** (250 mg) of metronidazole instead of the 500 mg dose to minimize the dry mouth and metallic taste
2. Alternate metronidazole prescription for bacterial infections:
   Rx: Metronidazole 7.5 mg/kg BW, maximum 1 g
   Sig: Take q6h × 7 days
3. Treatment of an initial or first recurrence of mild or moderate c. difficile–associated pseudomembranous colitis:
   Rx: Metronidazole (Flagyl), 500 mg/tab
   Disp: Variable
   Sig: 500 mg q8h × 10–14 days. Repeat treatment once more if infection persists after the initial 14-day treatment.
4. **Metronidazole (Flagyl) and Kidney Disease:**
   a. Predialysis: No dose adjustment is needed.
   b. Renal failure/dialysis: Dose adjustment is required only in the presence of renal failure/dialysis. Metronidazole should be dosed at 500 mg PO **q12h** instead of q8h and given **after** the dialysis.
5. **Metronidazole (Flagyl) and Liver Disease:**
   a. Mild liver disease: Prescribe the normal metronidazole dose.
   b. Moderate to severe liver disease: Metronidazole dose should be decreased by at least **50%**.

Metronidazole can be used in the presence of **both** liver and kidney disease but with a **reduced dose**, 250 mg q12h.

TETRACYCLINES

Tetracyclines Spectrum of Activity and Overview

Tetracyclines are broad-spectrum antibiotics that inhibit bacterial 30S ribosomal subunit. They may cause increased photosensitivity. They cause tetratogenic changes in the newborn when given during pregnancy, and pregnant women should never be prescribed tetracyclines. Children under the age of eight should also not use tetracyclines, especially during periods of tooth development because tetracyclines cause bone deformity and permanent staining of the teeth.

All tetracyclines are concentrated in the liver and excreted via bile into the intestine where they are reabsorbed to ultimately be eliminated through the kidneys.

Recent studies indicate that there is no truth to the past concept held about doxycycline being partially metabolized by the liver. The studies have confirmed that doxycycline is **not** metabolized but rather **deactivated** partially in the intestines by chelate formation and then excreted in the feces. Doxycycline does not require any renal clearance. Tetracycline HCL, on the other hand, has a large renal clearance. Tetracycline HCL is contraindicated in a patient with liver disease, kidney disease, or both liver and kidney disease. Tetracycline HCL should be taken on an empty stomach, but doxycycline can be taken with nondairy foods a few hours before bedtime.

Tetracyclines Adverse Effects and Drug-Drug Interactions

The following are adverse effects and DDIs for tetracyclines:

1. The beneficial bacteria in the gut are destroyed and secondary infection with candidiasis can occur.
2. All oral antacids—milk of magnesia, Tums, Mylanta, bismuth subsalicylate, zinc sulfate, and iron—impair the absorption of the tetracyclines, causing the tetracyclines to precipitate on ingestion. Maintain a gap of at least **2 hr** between the ingestion of a tetracycline with any of the above-mentioned metal cations.
3. The tetracyclines potentiate the effects of warfarin (Coumadin) and prolong the PT/INR.
4. Decreased doxycycline effect occurs with barbiturates, carbamazepine (Tegretol), and phenytoin sodium (Dilantin).
5. Tetracyclines decrease the effects of oral contraceptives and increase the effects of digoxin, lithium, and methotrexate.

   Tetracycline and Doxycycline Pregnancy Risk Factor: D

Tetracyclines Prescriptions

1. **Rx: Doxycycline**, 100 mg/capsule
   Disp: 11 capsules
   Sig: 200 mg PO 2 hr prior to bed, on day 1, and then 100 mg 2 hr prior to bed/day: days 2–10
2. **Rx: Doxycycline**, 50 mg/capsule
   Disp: 11 capsules
   Sig: 100 mg PO 2 hr prior to bed, on day 1, and then 50 mg 2 hr prior to bed/day: days 2–10

3. **Doxycycline and Kidney/Liver Disease:**
   a. No Doxycycline dose change is needed with kidney or liver disease.
   b. Doxycycline can be used **without** dose alteration in a patient who has both kidney and liver disease.
4. **Rx: Tetracycline HCL** 250 mg/capsule, on an **empty** stomach
   Disp: Variable
   Dose: 250 mg qid × 5–7 days
5. **Tetracycline HCL and Kidney Disease:** Avoid tetracycline HCL use with kidney disease, but if absolutely needed, use the following creatinine clearances/creatinine guidelines:
   a. **CrCl 50–80 mL/min or serum creatinine between 1.25–2.0 mg/dL:** Dose tetracycline HCL **q8–12h**
   b. **CrCl 10–50 mL/min or serum creatinine between 2.0 mg/dL to Predialysis:** Dose tetracycline HCL **q12–24h**
   c. **CrCl <10 mL/min or Dialysis:** Dose tetracycline HCL q24h

VANCOMYCIN (VANCOCIN)

Vancomycin Spectrum of Activity

Vancomycin is an effective alternative to the penicillins for prophylaxis against endocarditis caused by streptococcus viridans or enterococci, for severe staphylococcal infections, and for penicillin-resistant pneumococcal infections. Vancomycin is also the drug of choice for the treatment of infections caused by methicillin-resistant staphylococcus aureus (MRSA) and epidermidis.

The intravenous (IV) form of vancomycin is used for the management of all these infections. Intravenous (IV) vancomycin dose should be significantly reduced but, better yet, **avoided** in the presence of renal disease because there is rapid accumulation of metabolites. Vancomycin is minimally metabolized by the liver and no change in drug dose is needed for liver disease.

Oral vancomycin can be life-saving in patients with antibiotic-associated colitis due to clostridium difficile. Oral vancomycin is used when metronidazole (Flagyl) use is contraindicated in the presence of liver disease or alcoholism or when two, 14-day courses of metronidazole have been ineffective. Oral vancomycin is the **first** drug of choice for a **second** recurrence or **severe** c. difficile infection (CDI)–associated pseudomembranous colitis.

Vancomycin Adverse Drug Reactions

The following are adverse drug reactions for vancomycin:

1. **Frequent:** Thrombophlebitis, fever, chills.
2. **Occasional:** Eighth-nerve damage can occur, especially with large or continuous doses of more than 10 days, in the presence of renal damage, in the elderly, or in the presence of neutropenia.
3. **Rare:** Peripheral neuropathy, urticaria. If vancomycin is injected into a vein too quickly, it can cause the "red-neck"-syndrome–associated flushing; a rash over the neck, face, and chest; wheezing or difficulty breathing; and a dangerous decrease in blood pressure.

Vancomycin Drug-Drug Interactions

Increased nephrotoxicity occurs when used with aminoglycosides and cephalosporins.

Vancomycin Pregnancy Risk Factor: C.

Vancomycin Prescriptions

1. **Vancomycin HCl Pulvules/Oral Vancomycin:** The **first-line** therapy for an **initial** or recurrence of **severe** CDI disease.
   Rx: Vancomycin 125 mg/pulvule
   Dose: 125 mg qid ×10–14 days.This regimen is ineffective for any other infection.
   Second recurrence is treated with oral vancomycin tapered over 4 weeks, with or without pulse dosing, when 125 mg oral vancomycin is given q2–3 days, for 2–8 weeks.
2. **Systemic Infection:**
   Rx: Vancomycin 7.5 mg/kg BW or 500 mg–1 g injected IV, every 6–12 hr

7

Antifungals Commonly Used in Dentistry: Assessment, Analysis, and Associated Dental Management Guidelines

POLYENE AND AZOLE ANTIFUNGALS OVERVIEW

Two distinct classes of antifungal medications used are the polyenes and the azole antifungals.

Polyene Antifungals Mechanism of Action

Polyenes bind with ergosterol in the fungal cells and form holes, causing cell death due to the leaking out of the cell contents.

Polyenes Drugs Classification

Polyenes drugs are classified as the following:

1. Nystatin (Mycostatin): topical and oral nystatin
2. Amphotericin B (Fungizone): oral and IV amphotericin B

Azole Drugs Classification

Azole drugs are classified as the following:

1. **Imidazole antifungals:** Clotrimazole (Mycelex) and ketoconazole (Nizoral)
2. **Triazole antifungals:** Fluconazole (Diflucan) and itraconazole (Sporanox)

Imidazole and Triazole Antifungals Mechanism of Action and Facts

Imidazole and triazole antifungals inhibit the CYP450 enzyme, thus preventing the formation of ergosterol and fungal cell membrane synthesis.

Fluconazole and itraconazole, the **newer** azole antifungals generally have **fewer** side effects. They are used a lot more for treatment of fungal infections in the immune-compromised patient compared to ketoconazole. They both affect the fungal cell membrane a lot more than ketoconazole, thus needing lower doses, for effectiveness.

Topical and Oral Nystatin

Nystatin Facts

The topical and oral forms of nystatin are **not** absorbed on ingestion and consequently do not have DDIs. The oral form is used to treat oral or esophageal fungal infections. Both forms of nystatin are commonly used in HIV/AIDS patients with a low CD_4 count, in patients undergoing chemotherapy, and in patients in whom azole antifungals are contraindicated.

Nystatin suspension is the drug of choice for patients experiencing xerostomia.

Nystatin (Mycostatin) Prescriptions

1. **Nystatin Oral Suspension for Oral Candidiasis:**
   Rx: Nystatin Oral Suspension 100,000 units/ml
   Disp: 473 mL (1 pint) bottle (14-day supply)
   Sig: Use 1 tsp or 5 ml, qid. Rinse and hold in the mouth as long as possible before swallowing. There should be **no** eating or drinking for 30 min after use.
   Note: Nystatin suspension is also dispensed as a 60 mL bottle.
2. **Nystatin Oral Suspension for Soaking of Dentures/Partials:**
   Rx: Nystatin Oral Suspension 100,000 units/ml
   Disp: 473 mL (1 pint) bottle
   Sig: Add 5–10 mL of 1:100,000 units nystatin to half cup of water and soak the dentures overnight daily, for 14 days. Rinse the dentures before use.
3. **Nystatin Pastille Prescription for Oral Candidiasis:**
   Rx: Nystatin 200,000 units/pastille
   Disp: 70 pastilles
   Sig: Dissolve 1 pastille in the mouth 4–5 times/day for 14 days. Do not eat for 30 min after use.
4. **Nystatin (Mycostatin) Cream:** The cream can be applied to the dentures before insertion or can be used for angular chielitis.
   Rx: Nystatin 100,000 units/g
   Disp: 15 or 30 g tube
   Sig: Apply to affected area 4–5 times/day for 2 weeks and do not eat or drink for 30 min after use.

Amphotericin B (Fungizone)

Amphotericin B Facts

Amphotericin B is available for oral and intravenous (IV) use. The oral form is used for the management of oral candidiasis. As an oral preparation it is nontoxic. IV amphotericin B is used for systemic fungal infections.

Amphotericin B Mechanism of Action (MOA)

The MOA is almost similar to but more complex than nystatin. IV use can cause a histamine-like reaction causing nausea, vomiting, headaches, hypotension, and chills.

Amphotericin B Metabolism

The half-life of amphotericin B is 24 hr and it is metabolized in the kidneys. Amphotericin B can be associated with severe or irreversible nephrotoxicity. Avoid all nephrotoxic drugs and corticosteroids with amphotericin B.

Hepatotoxicity, leukopenia, thrombocytopenia, arrythmias, and cardiac failure can occur with amphotericin.

Amphotericin B Prescriptions

1. **Topical Amphotericin B:**
   Rx: 3% Topical Amphotericin B
   Disp: 20 g tube
   Sig: Apply to the affected area 3–4 times/day for 2–4 weeks.
2. **Oral Amphotericin B**
   The oral forms are poorly absorbed. Oral amphotericin B is dispensed in capsule or suspension form.
   Rx: Amphotericin B 500 mg/capsule or Amphotericin B suspension: 500 mg/mL
   Disp: 56 capsules or 56 mL suspension
   Sig: Take 500 mg capsule PO qid for 2 weeks or use 1 mL of the suspension, swish and swallow qid for 2 weeks.
3. **Intravenous (IV) Amphotericin B:**
   a. **IV Amphotericin B Normal Dose:** 0.25–1.5 mg/kg, q24h for 2 weeks
   b. **IV Amphotericin B Dose for GFR <10 mL/min or Dialysis:** Prolong the interval and dose at q24–36h.
   c. **IV Amphotericin B and Liver Disease:** No dose adjustment needed.

Clotrimazole (Mycelex)

Clotrimazole Facts

Clotrimazole is available as a cream and a troche and is a category **C** drug. The oral absorption of the drug is erratic. It is metabolized in the liver and alcohol use is discouraged with the drug. It is contraindicated in the presence of liver disease. Benzodiazepine use with clotrimazole should be avoided as it can cause significant elevation of benzodiazepine level because of the inhibitory action of CYP450 enzyme by clotrimazole.

Clotrimazole (Mycelex) Prescriptions

1. **Rx: Clotrimazole (Mycelex) Cream:**
   Disp: 15 g tube
   Sig: Rub into the affected area 2–3 times daily for 2 weeks.
2. **Rx: Clotrimazole (Mycelex) Troches,** 10 mg/Troche
   Disp: 70 troches (14-day supply)
   Sig: Dissolve 1 troche in the mouth 5 times daily and *swallow the saliva*. There should be no eating or drinking for 30 min after use.

Ketoconazole (Nizoral)

Ketoconazole is an imidazole antifungal that has a strong affinity for fatty tissue. It is a pregnancy category C drug.

Ketoconazole Mechanism of Action

Ketoconazole interferes with the synthesis of fungal ergosterol by inhibition of CYP3A4 enzyme.

Ketoconazole and H_2 Blockers, Antacids, or Vitamin Supplements

Ketoconazole needs an acidic pH for absorption and H_2 blockers or proton pump inhibitors impair the absorption of ketoconazole. Keep a **2-hr** interval between ketoconazole and the H_2 blocker/proton pump inhibitor, for optimal effectiveness. Antacids and vitamin supplements chelate ketoconazole and impair absorption. Keep a **2-hr** interval between these agents and ketoconazole.

Ketoconazole Dosing

1. **Normal Dose:** 200–400 mg q24h
2. **Dose with Kidney Disease:** No dose alteration is needed with kidney disease.
3. **Dose with Liver Disease:** 50% dose reduction is needed with liver disease.

Fluconazole (Diflucan)

Fluconazole (Diflucan) Facts

Fluconazole (Diflucan) is a triazole antifungal that is metabolized in the liver and significantly excreted through the kidneys. It is used for the treatment of local and systemic fungal infections. It is available as a topical agent, a capsule for oral use, and an intravenous (IV) preparation for systemic use. It inhibits the CYP450 enzyme and benzodiazepines should not be used with fluconazole. It can be taken with meals.

Fluconazole and Pregnancy/Breast-Feeding

Fluconazole is a category C drug and very high concentrations of the drug appear in breast milk. It is contraindicated if the patient is pregnant or breast-feeding.

Fluconazole and Kidney or Liver Disease

Decrease the dose by 50% in patients with GFR <50 mL/min or s. creatinine >2 mg/dL-predialysis. Decrease the dose by 50% in mild liver disease. Avoid fluconazole in patients with moderate or severe liver disease.

Fluconazole and Cardiac Conduction

Fluconazole is contraindicated in patients with impaired cardiac conduction:

1. **Fluconazole (Diflucan) Prescription for Refractory Oral or Systemic Candidiasis:**
   Rx: Fluconazole (Diflucan) 100 mg/capsule
   Disp: 15 capsules
   Sig: Day 1: Take 2 capsules. Days 2–14: Take 1 capsule daily.
2. **Fluconazole (Diflucan) Treatment for Esophageal Candidiasis:**
   Rx: Fluconazole (Diflucan) 100 mg/capsule
   Disp: Variable
   Sig: 100 mg qd (maximum 400 mg qd) for 14–21 days

Itraconazole (Sporanox)

Itraconazole Facts

Sporanox has a wider range of activity compared to fluconazole. The oral solution is better absorbed compared to the capsules. The oral or the IV form can be used for the treatment of blastomycosis, aspergillus infection, histoplasmosis, and onychomycosis. Only the IV form is used for the treatment of life-threatening fungal infections.
   Sporanox Dose: 200 mg/day.

Antivirals Commonly Used in Dentistry: Assessment, Analysis, and Associated Dental Management Guidelines

ACYCLOVIR AND VALACYCLOVIR OVERVIEW AND FACTS

Common Features

Acyclovir and valacyclovir are purine nucleoside analogues and both drugs act against herpes simplex 1 and 2 (cold sores and genital herpes respectively), varicella zoster (shingles and chicken pox), and the Epstein-Barr virus (infectious mononucleosis).

Neither drug cures the viral infection, but they do decrease the symptoms and signs associated with the viral infection. Both drugs can be taken with or without food and it is best to take the drug around the same time every day. The elderly patient should be given a lower dose of either drug, compared to the normal patient.

Acyclovir (Zovirax) and Valacyclovir (Valtrex) Mechanism of Action

Both drugs impair viral growth by inhibiting replication of the viral DNA. The virus-infected cells absorb more of the drugs, compared to the normal cells. Thus, the active form of the drug is available longer where needed, enhancing the efficacy of the drugs.

Acyclovir (Zovirax) and Valacyclovir (Valtrex) Clearance

Kidney

Both drugs are excreted mainly by the kidneys and the dose should be decreased in the presence of renal dysfunction. The dose of acyclovir or valacyclovir should be repeated after hemodialysis.

Liver

No dose modification is needed with any form of liver disease.

Acyclovir (Zovirax) and Valacyclovir (Valtrex) Drug Resistance and Side Effects

Resistance can occur with overuse of acyclovir or valacyclovir and it is best to use these drugs short-term and only when needed. Nausea, vomiting, and diarrhea can occur with both drugs.

Acyclovir

Acyclovir (Zovirax) Facts

Avoid acyclovir with amphotericin B, bactrim, aspirin NSAIDS, zidovudine (AZT/Retrovir), or prograf.

Acyclovir Preparations

- Acyclovir tablet: 400 mg/800 mg per tablet
- Acyclovir capsule: 200 mg/capsule
- Acyclovir suspension: 200 mg/5 mL: 473 mL/bottle
- Acyclovir ointment: 5% cream: 15 g tube

Acyclovir Prescriptions

1. **Acyclovir for Herpes Simplex Infection:**
   Rx: 200 mg 5 times per day × 10 days
2a. **Acyclovir for Herpes Zoster Infection:**
   Rx: 800 mg 5 times per day × 10 days
2b. **Acyclovir for Herpes Zoster Infection with Kidney Disease:**
   Rx: GFR 10–25 mL/min or s. creatinine >3 mg/dL to Predialysis: Dose 800 mg q8h
   Rx: GFR <10 mL/min or Dialysis: Dose 800 mg **q12h**
3a. **Five-Day Acyclovir Intermittent Therapy:**
   Rx: 200 mg **q4h** or 5 times per day × 5 days
3b. **Five-Day Acyclovir Intermittent Therapy with Kidney Disease:**
   Rx: GFR <10 mL/min or dialysis: Dose 200 mg **q12h**
4a. **One-Year Acyclovir Chronic Suppressive Therapy with Normal Kidney Status:**
   Rx: 400 mg bid or 200 mg tid × 1 year; Reevaluate after 1 year
4b. **One-Year Acyclovir Chronic Suppressive Therapy with Kidney Disease: GFR <10 mL/min or Dialysis:**
   Rx: Dose 400 mg **q12h** or 200 mg **q12h**

Valacyclovir

Valacyclovir (Valtrex) Facts

Valacyclovir is a "prodrug" that gets converted to acyclovir, its active form. It has a longer duration of action compared to acyclovir; thus, the drug is taken more infrequently. Avoid using valacyclovir with cimetidine (Tagamet) or probenecid (Benemid).

Valacyclovir Preparations

- 500 mg/caplet
- 1 g/capsule

Valacyclovir Prescriptions

1. **Valacyclovir Prescription for Herpes Simplex:**
   Rx: 2 g bid × 1 day

2. **First/Initial Herpes Infection Treatment with Valtrex:**
    Rx: 1 g bid × 10 days
3. **Recurrent Herpes Infection Treatment with Valtrex:**
    Rx: 500 mg bid × 5 days
4a. **Herpes Zoster Infection Treatment with Valtrex:**
    Rx: 1 g tid × 7 days. Begin Valtrex when symptoms begin or within 48 hr of the rash.
4b. **Herpes Zoster Treatment with Valtrex in the Presence of Kidney Disease:**
    Rx: GFR <30 mL/min or s. creatinine >3 mg/dL to predialysis: 1 g q24h

Acute Care and Stress Management

Management of Medical Emergencies in the Dental Setting: Assessment, Analysis, and Associated Dental Management Guidelines

MEDICAL EMERGENCIES OVERVIEW, FACTS, AND TOOLS

Every practitioner is aware that at one time or another, medical emergencies can happen. With proper assessment and care, however, the emergency can be successfully triaged and resolved. Prevention of medical emergencies is the key, and every effort should be made to assess each patient thoroughly prior to treatment. Steps should be incorporated to prevent emergencies from happening; this section discusses and details how to deal with these emergencies.

Prevention of Medical Emergencies

Preventive measures implemented to avoid medical emergencies in the dental setting are thorough assessment of the medical history, thorough physical examination, and appropriate treatment planning.

Thorough Medical History Assessment

Thorough medical history assessment should establish the following:

- The patient's current medical status
- The current list of medications used daily or PRN (as and when needed): prescribed and over-the-counter (OTC) medications
- The patient's compliance with medications
- Any history of medical or surgical complications requiring hospitalization within the previous 2 years
- Any history of allergies
- Any history of corticosteroid intake, currently or within the previous 2 years
- Any history of adverse reactions or feelings about visiting a dentist: anxiety, fear, or avoidance
- Personal habits, alcohol intake, "recreational" drug use

Thorough Physical Examination Assessment

A thorough physical examination should include an assessment of the following:

- General physical appearance
- Vital signs: pulse, blood pressure, respiration rate, temperature, height and weight
- Examination of the head and neck
- Assessment of the cardiovascular system
- Assessment of the respiratory system

Assessment of the Treatment Plan

Assessment of the treatment plan should include the following:

- Assessment of the type of anesthetics, analgesics, and antibiotics that can be safely used during dentistry
- Assessment of whether the patient needs to be premedicated
- Assessment of whether shorter appointments or appointments 7 days apart are needed
- Assessment of whether the patient has presented with a full stomach; the appointment should occur only after the patient eats
- Assessment of whether the patient needs to bring emergency medications for all dental visits: nitroglycerin, inhalers, sugar pills
- Assessment of whether stress management is needed

Preparation or Training for Medical Emergencies

Preparation or training for medical emergencies should include the following:

- Acquire CPR certification or ACLS training.
- Participate in continuing education courses in emergency medicine, annually.
- Know how to access/contact the emergency medical system (EMS) for the dental office during an emergency.
- Conduct practice drills in the dental office, making it a team effort.
- Have an emergency kit in the dental office with updated medications; know the location and contents of the emergency kit.

Common Medications Used During Medical Emergencies

The following medications are used in a medical emergency (list given in alphabetical order):

- Aminophylline (250 mg/10 ml)
- Ammonia vaporole: the white wrap turns pink when ammonia vapors form after the vaporole is cracked open
- Cimetidine (Tagamet): H_2 Blocker: 300 mg IV/IM/PO
- Dextrose ($D_{50}W$): 50 ml, 50% dextrose
- Diazepam (Valium): 5 mg/ml
- Diphenhydramine (Benadryl): H_1 Blocker: 50 mg/ml
- Epinephrine: 1:10,000: Administer 0.3 mg IV *slowly* in a hypotensive patient. ***This should be given by the emergency room physician or emergency personnel responding to the emergency.***
- Epinephrine: 1:1,000 dilution: Administer 0.3–0.5 mL SC/IM
- Famotidine (Pepcid): H_2 Blocker: 20 mg IV/PO

- Glucagon: 1 mg injected IM in the Deltoid muscle
- Glucose: Oral glucose
- Hydrocortisone sodium succinate (Solu-Cortef): 100–200 mg IV/IM
- Lidocaine
- Morphine sulfate
- Naloxone (Narcan): 0.4 mg IV
- Nitroglycerine: 0.3 mg Sublingual (SL): This is given every 5 min up to a maximum of 3 tablets after confirming that *each time*, the systolic BP is maintaining above 115 mmHg.

Emergency Equipment and Adjuncts

Emergency equipment and adjuncts should consist of the following:

- Artificial airways: Oropharyngeal and nasopharyngeal airways
- Airway adjuncts: Endotracheal tubes, laryngoscope
- Ambu-bag: Self-inflating bag-valve-mask: Provides 100% oxygen
- Syringes
- Tourniquets

Oropharyngeal Airways

Measure from lips to the angle of jaw to determine the size of oropharyngeal airway needed. Insert the airway inverted and turn it upright as you reach the back of the tongue. This holds the tongue off the throat. Oropharyngeal airways are tolerated only by the unconscious patient without a gag reflex.

Cricothyrotomy Needle

A 13-guage cricothyrotomy needle is occasionally inserted to access the airway at a point *below* an upper airway obstruction. It is done by inserting the wide-bore needle through the cricothyroid membrane. This form of care should be provided *only* by emergency personnel.

Endotracheal Intubation

A cuffed tube is passed through the vocal cords utilizing direct laryngoscopy and the tube is placed in the trachea.

Oxygen

With a nasal cannula you can give 1–6 L/min of oxygen. This provides the patient with 24–44% oxygen. Through a simple mask you can deliver 40–60% oxygen, and a nonre-breather mask can deliver 90–100% oxygen.

The Basics of Support: Airway, Breathing, and Circulation (The ABCs)

A: Airways: Do the head-tilt–chin-lift and reposition.
B: Breathing: Do rescue breathing; use the bag and mask.
C: Circulation: Do assessment of circulation; do CPR.

This should be followed by reassessment of the patient's status; use of medications; and transfer to the hospital if needed, for definitive therapy.

CLASSIFICATION OF MEDICAL EMERGENCIES

It is always best to classify medical emergencies according to the patient's presenting symptoms. Once you focus on the specific presenting symptoms you are able to triage the proper care for the patient immediately.

Syncope Attack

Multiple factors can cause syncope, and some factors can cause syncope more commonly compared to others:

- **Common Causes:** The more common causes of syncope attacks are vasovagal syncope orthostatic hypotension, hyperventilation syndrome, and hypoglycemic reaction or coma.
- **Less Common Causes:** The less common causes of syncope are transient ischemic attack (TIAs), cerebrovascular accident (CVA/stroke); cardiac arrest; hyperglycemia, and acute adrenal insufficiency.

Chest Pains

Chest pains can occur with angina, myocardial infarction, or hyperventilation syndrome. Angina can be stable angina/angina of effort, unstable angina, acute coronary insufficiency (preinfarction angina), and atypical/coronary artery spasm/Prinzmetal's angina.

Respiratory Distress

Respiratory distress can occur with foreign body obstruction, asthma, or hyperventilation syndrome.

Adverse Drug Reactions

Adverse drug reactions can be associated with anaphylaxis/allergy, local anesthetic, **and/or** epinephrine overdose.

Seizures

Seizures can be due to grand mal epilepsy, hypoglycemia, or hyperventilation syndrome.

VASOVAGAL SYNCOPE

Vasovagal Syncope Predisposing Factors

Predisposing factors for vasovagal syncope often are anxiety, fear, and sight of blood; hot and humid surroundings; upright position without movement; prolonged motionless standing for a period of time; and age (young patients in their teens to early 40s). Males are more often affected than females.

Vasovagal Prodrome Stage

There is a definite prodrome stage when the patient feels that a collapse is imminent: This is the fright and flight response. It lasts for 10 sec to a few minutes. Anxiety, tachycardia, perspiration, light-headedness, and blurred vision are commonly experienced.

Vasovagal Syncope Stage Vital Signs

Bradycardia with hypotension is *the* classic finding on physical examination. This is the only syncope where a *drop* in the blood pressure (BP) is associated with bradycardia and *not* tachycardia. Tonic-clonic activity may occur.

Vasovagal Postsyncope Stage

Recovery occurs within a few seconds. There may be some headache, dizziness, nausea, vomiting, pallor, and perspiration that may persist for a few minutes to a few hours. The patient may try to sit up on recovery. Discourage this from happening.

There is no postsyncope confusion. Confusion could occur if the patient falls during the emergency and knocks his/her head. This should prompt you to activate the emergency medical system (EMS) and transfer the patient to the nearest emergency room (ER) for evaluation of a head injury.

Vasovagal Syncope Treatment

Immediately put the patient in a supine position. Crack open a vial of ammonia (smelling salts) and hold it away from your face, to prevent you from inhaling the vapors! The white covering of the vial turns pink once the ammonia vapors are released. Next, lean forward and have the patient inhale the vapors. Reassure the patient on recovery. Assess the clarity of the mental status by having the patient respond to some common-knowledge questions. Observe for 1/2–1 hr, with the patient lying down.

Vasovagal Syncope and Suggested Additional Steps of Care

During an emergency always monitor the pulse using one of the most accessible arteries: radial, brachial (in children), or carotid. Use the following guidelines to get an instant perception of the blood pressure level:

1. Inability to feel the radial pulse during an emergency indicates that the systolic blood pressure (SBP) is *less* than 80 mmHg
2. Inability to feel the brachial pulse indicates the SBP is *less* than 70 mmHg.
3. Inability to feel the carotid pulse indicates the SBP has dropped *below* 60 mmHg.

Steps to Interrupt a Vasovagal Syncope Attack

Occasionally you will find yourself facing a patient who has denied anxiety and the need for stress management during an initial medical history assessment visit. Now when you are ready to inject the local anesthetic, you may find this patient clenching the sides of the dental chair and looking quite pale.

Immediately stop the treatment and put the chair in a horizontal or slight head-down position. Have the patient open and close the fists and perform bicycling movements with the legs. This will move the blood from the extremities and toward the heart.

Stress management should always be provided for future visits in patients who have experienced vasovagal syncope in the dental setting.

ORTHOSTATIC HYPOTENSION (OH)

Orthostatic Hypotension Predisposing Factors

An elderly patient is more likely to experience orthostatic hypotension because in the elderly patient, the erect vasoconstrictor action on standing up is slow in onset. Patients on antihypertension, antidepression, and anti–Parkinson's disease drugs often experience orthostatic hypotension as a side effect of the medications. OH can occur due to increased vasodilation right after IV sedation or nitroglycerine use and it is more common in diabetics with autonomic neuropathy.

Orthostatic Hypotension Prodrome Stage

There is no prodrome stage with OH and the patient feels **normal** prior to the syncope.

Orthostatic Hypotension Syncope Stage Vital Signs

The syncope occurs with rapid change from a lying-down position to an upright position. There is a precipitous drop in the blood pressure. The pulse is normal or slightly elevated from baseline values. The patient regains consciousness on becoming horizontal when circulation to the brain is maintained.

Orthostatic Hypotension Pretreatment Diagnosis

In a suspect case for orthostatic hypotension, monitor the BP and pulse in a lying-down and **immediate** upright position. You can diagnose OH if the systolic blood pressure (SBP) drops by 20–30 mmHg or the diastolic blood pressure (DBP) drops by 10–15 mmHg on standing up and the pulse rate increases by 10–15 beats/min.

Orthostatic Hypotension Prevention Strategy

At the end of the appointment have the patient sit upright in the dental chair for a few minutes and then assist the patient out of the chair. Hold onto the patient until the patient feels stable standing upright.

HYPERVENTILATION SYNDROME

Hyperventilation Syndrome Predisposing Factors

Anxiety and fear are the most common predisposing factors.

Hyperventilation Syndrome Pathophysiology and Clinical Features

Rapid and deep breathing occurs because of severe anxiety and fear. This causes a washout of CO_2 and the PCO_2 goes below normal (35–45 mmHg). The PO_2 stays in the normal range. Generalized vascular involvement, affecting the cerebral, coronary, and gastrointestinal circulation occurs.

Hyperventilation Syndrome Effect on the Cerebral Circulation

Involvement of the cerebral circulation causes the patient to experience headache, confusion, and visual disturbances. The patient feels as if a collapse is imminent, but it isn't.

Hyperventilation Syndrome Effect on the Coronary Circulation

Involvement of the coronary circulation causes the patient to experience severe tightness of the chest and angina-type pains.

Hyperventilation Syndrome Effect on the Gastrointestinal Circulation

Involvement of the gastrointestinal circulation causes the patient to experience nausea, vomiting, and a lump in the throat (globus hystericus).

Hyperventilation Syndrome Additional Clinical Features

The patient never loses consciousness, although the feeling of light-headedness persists. Tingling, numbness, and paresthesia in the perioral area and the extremities are experienced. Carpopedal spasm, tremors, and muscle twitching occur because of a fall in the ionized serum calcium in the arterial blood.

Hyperventilation Syndrome Vital Signs

The pulse, blood pressure, and respiration rate are markedly elevated and the respiratory rate is >25–30/min.

Hyperventilation Syndrome Treatment

Activate the EMS (emergency medical system) if the vital signs are extremely elevated and you have an uncooperative patient.

Give the patient an upright or a semi-sitting position in the chair, fan the patient, and loosen the clothing. Encourage rebreathing with the patient's cupped hands over his/her mouth and nose or breathing into a paper bag. Never use a plastic bag because it can suffocate the patient. Breathing into cupped hands or a paper bag will help the patient rebreathe the exhaled CO_2. Approximately 10–15 mg diazepam is administered IV if rebreathing is not helpful or the patient is uncooperative. Do not give more than 0.1 mg/kg body weight of Valium during the emergency. Never use any oxygen during a hyperventilation emergency.

HYPOGLYCEMIA

Hypoglycemia can occur in both the diabetic and the nondiabetic patient. The brain is totally dependent on an adequate glucose supply for its energy requirements.

Hypoglycemia Predisposing Factors

Hypoglycemia can be caused by acute starvation, alcohol bingeing, increased insulin, or oral hypoglycemic drugs intake.

Hypoglycemia Clinical Features

Hypoglycemia reaction is very rapid in onset and it can progress from a mild to moderate or severe stage in seconds to minutes.

Hypoglycemia Mild Stage

During this stage the patient experiences restlessness, irritability, and excitement and shows lack of cooperation. Nausea is quite pronounced and there is an extreme feeling of hunger.

Hypoglycemia Moderate Stage

Perspiration is very apparent now and the palms and soles are wet, cold, and clammy. Shivering with hair on end occurs.

Hypoglycemia Vital Signs

Tachycardia associated with a bounding pulse occurs in the initial stages of excitement and irritability. The respiration rate is normal, or it could be slightly increased in the mild stage. The blood pressure is elevated initially, but then it starts to drop when no treatment is initiated. The gag reflex is very prominent in the late moderate stage. If left untreated the patient goes into the severe stage of hypoglycemia, becoming glassy-eyed and quite unresponsive. Tonic-clonic seizures may occur and the patient becomes unconscious. During the unconscious stage the BP drops and hypotension occurs with bradycardia and hypothermia.

Hypoglycemia Treatment

Assess the ABCs and position the patient accordingly. Give a semi-sitting position if the BP is **maintained** and the patient stays **connected** with you in conversational response. Give a horizontal position when, in spite of being conscious, the patient **fails to communicate well** with you.

Administer oral glucose gel, liquid sugar, Glucola, or apple or orange juice in the mild stage. It is best to use baby apple juice because it does not need to be refrigerated. The juice has a long shelf life as long as it is unopened. A baby juice product is also less likely to suddenly disappear because someone was thirsty! The use of orange juice is not advised in an uncontrolled diabetic with preexisting kidney disease because of the high potassium content in orange juice. The potassium from the orange juice can worsen the hyperkalemia associated with kidney disease. Orange juice, however, can be used in the nondiabetic patient experiencing hypoglycemia.

Once the patient has recovered from a mild reaction, have the patient eat some complex carbohydrate foods such as whole wheat/rye crackers with cheese or whole wheat/rye crackers with peanut butter. The fiber in the complex carbohydrates helps keep the sugars in the stomach longer and prevent a relapse.

Administer 50 mL of $D_{50}W$ IV *slowly,* at the rate of 10 mL/min, in the moderate to severe stage. If you are unable to establish an IV line, give 1 mg glucagon IM in the deltoid muscle.

Administer oxygen by mask at a flow rate of 4–6 liters/min. Activate EMS if you have not yet done so, particularly when seizures occur or if the recovery is sluggish.

Hypoglycemia Additional Suggested Recovery Facts and Alerts

Once an insulin-dependent diabetic has completely recovered from a hypoglycemic reaction, dental treatment can continue if the patient feels comfortable going ahead with the dentistry planned for the day. Dental treatment must be *discontinued* if a diabetic on oral hypoglycemic drugs develops a hypoglycemic reaction. Oral hypoglycemic drugs can cause the patient to have **rebound hypoglycemia** 4–6 hr after an initial hypoglycemic reaction. Once the initial reaction is treated in the dental office, the patient should be sent to the ER for monitoring and steady maintenance of the blood sugar levels. If the patient is taking β-blockers for hypertension or benign tremors, etc., all the symptoms of hypoglycemia usually are absent **except** for perspiration because β-blockers blunt hypoglycemic symptoms. The blunting effect is more severe with the nonselective β-blockers compared to selective β-blockers.

TRANSIENT ISCHEMIC ATTACKS (TIAs)

The hallmark feature of TIA is that the patient never really loses consciousness. TIAs are associated with temporary cerebral ischemia and no permanent brain damage. Symptoms experienced last for a few seconds to a few minutes, occasionally for a few hours, and resolution of all symptoms occurs within 24 hr.

Transient Ischemic Attacks Predisposing Factors

Predisposing factors for TIAs are hypertension, diabetes, hyperlipidemia, or atrial fibrillation.

Transient Ischemic Attacks Clinical Features

The patient experiences tingling, numbness, or weakness of the limbs or hands and feet. Slurred speech, loss of speech, drooling, blurring of vision, and disorientation can also occur.

Transient Ischemic Attacks Vital Signs

The pulse is rapid and bounding and the BP is elevated.

Transient Ischemic Attacks Treatment

Activate the EMS if this is the first TIA attack for the patient or if it is a worsening attack for a patient with a past history of TIAs. Give the patient an upright position and monitor the vital signs. Try to calm an agitated patient. Do not use oxygen if the patient has no breathing difficulty because the oxygen will promote vasoconstriction and worsen the TIA symptoms. If this is not the first attack, observe the patient for some time and determine by communicating with the patient if this attack is any different than the past attacks. Once the symptoms have subsided, send the patient home as long as the TIA is no different when compared to the ones experienced by the patient in the past. If, however, there is a change in the severity or the symptoms experienced are new, the patient must be sent to the ER for further evaluation and monitoring for potential stroke/CVA.

CEREBROVASCULAR ACCIDENT (CVA)

Cerebrovascular accident/stroke is associated with permanent neurological damage. CVA may be due to cerebral ischemia, infarction, or intracranial hemorrhage. True syncope is rare. However, intracranial hemorrhage invariably results in sudden loss of consciousness and is associated with an increased morbidity and mortality rate.

Cerebrovascular Accident Predisposing Factors

Predisposing factors to CVA are similar to those for TIAs.

Cerebrovascular Accident (CVA) Clinical Features

Fear and anxiety in the dental setting may lead to the elevation of the BP in susceptible patients. All stroke patients experience headaches that may be mild, moderate, or severe. CVA due to ischemia or infarction is associated with mild to moderate headaches. True syncope rarely occurs at the onset with ischemia or infarction. Intracranial hemorrhage or ruptured aneurysm–associated CVA causes excruciating headaches and sudden loss of consciousness. This type of CVA is associated with increased morbidity and mortality. Dizziness, vertigo, nausea, vomiting, and progressive sensory and/or motor dysfunction are experienced with all forms of strokes.

Cerebrovascular Accident Vital Signs

The pulse is usually bounding with a thrombus or an embolism and may be normal or slow in association with an intracranial hemorrhage. The BP is elevated. Respiration is slow and shallow.

Cerebrovascular Accident Treatment

Activate the EMS. Maintain an upright position for the conscious patient and a supine position with the head **slightly elevated** with a neck role (to prevent a further increase in the intracranial pressure) for the unconscious patient.

Monitor vital signs and maintain the ABCs. Do not use oxygen if the patient is breathing adequately. Increased levels of oxygen can cause further vasoconstriction and worsening of symptoms. Oxygen should be given **only** to an unconscious patient experiencing true breathing difficulty. Always rule out airway obstruction due to improper positioning prior to administering oxygen. Once stable, immediately transfer the patient to the hospital.

CARDIAC ARREST OF UNKNOWN ORIGIN

The patient is unresponsive with no palpable pulse.

Cardiac Arrest Predisposing Factors

The predisposing factors are ventricular fibrillation or arrhythmia, severe myocardial infarction, drug overdose, or foreign body airway obstruction.

Cardiac Arrest Clinical Features

Loss of consciousness occurs within 3 to 5 sec, and brain damage can occur within 4 to 6 min without treatment.

Cardiac Arrest Unresponsive Patient Management

Activate the EMS and promptly institute the "ABCs"—plus "D," if necessary:

Step A: Identify for yourself: Does the patient have an airway? If the response is "yes," proceed to Step B. If the response is "no," do the head-tilt–chin-lift, and then proceed to Step B.

Step B: Identify for yourself: Are there any indications of spontaneous breathing? If the response is "yes," apply the oxygen mask and proceed to Step C. If the response is "no," ventilate with the bag-valve-mask apparatus using 100% O_2 at the rate of 12–20/min.

Step C: Identify for yourself: Can you palpate the carotid pulse? If the response is "yes," proceed to Step D. If the response is "no," start CPR and proceed to Step D.

Step D: Establish an IV line with normal saline. Give $D_{50}W$ IV and naloxone (Narcan), 0.4 mg IV.

Whenever you are unaware of the exact etiology of the collapse and unresponsiveness, you need to treat it as if it were a hypoglycemia reaction and narcotic overdose. These are two states that can cause brain damage if not treated promptly. In the event the cause is something different, the $D_{50}W$ IV and naloxone will not adversely affect the patient. Repeat the Narcan injection and the dextrose drip if you see a clinical response. If you are unable to establish an IV line, give Narcan IM, 0.4 mg, and if hypoglycemia is strongly suspected, give glucagon 1 mg IM in the deltoid muscle.

HYPERGLYCEMIA

Hyperglycemia affects diabetic patients only. Poor control and/or poor compliance leads to hyperglycemia. Infection, inflammation, trauma, and bleeding can exacerbate the hyperglycemia and cause precipitation of a hyperglycemic coma.

Hyperglycemia Clinical Features

Hyperglycemia takes a few hours to a few days to develop. The patient is red in the face, the skin is warm and dry due to dehydration, plus the patient has a ketotic smell. The mouth is dry and the patient experiences intense thirst. Abdominal pain often occurs.

Hyperglycemia Vital Signs

The pulse is rapid but weak. The BP is decreased. The respiration is deep and rapid. This is the classic Kussmaul's breathing, which is an abnormal breathing pattern characterized by rapid and deep breathing. It is often seen in patients with metabolic acidosis. The patient has a ketotic, fruity smell.

Hyperglycemia Treatment

Activate the EMS. Management of the syncope is supportive while the patient is in the dental office. Give the patient a horizontal position in the chair. Monitor the vital signs. Start an IV line with normal saline and give 4–6 L/min oxygen. The EMS and ER will manage the hyperglycemia with insulin.

ACUTE ADRENAL INSUFFICIENCY

Acute Adrenal Insufficiency Etiology

Acute adrenal insufficiency occurs with acute infection, inflammation, trauma, massive bleeding, or **failure to give** steroids in susceptible patients when there is a **need** to follow "the rule of twos."

The rule of twos: Ask whether the patient is currently on steroids or has been on corticosteroids for 2 weeks or longer within the past 2 years. You must go back 2 years in the history because it can take **2 weeks to 2 years** for the adrenal glands to bounce back to **normal** function.

Acute Adrenal Insufficiency Clinical Features

The patient experiences extreme fatigue; muscle cramps and muscle weakness; mental confusion (due to hypoglycemia); and nausea, vomiting, and severe abdominal pain. The deteriorating condition progresses rapidly without treatment, leading to coma.

Acute Adrenal Insufficiency Vital Signs

The respiration is slow and shallow. The BP falls very rapidly and the pulse is rapid and very weak.

Acute Adrenal Insufficiency Treatment

Activate the EMS and immediately give the patient a supine position. Assess the airway, breathing, and circulation (ABCs) and monitor the vital signs. Establish an IV line and start 5% glucose in normal saline. Give 100 mg hydrocortisone IV STAT (immediately) followed by hydrocortisone q6h (every 6 hr): Total dose given is 100–200 mg/24 hr. The hydrocortisone is given until the patient is stable. Give oxygen at a flow rate of 4–6 L/min.

ANGINA PECTORIS

Angina Pectoris Clinical Features

Activity precipitates an attack. With the start of the attack the patient is unable to continue with activity, immediately stands still, and is hunched over with the fist across the chest. Tightness or discomfort experienced in the chest occurs for less than 10–15 min, about 2–5 min in most cases. The discomfort experienced may or may not radiate. If it does radiate, it could go toward the jaw, left arm, back, or upper abdomen. This pain radiation can happen with unstable angina, too. The patient can be quite apprehensive if this is a first angina attack, but apprehension is less otherwise. Sweating can be significant depending on the intensity of the attack.

Angina Pectoris Vital Signs

The pulse is markedly increased and bounding and the BP is elevated. Some dyspnea or respiratory difficulty may occur.

Angina Pectoris Treatment

Activate the EMS if this is a first attack for the patient or it happens to be a worsening attack for a patient with a past history of angina attacks. Place the patient in an upright position.

Treat with nitroglycerine (NTG) tablets. Start with one 0.3 mg nitroglycerine tablet sublingual (SL). Always confirm that the tablet produces a burning sensation under the tongue and a flushed feeling going to the head. This indicates that the pill is potent. Repeat with a second or third nitroglycerine tablet at 5-min intervals, as long as the patient experiences pain and the systolic BP is *above* 115 mmHg prior to each tablet use.

You can give a total of three 0.3 mg nitroglycerine tablets at 5-min intervals. Do not go beyond three nitroglycerine tablets even if the pain continues and the BP is elevated. This patient needs to be sent to the ER immediately for further evaluation and care. Give oxygen 4–6 L/min with the start of the treatment because this facilitates recovery.

Angina Treatment Alerts

The shelf life of nitroglycerine tablets is 6 months, unopened, and 6 weeks, once the bottle is opened. The shelf life is further shortened when the pills are exposed to light and agitated constantly in the bottle. Always confirm that the patient experiences a burning and tingling sensation on using nitroglycerine.

Check the BP and confirm that the systolic blood pressure is elevated. If the systolic blood pressure goes **below** 115 mmHg with nitroglycerine, activate the EMS and stop using any further NTG. This BP drop typically occurs with unstable angina and one should always consider progression to myocardial infarction (MI). With conversion to MI the blood pressure drops and the pulse becomes rapid and thready (low volume). The pulse may become irregular. In this situation, place the patient in a horizontal position, maintain the ABCs, supply oxygen, and wait for the EMS to arrive. Management of this state is the same as for an MI attack.

Note: If there has been no response to nitroglycerine in the past, the patient could be given 10–20 mg niphedipine (Procardia) sublingual (SL) because this could be Prinzmetal's Angina.

Nitroglycerine and Erectile Dysfunction (ED) Drug Combination Alert

Erectile dysfunction(ED) drugs—sildenafil citrate (Viagra), tadalafil (Cialis), and vardenafil HCL (Levitra)—cause significant vasodilatation. Profound vasodilatation can occur when even a single nitroglycerine tablet is given to a patient who has used an ED drug in the past 24–48 hr, and this significant vasodilatation can cause a precipitous drop in the BP. This patient must therefore be sent to the ER for proper assessment, management, and triage for successful outcome of care. The vasodilatation caused by Viagra lasts for 24 hr and that caused by Cialis and Levitra lasts for 48 hr.

MYOCARDIAL INFARCTION (MI)

Myocardial Infarction (MI) Risk Factors

Risk factors include past history of angina or coronary artery disease, uncontrolled hypertension, any past history of thrombotic episodes (stroke or a previous MI), heavy smoking and excessive alcohol consumption, obesity, or hypercholesterolemia.

Myocardial Infarction (MI) Clinical Features

MI pain lasts for more than 10–15 min and it is a "crushing" type of chest pain. The pain can be precipitated with or without activity. The patient looks pale and acutely distressed. There is tightness of the chest and excruciating pain that may or may not radiate. If it does radiate it can go toward the lower jaw or left arm, and sometimes the right arm, back, or upper abdomen. Along with the chest pain, the patient often experiences palpitations, profuse sweating, restlessness, anxiety, lightheadedness, cold clammy skin, a feeling of impending doom, nausea, vomiting, and abdominal bloating. The patient may attribute the nausea, vomiting, and abdominal bloating, to a gastrointestinal problem and not seek help in a timely manner.

MI Vital Signs

The patient is short of breath and the respiration is shallow. The pulse is rapid, thready (low volume), and highly irregular. Occasionally bradycardia can occur. The BP is decreased when compared to normal base line readings.

Myocardial Infarction (MI) Medical Management

Activate the emergency medical system (EMS). Lay the patient down to assess the airway, breathing, circulation (ABCs), and monitor the vital signs. The first line of management for a suspected case of MI is morphine, oxygen, nitroglycerine, and aspirin (MONA).

Start 4–6 L/min of oxygen by mask. Immediately give one 0.3 mg tablet nitroglycerin as long as the SBP is **above** 115 mmHg. Also give 162 mg or 325 mg aspirin crushed under the tongue or have the patient chew or swallow the aspirin. The aspirin will thin the blood by decreasing the platelet cohesiveness. Do not use enteric-coated aspirin as that will delay absorption.

The EMS will establish an IV line, start 5% dextrose in water, and give 2–5 mg morphine every 5–15 min until the pain subsides. Respiration rate during morphine administration must always be maintained at >12 breaths/min. Once the pain is stabilized with morphine, the patient is moved to the hospital.

At any time during transportation or otherwise, cardiac arrest can occur with acute MI. Cardiopulmonary resuscitation (CPR) will maintain the patient till an automated electrical defibrillator (AED) can be used to evaluate ventricular tachycardia or ventricular arrhythmia. The AED will revive the cardiac rhythm in such circumstances.

FOREIGN BODY OBSTRUCTION (FBO)

Foreign Body Obstruction Facts

No noise or respiratory sound is heard in total laryngotracheal obstruction. Stridor, cough, cyanosis, and wheezing occur in partial laryngotracheal obstruction or bronchial obstruction. The victim grabs at the throat and experiences intense fear.

Foreign Body Obstruction (FBO) Treatment

Activate the EMS immediately. Perform the Heimlich maneuver and continue doing it till the FBO is relieved or the patient becomes unconscious. Straddle over the supine patient and do 6–10 abdominal thrusts, after doing a head-tilt–chin-lift, if the patient becomes unconscious.

Next, proceed to do a finger sweep followed by ventilation of the patient. Repeat the thrusts, sweep, and ventilation until you are successful or the EMS has arrived.

Additional care can be provided with epinephrine, steroids, or metaproterenol to open the airways and decrease inflammation. Cricythyrotomy with the cricothyrotomy device or 13-guage needle may be done if the Heimlich maneuver is unsuccessful.

ASTHMA

Asthma Types

Extrinsic asthma is typically the allergy-associated asthma. Intrinsic asthma is nonallergy-associated asthma and it is frequently precipitated by infection in the lung(s).

Acute Asthma Clinical Features

Acute asthma is typically associated with shortness of breath (SOB), wheezing on inspiration and/or expiration, cough with or without expectoration, and labored breathing. Cyanosis, intense fatigue, and mental confusion can occur in severe cases.

Asthma Vital Signs

Initially and very transiently the respiratory rate (RR) is normal, but as the asthma progresses the RR becomes rapid. The pulse and the BP are both elevated.

Asthma Treatment

Activate the EMS in severe cases or if this is an initial attack. Immediately give the patient an upright position in the chair. The patient will prefer to sit hunched over as this enhances the taking in of air for the patient.

As a first choice, use the patient's own bronchodilator. If this is not possible, have the patient use the metaproterenol (Alupent) spray from the emergency kit. Give 0.3–0.5 ml, 1:1,000 epinephrine, SC/IM if nothing else is available. If the patient's pulse is less than 120–130 beats/min and the BP is less than 140/90 mmHg, epinephrine may be repeated twice at 20-min intervals, following the pulse and BP guidelines. Give oxygen at a flow rate of 4–6 L/min. In refractory cases, slow infusion of 6 mg/kg IV aminophylline, diluted in 50–100 mL saline and 100–200 mg, IV hydrocortisone sodium succinate are also given.

ANAPHYLAXIS/ALLERGY

Anaphylaxis/Allergy Clinical Features

The patient experiences a sinking feeling, intense itching, hives, and flushing over the face and chest. Rhinitis, conjunctivitis, nausea, vomiting, abdominal cramps, and perspiration also occur. Additionally the patient experiences palpitation, tachycardia, substernal tightness, coughing, wheezing, and dyspnea. The patient initially looks pale and then cyanosis and laryngeal edema can occur. The blood pressure (BP) drops rapidly and loss of consciousness or cardiac arrest can occur in severe cases.

Anaphylaxis/Allergy Treatment

Give the patient a supine position. Establish an IV line with normal saline and give 0.3–0.5 mL 1:1,000 epinephrine, SC/IM. Epinephrine may be repeated every 3–5 min until improvement occurs. In the severely hypotensive patient, *emergency personnel only* can give 1:10,000 epinephrine, 0.3 mL IV *slowly*. Once epinephrine has stabilized the pulse and the BP, inject, 50 mg diphenhydramine (Benadryl) IV **plus** 300 mg cimetidine (Tagamet) **or** 20 mg famotidine (Pepcid) IV. Cimetidine and famotadine are H_2 blockers. Additionally give 100–200 mg hydrocortisone sodium succinate (Solu-cortef) IV. Metaproterenol spray can also be used for refractory cases to open the airways. Oxygen is given at a flow rate of 4–6 L/min.

When the acute phase is over, 50 mg diphenhydramine and/or 300 mg cimetidine/20 mg famotidine (Pepcid) are given **PO q6h for next 48–72 hr,** following recovery. Premature withdrawal of the H_1 with or without the H_2 blocker can cause a hypotensive reaction because excess histamine is still in the circulation. Nonsedating fexofenadine HCL (Allegra), cetirizine HCL (Zyrtec), or loratadine (Claritin) can be used instead of the sedating Benadryl for 48–72 hr in the postrecovery period.

LOCAL ANESTHETIC OVERDOSE

Duration of the local anesthetic overdose reaction is very short because of quick redistribution and biotransformation.

Local Anesthetic Overdose Clinical Features

The patient experiences agitation, confusion, excitement, talkativeness, apprehension, slurred speech, muscle twitching, and tremors. Headache, light headedness, visual disturbance, and a flushed feeling can also occur. Numbness of the tongue and around the perioral area may also occur. Disorientation, drowsiness, and tonic-clonic seizures may occur in progressive cases.

Local Anesthetic Overdose Vital Signs

The pulse, BP, and respiratory rate are all increased.

Local Anesthetic Overdose Treatment

Activate EMS in severe cases. Give the patient a semi-sitting position. Reassure, and ask the patient to hyperventilate. Inject 10 mg diazepam (Valium) IV slowly if seizure occurs. Give oxygen in severe cases. Perform CPR with cardiac arrest.

EPINEPHRINE OVERDOSE REACTION

Epinephrine Overdose Clinical Features

The patient experiences anxiety, fear, restlessness, throbbing headache, tremors, perspiration, weakness, dizziness, and pallor.

Epinephrine Overdose Reaction Vital Signs

The pulse is rapid and bounding. The respiratory rate is increased and respiratory difficulty is experienced. The BP is elevated.

Epinephrine Overdose Reaction Treatment

Position the patient in a semi-sitting or upright position. Reassure the patient and monitor the vital signs. Administer oxygen at a flow rate of 4–6 L/min.

SEIZURES

A typical grand mal seizure attack is always associated with the ictal/seizure phase. A prodromal phase may or may not precede the ictal/seizure phase.

Prodromal Phase

The prodromal phase occurs hours to days before the seizure and it can last for several minutes to several hours. The patient can experience increased anxiety, depression, a low feeling, or tunnel vision. This phase does not occur in every patient. However, if the patient does experience specific symptoms that herald a seizure, those specific symptoms *will always precede* the ictal/seizure phase in the patient.

Seizure or Ictal Phase

The seizure/ictal phase can have four components: The aura, tonic, clonic, and flaccid phase. A typical tonic-clonic seizure lasts for no more than 2 min.

Aura Phase

The aura is not present in every patient, but if it does exist the aura symptoms experienced **repeat** with every seizure that occurs. The aura lasts for a few seconds only. The patient can see, hear, taste, or smell something specific like a rotten egg taste or sulfur smell, etc., and verbalizes this during this phase. These are abnormal sensations experienced, but the patient is **unaware** of their presence when questioned later upon recovery. The patient could, however, recount their presence during history-taking if someone present during a past attack had informed the patient about experiencing the symptoms. Do not remove the patient from the chair during this phase. The patient is conscious but unaware of the surroundings. Immediately give the patient a horizontal position, push the tray away and call for help. You and an assistant should stand on either side of the chair and provide passive restraint to prevent the patient from falling.

Tonic Phase

In this phase the patient gives out a loud cry and becomes very rigid and hyperextended after taking in a deep breath. There is loss of consciousness and the patient turns blue from holding the breath. If standing, the patient falls to the ground. You may want to, but **do not** hold the patient down because you can injure the patient's spine. This phase lasts for less than a minute.

Clonic Phase

The clonic phase follows the tonic phase. The patient starts breathing and the limbs start to flay. The flailing is initially rhythmic and then becomes arrhythmic toward the end of the phase. Again, do not hold the patient down because fractures may occur. This phase **also** lasts for about 1 min or less and is then followed by the postictal or the flaccid phase.

Flaccid Phase

The entire body becomes limp during this phase. Frothing occurs at the mouth, the tongue falls back and the patient starts to "grunt". There is always incontinence of the bowel and/or the bladder during this phase. Incontinence does **not** occur with seizures due to other causes: drug reaction, hypoglycemia, etc.

Seizure Treatment

Activate the EMS. Keep the patient in a supine position. Prevent injury during the tonic, clonic, and flaccid phases. Once in the flaccid phase, monitor the vital signs. Perform a head-tilt–chin-lift and turn the head to the side. Use suction and actively remove all secretions to clear the airway. Give oxygen at a flow rate of 4–6 L/min, by mask. Once the airways have been cleared during the flaccid phase, confirm that the patient has regained consciousness. It is very important to shake the patient and have the patient respond to your questions. It is not uncommon for the patient to go into a deep sleep once the seizure ends. Pinch an unresponsive patient to see whether a painful stimulus can awaken the patient. If there is no response, the patient is in the *status epilepticus,* which is a phase of ongoing seizures where the patient continues to remain unconscious. The EMS has to transfer such a patient to the nearest emergency room after injecting diazepam (Valium) during one of the flaccid phases to stop the constant seizure activity. 5–10 mg diazepam (Valium) is injected IV, over 1–2 min. 50 mL of $D_{50}W$ IV is also given if hypoglycemia is suspected. There is a 15% mortality rate with status epilepticus.

Oral and Parenteral Conscious Sedation for Dentistry: Assessment, Analysis, and Associated Dental Management Guidelines

CONSCIOUS SEDATION OVERVIEW

Conscious sedation is what makes dentistry "painless" for the phobic patient or the patient fearful of the dental environment. Elimination of pain and anxiety control is usually the first option considered for patients experiencing fear or phobia toward dentistry. Conscious sedation is an extension of care, beyond these measures. Sedation dentistry helps make dental procedures virtually painless. Conscious sedation is not just reserved for the fearful patient. It is also an important option for patients with developmental disabilities and movement disorders so that dentistry can be completed effortlessly for these patients.

Anesthesiologist-administered general anesthesia for dentistry is not a part of conscious sedation and should be confined to only a hospitalized setting.

SEDATION CLASSIFICATIONS

Sedation is classified as the following:

1. Anesthesiologist-administered deep sedation
2. Intravenous (IV) sedation or deep conscious sedation
3. Inhalation conscious sedation
4. Oral conscious sedation

Anesthesiologist-Administered Deep Sedation

This type of sedation is administered only by an anesthesiologist. The patient has partial or complete loss of protective reflexes, and there is inability to maintain a patent airway independently and at all times. The patient is not easily aroused and is unable to respond to verbal commands or physical stimulation.

Intravenous (IV) Sedation or Deep Conscious Sedation

This technique is used by most oral surgeons and some trained dentists. It requires certification by the state board of dentistry. IV sedation is provided using a single drug, usually one of the benzodiazepines. The dose is titrated matching the patient's needs.

More can be injected for immediate effect when the dose wears off. Fixed dose or bolus dose drug use is highly discouraged. Drugs used for IV sedation are more effective than the same drugs taken orally. There is a more profound amnesia associated with this technique.

Inhalation Conscious Sedation

Inhalation sedation is provided by using titrated doses of O_2 + N_2O. The patient usually falls asleep during the procedure. There is some amount of amnesia and analgesia.

Oxygen/nitrous oxide sedation is the most frequently used sedation in dentistry. This type of sedation requires special delivery and scavenging systems. The patient should not have had any recent upper respiratory tract infections (URTIs).

All bodily functions remain normal with this type of sedation and the patient is able to breathe on his own. The patient will often fall asleep and experience some degree of amnesia. Dental inhalation sedation works well for mild to moderate anxiety. It has a rapid onset, there is flexibility of duration, and it can be used for any appointment length. The dentist has absolute control because it is easy to titrate the level of sedation, which may be altered moment to moment. The recovery is quick and there are very few side effects. There is an analgesic effect experienced and the patient can resume normal activities immediately.

The disadvantages of dental inhalation sedation include severe anxiety, which may require a deeper level of sedation, plus it is not indicated for patients with respiratory problems such as severe asthma, significant emphysema, or COPD.

Oral Conscious Sedation

This type of sedation is patient-administered, safe, and easy to monitor. The patient takes oral benzodiazepines prescribed by the dentist. The patient invariably falls asleep, and deep relaxation is experienced with this method of sedation. All body functions remain normal and the patient is able to breathe on his/her own, often falling asleep. Some degree of amnesia is common. The disadvantage of oral sedation, however, is that the level of sedation for each patient is not predictable. Someone must drive the patient to and from the dental appointment and there is no analgesic effect.

Inhalation and Oral Conscious Sedation Additional Facts

Oral conscious sedation and inhalation sedation are the two most common types of sedation techniques used by most dental practitioners doing sedation dentistry, outside of the oral surgery setting. Conscious sedation is not light general anesthesia. In fact there is a huge difference between conscious sedation and the unconscious state associated with general anesthesia. In conscious sedation the patient maintains all bodily functions independently, including airway, circulation, and responsiveness to verbal commands and/or stimulation. The sedation level is reached when slurring of speech occurs.

The type of conscious sedation used may sometimes be dictated by the types of phobias experienced by the patient. A patient experiencing injection-needle phobia may need to be induced with O_2 + N_2O prior to IV sedation.

PATIENT SELECTION AND INSTRUCTIONS FOR CONSCIOUS SEDATION

Proper patient selection is very important when deciding on sedation. Sedation may not work for all patients. You must do a thorough history and physical examination on the patient and assess the patient's weight, baseline vital signs, mental status, allergy status, airway status, past history of significant anesthesia and outcome, current medical conditions, current medications (many drugs may interfere with the metabolism of sedatives, resulting in prolonged CNS effects), laboratory tests evaluation and assessment of the patient's vital organ status, drug-drug interactions (DDIs) between the patient's medications and the sedation medications, and the patient's ASA status.

The American Society of Anesthesiology (ASA) Status

The American Society of Anesthesiology (ASA) status establishes the patient's overall cardiopulmonary status (Table 10.1). The ASA status is determined in all patients undergoing surgery using local or general anesthesia. The cardiopulmonary status is determined by assessing the patient's capacity to walk up a flight of stairs or walk two blocks. *Note:* Patients with arthritis may not be able to climb stairs. The ASA status in these patients is established by determining the patient's capacity to walk a block or two.

Sedation and the Medically Compromised Patient (MCP)

When deciding on sedation for a medically compromised patient the dentist must know the total number of medical conditions for which the patient is being treated, the level of control of each disease state and the patient's ASA status. These facts need to be accounted for when assessing the type of conscious sedation that will be safe for the patient (Table 10.2).

Conscious Sedation Contraindications

Conscious sedation is contraindicated in patients with moderate to severe liver or kidney disease; patients with moderate to severe respiratory disease and COPD; patients with acute narrow angle glaucoma; patients with unstable arrhythmias; frail, debilitated, and elderly patients; pregnant patients or nursing mothers; and significantly compromised developmentally disabled patients.

Table 10.1.   The ASA classification

ASA Status	Task Performance Climbing a Flight of Stairs
ASA I	The normal or well-controlled patient reaches the top of the stairs effortlessly.
ASA II	The patient is winded on reaching the top and has to rest to feel comfortable.
ASA III	The patient gets winded and stops frequently while climbing, but does reach the top.
ASA IV	The patient is very winded and unable to climb.

Table 10.2.   Medically compromised patient: Disease-associated ASA status and conscious sedation (CS) guidelines

ASA Status	Disease Status	Comments
ASA I	No known systemic disease	Conscious sedation is OK. No Primary Care Physician (PCP) consult is required.
ASA II	Single mild or well-controlled systemic disease	Same as ASA I, but get laboratory tests to confirm disease control.
ASA III	Multiple or moderately controlled systemic diseases	Get PCP consult. Review patient's lab tests, medications, and DDIs with the conscious sedation medication(s).
ASA IV	Poorly controlled systemic diseases	CS done by anesthesiologist in a hospitalized setting.

Conscious Sedation Patient Instructions

Each patient must be completely evaluated prior to conscious sedation and conscious sedation is not for *all* patients. ASA I and ASA II patients are the lowest-risk populations; ASA III patients need to have a PCP consult to determine whether conscious sedation can be given. The informed consent must be obtained prior to the procedure and the start of conscious sedation. Prior to conscious sedation inform the patient, and the person transporting the patient, about postsedation discharge and give follow-up instructions.

There should be no intake of solid food or full liquids for at least 6–8 hr prior to sedation. No clear liquids should be consumed for at least 3–4 hr prior to the sedation. It is best, however, to have the patient fasting or nil-by-mouth (NPO) for conscious sedation. Patients must be monitored before, during, and after a procedure.

VITAL PARAMETERS AND CONSCIOUS SEDATION

The vital parameters that need to be monitored during conscious sedation are baseline vital signs, oxygen saturation level, heart rate and rhythm, and level of consciousness.

Vital Parameters Timeline Protocol

The timeline protocol for monitoring of vital parameters is as follows:

1. **Monitor and document the vital parameters every 5 min:** during administration of the medication(s), during the sedation period, and during the recovery period.
2. **Monitor the vital parameters every 15 min:** once the parameters return to baseline in the postsedation period or if it has been 30 min since the last medication was given. The endpoint for monitoring is when the patient regains consciousness and achieves presedation status.

Conscious Sedation Recovery Alerts

Take immediate action when there is

1. A ±20% change in the pulse or blood pressure (BP).
2. Change in the cardiac rhythm.

3. Drop in the oxygen saturation by ≥5% below baseline.
4. Dyspnea/apnea/hypoventilation experienced by the patient.
5. Patient experiences sweating.
6. Inability to arouse the patient.
7. A need to maintain the patient's airway mechanically.

Conscious Sedation and the Aldrete Scoring System

The Aldrete scoring system should be used during conscious sedation to determine the patient's ability to follow commands, to maintain respiratory and circulation status, to determine consciousness level, and to determine the patient's ability to maintain color (Table 10.3).

Patient Assessment Alerts

The following are patient assessment alerts:

1. Document the patient's ability to maintain an open airway; this is established by checking the level of consciousness and arousability.
2. Breathing should be assessed through the use of continuous pulse oximetry and by observation of the respiratory rate, depth of respiration, and breathing effort.
3. Maintain an IV line throughout the recovery stage of sedation.
4. You must have ACLS training and resuscitation equipment available and functional at all times (Table 10.4).

Table 10.3. The Aldrete scoring system

Function	Aldrete Scoring System Points
Activity	Voluntary movement of all limbs to command: 2 points Voluntary movement of two extremities to command: 1 point Inability to move: 0 points
Respiration	Patient breathes deeply and coughs: 2 points Dyspnea or Hypoventilation: 1 point Apnea: 0 points
Circulation	BP ±20 mmHg from preanesthesia BP: 2 points BP >20–50 mmHg from preanesthesia BP: 1 point BP >50 mmHg from preanesthesia BP: 0 points
Consciousness	Fully awake: 2 points Arousable patient: 1 point Unresponsive patient: 0 points
Color	Pink: 2 points Pale or Blotchy: 1 point Cyanotic: 0 points
On Discharge	Total score must be 9–10 at end of monitoring. Patient must retain oral fluids on discharge. Patient should be able to void on discharge.

Table 10.4. Emergency resuscitation equipment

Emergency Equipment	Emergency Equipment Specifics
Oxygen	System capable of delivering 100% at 10 L/min, for 30 min
Suction	Powerful suction
Airway Management	All sizes face masks, endotracheal tubes, laryngoscopes, oral and nasal airways
Monitors	Pulse oximeter, cardiac monitor, blood pressure (BP) device
Resuscitative Equipment/ Medications	**Emergency equipment:** Emergency drug card, ACLS protocols, ambu-bag, defibrillator with EKG recording capability
	Emergency drugs: Naloxone (Narcan), Flumazenil (Mazicon), and Epinephrine

COMPLICATIONS OF CONSCIOUS SEDATION

Complications associated with conscious sedation are:

- Respiratory depression and hypoventilation
- Cardiac complications and hypotension
- Inadequate amnesia/analgesia

Respiratory Depression and Hypoventilation

This complication presents as shallow respirations and decreased oxygen saturation. It is treated with oxygen and airway management. Perform the head-tilt–chin-lift. This will often improve ventilation and oxygen saturation. Provide oxygen by nasal cannula throughout the procedure and increase the flow when the oxygen saturation is low. Encourage the patient to take deep breaths.

If the oxygen saturation remains low, use the 100% non-rebreathing face mask. Bag the patient with an ambu-bag if the respiratory status is compromised. Continue to bag the patient until the oxygen saturation improves. Use an artificial airway (nasal or oral), if the patient is unable to maintain an airway. This ensures that the patient is breathing and that there is adequate oxygen saturation. The nasal airway may be more tolerable than an oral airway. To determine the airway size, use the following guidelines:

1. **Nasal airway size:** Measure distance from the tip of patient's nose to the earlobe.
2. **Oral airway size:** Measure distance from the corner of patient's mouth to the earlobe.

Respiratory depression can progress to respiratory arrest. If the patient stops breathing, begin artificial respirations immediately and intubate the patient.

Cardiac Complications and Hypotension

Hypotension is corrected by putting the patient in the "Trendelenburg" (head-down) position. Hypotension is also corrected by giving IV fluids. Aggressive drug treatment will be needed if there is no improvement. Call for *HELP* if there is no improvement. Cardiac arrythmias can potentially occur as a complication of conscious sedation. Cardiac arrythmias must be recognized and treated ASAP. Call the emergency medical system (EMS) if you have not done so. Begin CPR immediately if the patient arrests. Use the Aldrete scoring scale to determine the patient's status.

Inadequate Amnesia/Analgesia

The dose of amnesic or analgesic drugs is based on the patient's weight. As a general rule, the elderly need less of these drugs and muscular young men need more of these drugs. Allow sufficient time for the drugs to work.

CONSCIOUS SEDATION DRUGS CLASSIFICATION AND FACTS

The most common drugs used for conscious sedation are the benzodiazepines, opioid narcotics, and barbiturates (Table 10.5).

Benzodiazepines Classification

- Midazolam (Versed): IV or Oral. The liquid form is most used in children.
- Triazolam (Halcion): The oral form is most used in adults.
- Diazepam (Valium): IV or oral.
- Lorazepam (Ativan): IV or oral.

Triazolam (Halcion), diazepam (Valium), and lorazepam (Ativan) are the most-used bendodiazepines for oral conscious sedation.

Benzodiazepines are contraindicated in the morbidly obese patient, the pregnant patient, the fragile elderly patient, patients receiving treatment for gastroesophageal reflux disease (GERD)/peptic ulcer with H_2 blockers, and patients who are on psychiatric medications for depression or schizophrenia.

Opioid Narcotics Classification

The most common opioids used are

- Morphine, hydromorphone (Dilaudid)
- Fentanyl (Sublimaze)
- Meperidine (Demerol)

Opioids produce the most reliable pain control. Always determine the patient's history of drug use prior to giving opioids. Chemically dependent patients need higher doses of opioids. Doses are adjusted to meet the patient's individual needs.

Avoid opioids in moderate to severe asthma or airway obstructive states. Start low, go slow, and avoid large bolus doses. Dose levels are maintained after desirable levels of analgesia and sedation are achieved. Narcotic opioids provide analgesia, sedation, and elevation of pain threshold.

Barbiturates Classification

The drugs most often used are:

- Pentobarbital (Nembutal)
- Secobarbital (Seconal)

MIDAZOLAM (VERSED)

Midazolam is the more commonly used short-acting drug, compared to diazepam (Valium), due to its water solubility. It is 3–4 times more potent per milligram than

Table 10.5. Dosages: Stress management medications and reversal drugs

Medication	Dosages: Oral (PO), Intramuscular (IM), Intravenous (IV)
BENZODIAZEPINES	
Midazolam (Versed)	Most common route: IV **Initial IV Dose:** 0.5–l.0 mg; initial adult dose should **not** exceed 2.5 mg **Maintenance Dose:** 0.25–1.0 mg **Total IV Dose:** 5.0 mg **IM Dose:** 0.075 mg/kg IM, maximum 30 mg **Single Oral Dose:** 0.25–0.5 mg/kg 30–40 min prior to treatment. Max: 20 mg
Triazolam (Halcion)	**Adult Oral Dose:** 0.25 mg hs (bedtime) the night prior **and** 0.25 mg 1 h before the dental treatment (Rx) **Healthy Older Patient Oral Dose:** 0.125 mg hs and 1 h prior to Rx. Max: 0.25 mg/day
Diazepam (Valium)	**IV Dose:** Initial dose: 2.5–5 mg; Titrate in 1.5 mg increments till desired effect. **Healthy Elderly IV Dose:** 1.25–2.5 mg. Titrate in increments of 1.0 mg **Oral Dose Under Age 50:** 5–10 mg hs; 5–10 mg PO 1 h prior to Rx. Max. dose 10 mg PO **Lean and Petite Patient OR Healthy Person Above Age 50:** 2–5 mg hs; 2–5 mg PO 1 h prior to Rx Max. dose 5 mg or less.
Lorazepam (Ativan)	**Adult Dose:** 1–2 mg PO hs the night prior; 1–2 mg PO 30 mins–1 h prior to Rx
OPIOID NARCOTICS	
IV Morphine	**Dose:** 2–5 mg IV. Give 1–2 mg increments over 30 sec every (q) 5–10 min.
Hydromorphone (Dilaudid)	**IV Dose:** 0.1–0.5 mg increments over 30 sec q5–10 min. Max dose: 1.5 mg **PO Dose:** 2 mg 1 h prior to procedure.
Fentanyl (Sublimaze)	**Adult dose:** IV/IM 75–150 μg, start dose at 1–2 μg/kg if used alone
Meperidine (Demerol)	**IV Dose:** 25–100 mg: Give in 10 mg increments over 30 sec q5–10 min. **IM Dose with IM Hydroxyzine (Vistaril):** 50–75 mg Meperidine + 25 mg Vistaril
BARBITURATES	
Pentobarbital (Nerabetal)	**Oral Dose:** 100–200 mg hs **IM Dose:** 150–200 mg **IV Dose:** 100 mg q 1–3 min. Maximum IV dose: 200–500 mg
Secobarbital (Seconal)	**Oral Dose:** 100 mg hs **IM Dose:** 100–200 mg **IV dose:** 50–250 mg
BENZODIAZEPINES ANTIDOTE	
Flumazenil (Romazicon)	**IV Dose:** 0.1–0.2 mg IV over 15 sec **Follow-up Dose:** 0.2 mg IV Repeat at 1-min intervals till l mg is given.
NARCOTIC ANTIDOTES	
Naloxone (Narcan)	**IV Dose:** 0.1–0.2 mg. Repeat in 3 min with no improvement. Use no more than 0.5 ml over 2 min. Max dose: 0.8 mg.

diazepam. It can be used alone or with a narcotic. Reduce the dose of Versed by a third when combining it with an opioid. It can be given IV, IM, PO, or nasally. The most common route used is IV.

Midazolam is given slowly over 2 or more min. Never give it as a single large bolus dose. Rapid or excessive IV doses can cause respiratory depression or arrest, and the use of this drug requires special training. Active metabolites of midazolam can accumulate in patients with kidney disease, causing prolonged sedation.

Midazolam (Versed) Dose

Initial IV Versed Dose

0.5–1.0 mg. The initial dose should not exceed 2.5 mg in a healthy adult and it should be titrated to the desired effect. Slurring of speech is an excellent indicator of an adequate dose.

Versed Maintenance Dose

0.25–1.0 mg. Once sedation is achieved, additional doses should be 25% of the dose required to produce the sedation end point.

Total IV Versed Dose

Total dose should not exceed 5.0 mg.

Intravenous (IV) Versed Pharmacology Facts

Sedation will occur within 3 to 5 min and the duration of action is 1 to 6 hr. The half-life ranges from 1.2 to 12.3 hr. Patients should not drive on recovery.

Intramuscular (IM) Midazolam (Versed)

Give 0.075 mg/kg Versed IM. The maximum dose should not exceed 30 mg. Onset of action occurs in 15 min and the duration of action is 2–3 hr.

Oral Midazolam (Versed)

Adult Oral Midazolam (Versed) Dose

Give 0.25–0.5 mg/kg Versed as a single dose preprocedure, up to a maximum of 20 mg and administer it 30–45 min prior to the procedure.

Pediatric Oral Midazolam (Versed) Dose

Children under 6 years or patients that are less cooperative may require as much as 1 mg/kg as a single dose. 0.25 mg/kg Versed may be sufficient for children 6–16 years of age.

IV Midazolam (Versed) Adverse Reactions

Adverse reactions from IV midazolam (Versed) are hiccups, nausea, vomiting, oversedation, headache, coughing, and pain at the injection site.

Midazolam (Versed) Lower Dose Alert

Give the lower dose of midazolam (Versed) to: patients over 60 years of age, as long as they are healthy, and patients receiving narcotics. Avoid in patients with acute narrow-angle glaucoma.

Midazolam (Versed) and Diazepam (Valium) Shared Properties

Both these drugs have antianxiety, anticonvulsant, sedation, muscle relaxant, and amnesic properties.

TRIAZOLAM (HALCION)

Triazolam is available as 0.125 mg and 0.25 mg tablets. Onset of action is rapid and occurs in 15–30 min. Halcion has the shortest half-life when compared to Valium or Ativan. It is ideal for sedative hypnotic use. Active metabolites of triazolam can accumulate in patients with kidney disease, causing prolonged sedation.

Halcion and Drug-Drug Interactions

Halcion should not be combined with the following drugs:

- Tegretol, Dilantin: These drugs are CYP3A4 inducers and they decrease Halcion levels.
- Azole antifungals, ciprofloxacin, biaxin, and doxycycline: These drugs are CYP3A4 inhibitors and they increase Halcion levels.

Triazolam (Halcion) Adult Oral Dosage

Give the patient 0.25 mg triazolam hs (bedtime) the previous night and give 0.25 mg, 1 hr before the dental procedure. The half-life of Halcion is 1.5–5.5 hr and the maximum adult dose is: 0.5 mg/day.

Triazolam (Halcion) Healthy Older Patient Oral Dose

Give 0.125 mg hs the previous night and the same dose 1 hr prior to the procedure. The maximum dose for a healthy older adult is 0.25 mg/day.

DIAZEPAM (VALIUM)

Diazepam (Valium) Facts and Pharmacology

Diazepam can also be used alone or with a narcotic. Reduce the dose of diazepam by a third when combining with an opioid. Diazepam can be given IV or PO. Diazepam intramuscular (IM) is very painful and for this reason it is contraindicated. The IV dose can range from 2–20 mg in a healthy adult, but 10 mg or less is usually sufficient.

Initial IV Diazepam Dose

The initial IV dose of diazepam is 2.5–5 mg. Titrate in increments of 1.5 mg for desired effect. Slurring of speech is an excellent indicator of an adequate dose.

Healthy Older Patient IV Diazepam Dose

Dose is 1.25–2.5 mg. Titrate in increments of 1.0 mg. Sedation after IV injection occurs within 3 to 5 min. Peak action is seen in 15–30 min. Duration of action is 15–60 min and the half-life is 32–90 hr. Patients should avoid fine motor or cognition skills posttreatment. Diazepam is irritating to the tissues, so inject through a large vein. Do not dilute Valium or mix it with other medications because it will precipitate. Active metabolites of diazepam can accumulate in patients with kidney disease, causing prolonged sedation.

IV Diazepam (Valium) Adverse Reactions

Adverse reactions that can occur are venous thrombosis, phlebitis, apnea, and hypotension. Avoid diazepam (Valium) in patients with narrow-angle glaucoma.

Oral Diazepam (Valium)

Diazepam is a very effective oral anxiolytic for stress management.

Oral Premedication Diazepam (Valium) Dosage

Diazepam Average Adult Sedation Dose

5–10 mg hs, the night before the appointment and 5–10 mg, 30 min–1 hr prior to the appointment. Use the 2–5 mg dose hs and 1 hr prior to treatment for the lean, petite, or healthy-over-age-50 patients. Use only if the patient can be *escorted* to the dental office. The conscious sedation policy does not apply for premedication doses. Avoid oral sedation with diazepam in the elderly debilitated patient.

Oral Diazepam Use for Anxiety, Sedation, and Skeletal Muscle Relaxation in Adults

Oral diazepam is available in the following strengths: 2 mg, 5 mg or 10 mg tablets.

Oral Diazepam Antianxiety Dose

2–10 mg 2–4 times per day.

Healthy Older Patient Antianxiety Dose

Initial oral dose for anxiety is 1–2 mg, once/twice per day; increase gradually as needed. Do not use >10 mg/day and watch for hypotension and excessive sedation.

Diazepam Contraindications

Avoid diazepam (Valium) in the pregnant patient, the obese patient, the elderly patient, patients taking CNS drugs and patients on H_2 blockers.

LORAZEPAM (ATIVAN)

Reduce dose by one-third when combining lorazepam with an opioid. Dilute 1:1 in compatible solution immediately before administering IV.

IV Lorazepam (Ativan)

0.05 mg/kg to 4 mg is the maximum total dose for IV lorazepam. Onset of action occurs in 5–15 min and duration of action is up to 48 hr. The half-life of lorazepam is 10–20 hr. The long half-life of lorazepam makes midazolam a preferable choice.

Lorazepam (Ativan) Dosages

Oral Lorazepam Adult Dose for Anxiety

1–10 mg/day in 2–3 divided doses; usual dose: 2–6 mg/day in divided doses.

Healthy Older Patient Oral Lorazepam Antianxiety Dose

0.5–4 mg/day; initial dose not to exceed 2.0 mg.

Oral Lorazepam for Insomnia in Adults

2–4 mg at bedtime. Oral lorazepam is available as a 0.5 mg or 1 mg or 2 mg tablet.

Oral Lorazepam Dose for Stress Management

1–2 mg hs the previous night and 1–2 mg 30 min–1 hr prior to the appointment.

Lorazepam Contraindications

Contraindications for lorazepam (Ativan) are the same as those for diazepam (Valium).

MORPHINE

Morphine (IV) Dose

2–5 mg. 1–2 mg increments are given over a 30-sec period every 5–10 min. Onset of action is rapid and peak effect occurs in 20 min. The half-life of morphine is 2–3 hr.

HYDROMORPHONE (DILAUDID)

IV Hydromorphone Dose

1.5 mg. 0.1–0.5 mg increments of hydromorphone are given over a 30-sec period every 5–10 min. Onset of action is rapid and peak effect occurs in 15–30 min. The half-life of hydromorphone is 2–4 hr.

PO (oral) Hydromorphone Dose

2 mg 1 hr prior to procedure.

FENTANYL (SUBLIMAZE)

Fentanyl is a synthetic opioid that provides excellent analgesia. It is indicated for its analgesic action for short procedures. If used alone, start the dosage at 1–2 µg/kg.

Average Adult IV Fentanyl (Sublimaze) Dose

75–150 µg. Use a smaller dose in conjunction with a benzodiazepine. The average patient usually requires 50–100 µg. Fentanyl produces an immediate response. Onset of action occurs in 1–2 min and peak effect occurs in 3–5 min. The half-life of fentanyl is 2–4 hr. Administer doses very slowly over 2–5 min.

Patients should avoid fine motor or cognition skills activity posttreatment. Rapid IV administration of fentanyl can cause difficulty breathing. Breathing difficulty can be reversed with naloxone (Narcan) or it may require a muscle relaxant and intubation.

MEPERIDINE (DEMEROL)

Meperidine IV Dose

25–100 mg. Administer in 10 mg increments over 30 sec every 5–10 min. Inject slowly as meperidine can be painful on injection. Onset of action is immediate and peak effect occurs in 5–7 min. The half-life of meperidine is 3–8 hr. Meperidine metabolites accumulate with kidney disease. Avoid Demerol use in the renal-compromised patient.

Intramuscular (IM) Meperidine (Demerol)

IM meperidine is usually combined with the antihistamine, hydroxyzine (Vitaril).

IM Meperidine + Hydroxyzine Dose

50–75 mg Meperidine IM and 25 mg Vistaril IM. Duration of action: 2–6 hr.

BARBITURATES

Both pentobarbital (Nembutal) and secobarbital (Seconal) are used primarily on the evening before the dental appointment.

Pentobarbital (Nembutal) Dosages
- Pentobarbital adult oral dose: 100–200 mg hs
- Pentobarbital adult IM dose: 150–200 mg
- Pentobarbital adult IV dose: 100 mg q 1–3 min
- Maximum IV dose for pentobarbital: 200–500 mg

Secobarbital (Seconal) Dosages
- Secobarbital adult oral dose: 100 mg hs
- Secobarbital adult IM dose: 100–200 mg
- Secobarbital adult IV dose: 50–250 mg

CONSCIOUS SEDATION OVERDOSE MANAGEMENT AND REVERSAL DRUGS

With excessive sedation with just an opioid, the opioid dose must be decreased. Combination of benzodiazepines and opioids may cause sedation and respiratory depression. Initial doses of both should be decreased when used in combination. With excessive sedation the dose of the benzodiazepine must be decreased before decreasing the dose of the opioid. Benzodiazepines have no analgesic properties so decreasing the dose of benzodiazepines will not affect pain control.

If the opioid dose is decreased first, pain control can be lost. Opioids provide sedation plus analgesia. A desirable level of sedation and pain control can often be achieved in this type of situation by simply decreasing the dose of benzodiazepine while maintaining the opioid dose.

Conscious Sedation Reversal Drugs
- Benzodiazepines overdose antidote: flumazenil (Romazicon)
- Narcotics overdose antidote: naloxone (Narcan).

FLUMAZENIL (ROMAZICON)

Flumazenil (Romazicon) is a benzodiazepine antagonist that competes for receptor sites, consequently reversing the effects of benzodiazepines. Start by giving 0.1–0.2 mg flumazenil IV over 15 sec. If reversal does not occur (the patient does not awake), give 0.2 mg IV and repeat at 1 min intervals until 1 mg is given. The flumazenil effect lasts for 1 hr. It can cause seizures in patients who have overdosed on barbiturates or TCAs.

Flumazenil Seizure Alert

Flumazenil, when used in patients receiving benzodiazepines chronically, are at risk for grand mal seizures. Patients with a history of seizures should receive flumazenil with extreme caution. Seizures have occurred after the reversal of benzodiazepines even with patients not dependent on benzodiazepines. Flumazenil should not be used as a matter of routine in such cases. If needed, it should be administered slowly and the patient should be carefully and continuously monitored.

NALOXONE (NARCAN)

Naloxone is a pure narcotic antagonist. It competes for the receptor sites reversing effect of the narcotic. All opioid effects are reversed in parallel: An injection of Narcan reverses sedation, respiratory depression, and analgesia. This sudden unmasking of pain may result in significant sympathetic and cardiovascular stimulation. This, in turn, can cause hypertension, stroke, tachycardia and arrythmias, pulmonary edema, congestive heart failure, and cardiac arrest.

Naloxone Dose

0.1–0.2 mg IV. Repeat naloxone (Narcan) after 3 min if the respiratory rate is <12/min and/or the level of consciousness is depressed. Give naloxone until the patient is alert, ventilating, and without significant pain or discomfort. Give no more than 0.5 mL over 2 min, up to 0.8 mg maximum.

The effects are seen in 1–2 min and the effects last from 1–4 hr. The half-life of naloxone is 60–90 min. Due to the short half-life, patients can become narcotized after the effects of naloxone have worn off. Patients should be closely monitored to watch for renarcotization.

IV

Hematopoietic System

Complete Blood Count (CBC): Assessment, Analysis, and Dental Management Guidelines

HEMATOPOIETIC SYSTEM OVERVIEW

The hematopoietic stem cell resides predominantly in the bone marrow and very particularly in the pelvis and the long bones. The hematopoietic stem cell differentiates and matures to form the three cell lines found in the blood: the white blood cells (WBCs); red blood cells (RBCs); and platelets (Plts). Discussion in this section centers on disease states associated with these cell lines.

THE COMPLETE BLOOD COUNT (CBC) COMPONENTS

The individual components of the CBC are

- The total white blood cell (WBC) and red blood cell (RBC) count
- Hemoglobin (Hb)
- Hematocrit (Hct)
- Mean corpuscular volume (MCV)
- Mean corpuscular hemoglobin (MCH)
- Mean corpuscular hemoglobin concentration (MCHC)
- Red cell distribution width (RDW)
- Platelet count
- WBC differential

The WBC differential count consists of neutrophils plus bands (immature neutrophils), lymphocytes, monocytes, eosinophils, and basophils.

The total RBC count, Hb, Hct, MCV, MCH, MCHC, and RDW help analyze some of the common RBC-related conditions encountered such as anemia, polycythemia, and hemochromatosis.

The reticulocyte count, which is not part of the CBC, is also evaluated to determine the status of anemia, polycythemia, and hemochromatosis.

The total WBC and the WBC differential counts help analyze infection, inflammation, underlying allergy states, leukemias, lymphomas, etc.

Serial WBC with differential (WBC w/diff.) helps determine the patient's response to treatment.

The platelet (Plt) count helps assess the number of platelets available for primary or platelet-related hemostasis. The Plt count also highlights any platelet-related disorders such as thrombocytopenia (decreased Plt count) or thrombocytosis (increased Plt count).

The bleeding time (BT), which is not a part of the CBC, shows the functioning capacity of the platelets. The function of the platelets is to stick together during primary hemostasis and arrest bleeding when injury occurs.

The Red Blood Cell (RBC)

The RBC count can be normal or decreased depending on the acuteness of the anemia. A decreased RBC count can occur because of decreased RBC production by the bone marrow or due to overdestruction of the RBCs, as with hemolysis. The average life span of the normal RBC is 120 days. The normal RBC count for male patients is 4.5–5.9 million/μL; for female patients it is 4.0–5.2 million/μL.

Hemoglobin (Hb)

All mature RBCs contain hemoglobin (Hb). Hemoglobin in the fetus is hemoglobin F, and following birth it changes to hemoglobin A. Hemoglobin A contains two alpha (α) chains and two beta (β) chains. Anemia is associated with a reduction in the hemoglobin content. A reduction in the hemoglobin content results in tissue hypoxia and poor wound healing. The normal hemoglobin value in males is 13.5–17.5g/dL; in females it is 12.0–16.0g/dL.

Hematocrit (Hct)

Hematocrit is expressed as a percentage and it reflects the red cell mass divided by the total blood volume. The hematocrit can also be estimated by multiplying the hemoglobin by 3. Anemia is associated with a decreased hematocrit. The hematocrit thus helps establish the extent of anemia. The normal hematocrit value is 37–47%.

Mean Corpuscular Volume (MCV)

MCV measures the size/volume of the **mature** RBC. The red cells are said to be *microcytic* when the MCV is below normal and *macrocytic* when the MCV is above normal. Microcytic cells occur when there is a problem with hemoglobin synthesis, affecting either the heme or globin components. Iron deficiency is the leading cause for microcytic cells, followed by thalassemia. Macrocytic cells occur when there are problems associated with DNA synthesis. Common causes for macrocytic cells are pernicious anemia, B_{12} or folic acid deficiency, HIV/AIDS medications, and some cytotoxic drugs. The normal MCV is 80–100 fL/RBC.

Mean Corpuscular Hemoglobin (MCH)

MCH measures the average amount of hemoglobin in each mature RBC. Microcytic anemias are associated with low MCH, and the macrocytic anemias are associated with "increased" MCH. The "increased" MCH in the macrocytic cell is a relative increase caused by an increase in cell size. That the increase is "relative" is further confirmed by the associated presence of a **normal** mean corpuscular hemoglobin concentration (MCHC). The normal MCH is 26–34 pg/RBC.

Mean Corpuscular Hemoglobin Concentration (MCHC)

MCHC measures the hemoglobin concentration in a given volume of packed RBC. The MCHC is labeled as *hypochromic* when the MCHC is decreased, and this hypochromic pattern is associated with the microcytic anemias. The MCHC is listed as *normochromic* when the MCHC is normal and this pattern is associated with the macrocytic anemias. MCHC is calculated as follows: MCHC = Hemoglobin ÷ Hematocrit. The normal MCHC is 31–37 g/dL.

MCV-MCHC Values and Associated RBC Types

The MCV and MCHC patterns on the CBC help categorize the RBC types as the following:

- Microcytic, hypochromic cells
- Macrocytic, normochromic cells
- Normocytic, normochromic cells.

Red Cell Distribution Width (RDW)

RDW measures the anisocytosis (RBCs of unequal size) associated with the RBCs. Increased anisocytosis is associated with an increased RDW. The greater the number of immature RBCs in the circulation, the greater will be the RDW.

Note: The immature RBCs are larger in size when compared to the mature RBCs and the immature RBCs **do not** carry oxygen.

The RDW also helps differentiate between iron deficiency anemia and thalassemia minor. The RDW is **increased** in iron deficiency anemia and **normal** in thalassemia minor. An increased RDW in the presence of a decreased RBC count indicates an **active** bone marrow: This pattern is frequently seen with many of the anemias, indicating that the body is trying to compensate. A decreased RDW along with a decreased RBC count indicates a depressed bone marrow. The normal RDW is 11.5–14.5%.

Reticulocyte Count

The reticulocyte count measures erythropoietic activity and the response of the bone marrow to anemia. Immature nucleated RBCs abound in the circulation when the reticulocyte count is increased. Hemolysis is associated with an increased reticulocyte count. Hemolysis can occur with any of the inherited or hemolytic anemias: sickle-cell anemia, thalassemia, G6PD deficiency anemia, and hereditary spherocytosis.

A decreased reticulocyte count can be associated with anemia of chronic disease, anemia due to renal failure because of decreased erythropoietin production, or anemia associated with bone marrow failure.

WHITE BLOOD CELL (WBC) COUNT AND WBC DIFFERENTIAL FUNCTION

Neutrophils

Neutrophils engulf bacteria and cellular debris.

Lymphocytes

Lymphocytes produce antibodies and regulate the body's immune response.

Monocytes

Monocytes engulf cellular debris and are involved in the processing of antigen.

Eosinophils

Eosinophils are associated with response to allergens and parasites.

Basophils

Basophils are associated with hypersensitivity and release histamine.
   Average WBC Count: $4\text{--}10\,\text{k}/\text{mm}^3$.

White Blood Cell (WBC) Disorders

The following are WBC disorders:

1.   **Leukocytosis (increased WBCs) causes:**
     - Increased production: leukemia, myeloproliferative diseases
     - Reactive leukocytosis: secondary to infection or inflammation
     - Drugs: prednisone-associated leukocytosis
2.   **Leukopenia (decreased WBCs) causes:**
     - Decreased WBC production: secondary to aplastic anemia or exhaustion of the bone marrow due to leukemia
     - Drugs: secondary to drugs causing an allergic reaction or chemotherapy drugs
     - Consumption: due to overwhelming bacterial or viral infections
     - Radiation: secondary to radiation therapy

Leukocytosis and WBC Differential Analysis

The WBC differential is used to follow the course of diseases, infections, or neoplastic conditions. When analyzing the WBC count w/diff, always focus on which specific cell line(s) show change, with respect to the increased WBC count. You also must check whether the CBC shows any "shift" patterns, as discussed next.

Immature WBCs

An acute influx of immature cells in the circulation can be from the following:

1.   The bone marrow's response to severe infection inflammation
2.   Arrest in the development process due to underlying hematologic disease.

   The CBC can show a "shift to the left" or a "shift to the right" when immature cells enter the circulation in abundance.

WBC Shift Patterns

A shift to the left or a myeloid reaction is associated with an influx of immature bands or granulocytes in the circulation; this occurs in response to an acute bacterial infection, such as pneumonia. A shift to the right or a lymphoid reaction is associated with an influx of immature lymphocytes in the circulation; this occurs in response to viral infections.

WBC Differential Patterns and Suggested Dental Guidelines

Listed in the following sections are suggested guidelines for each specific WBC line change along with an increased WBC count.

Common WBC Total and Differential Patterns

Common WBC total and differential patterns encountered are discussed in the following sections (Table 11.1).

Increased WBC Count + Increased Neutrophil Count Pattern

Increased WBC count plus an increased neutrophil count occurs with an acute bacterial infection. The treatment required with this pattern is antibiotics to ward off the infection.

Increased WBC Count + Decreased Neutrophil Count + Increased Lymphocyte Count Pattern

This pattern is associated with viral infections. Treatment required with this pattern is antiviral drugs—*not antibiotics*—to ward off the infection.

Increased WBC Count + Increased Monocyte Count Pattern

This pattern can be seen with chronic bacterial infections or acute exacerbation of chronic inflammation. Examples of chronic bacterial infections are subacute bacterial endocarditis (SBE) or mycobacterium tuberculosum (MTB).

Acute or chronic inflammation can be seen with systemic lupus erythematosus (SLE) or rheumatoid arthritis (RA).Treatment guideline for this pattern: Defer routine dental treatment for 4–6 weeks so the patient can be treated and fully recover from the underlying cause.

Increased WBC Count + Increased Eosinophil Count Pattern

This pattern is often associated with allergies, parasites, or Hodgkin's lymphoma. Treatment required for this pattern involves treating the underlying cause: allergy, parasites, or Hodgkin's lymphoma.

Table 11.1. Summary: Increased WBC count with associated differential patterns

Leukocytosis (Increased WBC Count)

WBC Differential analysis:
- **I:**   ↑ **WBC count and** ↑ **Neutrophils Pattern:** Seen with acute bacterial infection. Treatment: Antibiotics
- **II:**   ↓ **Neutrophils and** ↑ **Lymphocytes Pattern:** Seen with viral infections. Treatment: Antiviral drugs
- **III:**   ↑ **WBC count and** ↑ **Monocytes Pattern:** Seen with chronic bacterial infections: SBE; MTB **OR** with acute exacerbation of inflammation: SLE; RA. Defer routine dental treatment for 4–6 weeks.
- **IV:**   ↑ **WBC count and** ↑ **Eosinophils Pattern:** Seen with allergies; parasites; Hodgkin's lymphoma.
- **V:**   ↑ **WBC count and** ↑ **Basophils Pattern:** Seen with CML; polycythemia.

This patient will benefit with the use of antihistamine diphenhydramine (Benadryl): 25–50 mg qid × 2–3 days, if the history reveals mild to moderate allergy. Always inform the patient that drowsiness will occur with Benadryl.

Nondrowsy antihistamines, fexofenadine (Allegra): 60mg bid (twice/day) or Loratadine (Claritin): 10mg/day, on an empty stomach, can alternatively be prescribed for 2–3 days. The eosinophil count is increased during the active stage of Hodgkin's lymphoma. Routine dental treatment should be deferred during the acute stage. You must, however, provide supportive care for any associated xerostomia or mucositis that may develop as a consequence of the medical management.

Increased WBC Count + Increased Basophils Pattern

This pattern is usually seen with chronic mylocytic leukemia (CML) or polycythemia. The treatment for this pattern relies on determining the underlying causes, which need immediate medical attention before dentistry is planned for the patient.

LEUKOPENIA AND ABSOLUTE NEUTROPHIL COUNT (ANC)

When a patient presents with leukopenia or a decreased WBC count it is extremely important that you calculate the absolute neutrophil count (ANC) *before* you proceed with dentistry (Table 11.2). The ANC count helps assess the gravity of the leukopenia.

Table 11.2.   Summary absolute neutrophil count (ANC)

Neutropenia Type	Suggested Dental Management Guidelines
Mild Neutropenia: 1,000–1,500 Neutrophils/mm^3	Have patient use nonalcoholic mouth rinse prior to dentistry. Mild risk of infection exists. Patient can have major or minor dentistry. Premedicate for **major surgery only** with cidal or static **oral** antibiotics **plus** give cidal or static antibiotics for 3 or 5 days, **post major surgery only.**
Moderate Neutropenia: 500–1,000 Neutrophils/mm^3	Have patient use nonalcoholic mouth rinse prior to dentistry. Moderate risk of infection exists. Patient can have major or minor dentistry. Premedicate for major **and** minor dentistry using cidal or static antibiotics. Give cidal or static oral antibiotics for 3 or 5 days, post major surgery.
Severe Neutropenia: 0–500 Neutrophils/mm^3	Risk of life-threatening infection. Patient is isolated and hospitalized. Masking of oral infection symptoms and signs exists. Only palliative care is given. **Prior to Palliative Dentistry:** Determine whether a WBC transfusion (Neupogen) is needed. Use only systemic cidal antibiotics. Premedicate with systemic antibiotics as per AHA guidelines. Use a nonalcoholic mouth rinse. **Postpalliative Dental Treatment:** Use systemic antibiotics for 5, 7, or 10 days, postpalliative care. Provide systemic pain medication. Maintain nutritional support for adequate T cell function.

ANC Calculation Formula

The ANC is calculated as follows: ANC = Total WBC count × (% neutrophils + % bands). *Bands* indicate the percentage of immature neutrophils.

The normal ANC count equals 1,500–7,200 cells/mm³. As long as the ANC is above 1,500/mm³ the patient has a good capacity to fight acute bacterial infections. The risk for infection increases when the ANC drops below 1,500/mm³.

Decreased Absolute Neutrophil Count (ANC) Classification

To best analyze the risk for infection and leukopenia severity, it is suggested you divide the **low** ANC counts into three categories:

1. **0–500 neutrophils/mm³:** This range identifies severe neutropenia. An increased risk for life-threatening infections exists with this range.
2. **500–1,000 neutrophils/mm³:** This range identifies moderate neutropenia. Moderate risk of infection exists with this range.
3. **1,000–1,500 neutrophils/mm³:** This range identifies mild neutropenia: Mild risk of infection exists with this range.

Severe Neutropenia and Infection Associated Symptoms and Signs (S/S)

Fever is usually the only symptom present. Minimal or no pus formation occurs and consequently there is no fluctuation and/or exudates associated with any abscess formation in the oral cavity. Pain and erythema may be the *only* signs of infection.

Severe Neutropenia (0–500 Neutrophils/mm³) Management Protocol

The patient is always hospitalized because of the increased risk of infection. Prior to the initiation of palliative dentistry, determine whether a white blood cell transfusion (Neupogen) is needed to improve survival. Provide only palliative treatment (incision and drainage of an abscess, pain medications, antibiotics) for acute dental problems. The patient is handled with frequent hand washings and strict infection control procedures. Use a nonalcoholic mouth rinse prior to attending to the oral cavity. Provide *premedication* prophylaxis with *systemic bactericidal* antibiotics (IV/IM) as per AHA guidelines, 30 min prior to the handling of the oral tissues. Additionally, use systemic antibiotics for 5, 7, or 10 days following palliative dentistry. The duration for which antibiotics are given will depend on the extent of the underlying infection. Provide systemic pain medication and maintain nutritional support for adequate T cell function.

Mild (1,000–1,500 Neutrophils/mm³) or Moderate (500–1,000 Neutrophils/mm³) Neutropenia Management Protocol

These patients can have major or minor dentistry. *Oral, cidal, or static* antibiotics can be prescribed. The moderately neutropenic patient (500–1,000 neutrophils/mm³) gets *premedication prophylaxis* as per AHA guidelines *for all types of dental procedures.* The mildly neutropenic patient (1,000–1,500 neutrophils/mm³) gets *premedication prophylaxis for major procedures only.* Additionally, prescribe antibiotics for 3–5 days in the mild and moderate neutropenic patient *following major dental procedures.* Always have the patient use a nonalcoholic mouth rinse *prior to all* dental visits in the presence of mild or moderate neutropenia.

Red Blood Cells (RBCs) Associated Disorder: Anemia: Assessment, Analysis, and Associated Dental Management Guidelines

ANEMIA FACTS AND CLASSIFICATION

Anemia is a clinical condition associated with a reduction of the red blood cells and/or the hemoglobin in the blood. Hemoglobin consists of two protein molecules, heme and globin. Oxygen binds to heme, thus enabling hemoglobin to transport oxygen to the tissues. Anemia is associated with a reduction in the oxygen-carrying capacity of the blood, resulting in tissue hypoxia. This lack of tissue oxygenation accounts for the poor wound healing in anemic patients. Anemia can occur when the red blood cell (RBC) production is affected. It can also occur with excessive RBC destruction associated with the hemolytic anemias and excessive RBC loss associated with acute or chronic bleeding. A thorough medical history and physical examination will help assess the type and severity of anemia. The patient's dietary history, over-the-counter (OTC) and prescribed medications history, ethnicity, and family history will provide additional clues.

The complete blood count (CBC) is the basic test used to evaluate anemia. The CBC analyzes various characteristics of the RBCs along with the white blood cell (WBC) count, WBC differential count, and platelet count.

ANEMIA CLASSIFICATION BY ETIOLOGICAL FACTORS

Congenital/Hereditary/Hemolytic Anemia

Sickle-Cell Anemia

Sickle-cell anemia is associated with sickle-shaped RBCs.

Thalassemia Major/Minor

Major or minor thalassemia is associated with microcytic hypochromic RBCs.

Glucose-6-Phosphate Dehydrogenase (G6PD)–Deficiency Anemia

The MCV and MCHC are normal, and the reticulocyte count is increased.

Hereditary Spherocytosis

Hereditary spherocytosis is associated with large spherical RBCs. The MCV and MCHC are normal, and the reticulocyte count is increased.

Nutritional Anemia

Iron (Fe) Deficiency

Iron deficiency anemia is associated with a hypochromic, microcytic RBC pattern.

Folic Acid Deficiency

Folic acid deficiency anemia is associated with a macrocytic, normochromic pattern.

Vitamin B_{12} Deficiency

Vitamin B_{12} deficiency anemia is also associated with a macrocytic, normochromic RBC pattern.

Celiac or Crohn's Disease

Celiac or Crohn's disease is associated with nutritional malabsorption of iron, folic acid, or vitamin B_{12} resulting in iron, folic acid, or vitamin B_{12} anemias.

Acquired Iron Deficiency Anemia

Acquired iron deficiency anemia is due to chronic use of aspirin, NSAIDs, or cortico-steroids. Chronic use of these drugs can cause gastric mucosal irritation, ulceration, and bleeding. A microcytic, hypochromic RBC pattern is seen on the CBC.

Anemia of Chronic Disease/Malignancy-Related/Early Iron Deficiency/Acute Blood Loss/Chronic Renal Failure (CRF)–Associated Anemia

Normochromic, normocytic RBC pattern is seen on the CBC with all the causes listed. The reticulocyte count is decreased. Chronic renal failure (CRF) is associated with low levels of the erythropoietin hormone. Erythropoietin formed in the kidneys, is needed for RBC production.

Bone Marrow (BM) Infiltration–Associated Anemia

Cancer cell infiltration of the BM can cause a reduction in any or all of the cell lines: white blood cells (WBC), red blood cells (RBC), and/or platelets. When all cell lines are decreased the patient is said to have **pancytopenia**, a status of significant concern in the medical and dental setting. During pancytopenia, the low WBC count can increase the patient's susceptibility to infection. The low RBC count can cause tissue hypoxia and poor wound healing. The low platelet count can be associated with an immediate type of bleeding and excessive oozing at the time of surgery if the platelet count is significantly decreased.

CONGENITAL/HEREDITARY ANEMIA

Overview

The congenital types of anemias are associated with alteration in the alpha (α) or beta (β) chains of hemoglobin or both. The congenital types of anemias occur commonly in the African-American, Middle Eastern, and Mediterranean populations. The anemias appear early on in life. There is often a history of "crisis bouts" starting from childhood that occur through the years. As and when the patient gets exposed to factors that trigger hemolysis, the symptoms and signs of the crisis bouts occur. The patient experiences fever, pain in the long bones, malaise, and worsening of the anemia. Vascular infarction in the long bones causes the bone pains. This classic presentation pattern is most commonly seen with sickle-cell anemia. The spleen is a common site for sequestration of the abnormal red blood cells. With time, this causes the spleen to increase in size. The enlarged spleen causes pain in the upper-left abdominal quadrant, and this is often the reason for removal of the spleen in severe cases.

Complications Associated with Frequent Hemolysis

Frequent hemolysis increases the incidence of gallstones. Increased RBC breakdown can also increase the serum bilirubin level and the patient can appear jaundiced. Frequent crisis bouts can also cause renal damage. Always **check the serum creatinine** level prior to dentistry in the hemolytic anemia patients. The hemolytic anemia patient is treated with repeat blood transfusions and, in rare circumstances, by bone marrow transplant.

SICKLE-CELL ANEMIA

Sickle-cell patients have a variant of hemoglobin A called *hemoglobin S*. The S denotes *sickle*. Hemoglobin S and hemoglobin C are abnormal types of hemoglobin. Sickle-cell disease can present as sickle-cell anemia (SS) or sickle-hemoglobin C disease (SC). Sickle-hemoglobin C disease (SC) is the milder form.

Red blood cells that contain mostly **hemoglobin S** have a very short life span of about **20 days**. The abnormal hemoglobin causes the red blood cells to become sickle-shaped, and the sickling is exacerbated during the crisis bouts. Sickle cells have difficulty flowing through small blood vessels, thus causing obstruction to the flow of blood and this causes damage of the tissues beyond the obstruction. Patients with sickle-cell anemia are more prone to bacterial infections.

Sickle-Cell Anemia Major Manifestations

The major manifestations specific to sickle-cell anemia are:

- **Frequently recurring bone pain:** Opioid analgesics are the treatment of choice. Opioid analgesics must be used immediately and aggressively during dentistry.
- **Avascular necrosis of the bones:** Avascular necrosis of the bones especially involves the hips and shoulder. Joint prosthesis history is not uncommon, but, when present, premedication for the joint prosthesis prior to dentistry will be needed.
- **Sickle-cell anemia and kidney disease:** Always assess the serum creatinine level prior to dentistry in the sickle-cell anemia patient. When the serum creatinine is elevated, modify the use of anesthetics, analgesics, and antibiotics as outlined for the compromised kidney in Chapter 22, Hypertension and Target Organ Disease States: Assessment, Analysis, and Associated Dental Management Guidelines.
- **Congestive heart failure (CHF):** CHF can occur in the presence of severe anemia.
- **Retinopathy:** Retinopathy can occur due to intraocular bleeding or retinal detachment.

Sickle-Cell Anemia Medical Management

Medical management is provided with the following:

1. **Hydroxyurea (Droxia/Hydrea)** Hydroxyurea is often used in adult patients to decrease the frequency of severe pain and the need for blood transfusions. This drug results in the formation of a different kind of hemoglobin that then prevents sickling of the RBCs.
2. **Folic acid:** Folic acid helps generate new red blood cell formation.

Sickle-Cell Trait

The patient with sickle-cell trait has hemoglobin A and S, and hemoglobin A is always more prevalent than hemoglobin S. The patient with sickle-cell trait does not have the disease and goes on to live a healthy life. The patient, however, does pass the gene on to the children.

THALASSEMIA/COOLEY'S ANEMIA

Thalassemia is an inherited blood disorder wherein the chains of the hemoglobin molecule are decreased. Mutation can occur in the alpha or beta chain. A patient can thus have alpha or beta thalassemia. Alpha thalassemia is the milder form and beta thalassemia is the severe form of the disease.

Thalassemia Minor

The amount of beta globin in the cell is reduced by half.

Thalassemia Major

No beta globin protein is produced in the cell.

RBC Pattern

Thalassemia patients have hypochromic, microcytic RBC pattern on the CBC.

GLUCOSE-6-PHOSPHATE DEHYDROGENASE (G6PD) DEFICIENCY ANEMIA

G6PD anemia is an inherited condition associated with a reduction or absence of the enzyme G6PD in the red blood cells. The G6PD patient becomes symptomatic when the red blood cells are exposed to oxidant drugs, severe stress, or infections, causing immediate hemolysis. The G6PD patients cannot protect their RBCs against buildup of oxygen chemicals, and this causes RBC destruction and consequent anemia.

Oxidant Drugs and Associated Hemolysis

Oxidant drugs associated with hemolysis in the dental setting are acetaminophen (Tylenol), acetyl salicylic acid (ASA), Anacin, APC tablets, aspirin, celecoxib (Celebrex), Exedrin, NSAIDS, phenacetin, propoxyphene (Darvon), sulfa antimicrobial drugs, sulfite, and metabisulfite in the local anesthetics.

Oxidant Drugs Contraindicated in the Medical Setting

Drugs contraindicated with G6PD anemia are nitrofurantoin (Macrobid/Macrodantin), quinidine (Quinaglute/Dura-Tabs), quinine, and antimalarials.

Avoid all sulpha drugs in patients with G6PD deficiency. Be attentive and vigilant when assessing the patient's medical history about certain facts revealed by the patient. G6PD patients could indicate in the medical history that they are "unable to tolerate" trimethoprim-sulphamethoxazole (Bactrim).

Bactrim is not an effective antibiotic for oral infections. It is used to treat respiratory and urinary tract infections.

These patients will also tell you that they are not able to eat fava beans. Fava beans are oxidative in action and are a staple dietary item among Middle Eastern and Mediterranean descent populations.

G6PD CBC Pattern

The MCV and MCHC are normal, and the reticulocyte count is increased.

HEREDITARY SPHEROCYTOSIS

This type of anemia is associated with a congenital defect of the RBC membrane. Abnormal permeation of sodium causes the RBCs to be thickened, spherical, and fragile.

Hereditary Spherocytosis RBC Pattern

The MCV and MCHC are normal, and the reticulocyte count is increased.

IRON (Fe) DEFICIENCY ANEMIA

Iron deficiency anemia is the most common type of anemia seen the world over. Acute or chronic blood loss is the leading cause of iron deficiency anemia and women are more prone to this type of anemia.

A history of menorrhagia (heavy menstrual cycles); metrorrhagia (frequent menstrual cycles); gastrointestinal bleeding; hemorrhoids; or chronic intake of aspirin, NSAIDS, or corticosteroids should always be explored during patient assessment.

A positive stool **Guiac** test will identify the presence of microscopic gastrointestinal bleeding.

Iron deficiency can also trigger **pica**. Pica is an abnormal craving of nonfood items such as dirt, chalk, ice, etc. The thinking is that once the low iron level is corrected, it can reverse the pica. Pica is often seen in children with poor dietary intake of iron and in pregnant patients suffering from iron deficiency.

Iron deficiency causes significant cold intolerance and this presents as tingling and numbness of the extremities. Iron deficiency is the leading cause of cracking at the corners of the mouth or angular cheilitis.

Iron Deficiency Anemia Treatment

Treatment is as follows:

1. **Eliminate the etiological factors. Correct the low serum ferritin level.** The serum ferritin level indicates the patient's total iron stores and the serum ferritin level is decreased in iron deficiency anemia.
2. **Daily iron replacement in the form of ferrous sulfate pills.** Ferrous sulfate is easily absorbed from the upper gut. The pills should be taken with food, to decrease abdominal cramping. The ferrous sulfate pills can also cause green or black tarry discoloration of the stool.

Avoid the use of **macrolide antibiotics** erythromycin (no longer used in the dental setting), azithromycin, and clarithromycin in patients with iron deficiency anemia as these drugs can also cause abdominal cramping.

B$_{12}$ DEFICIENCY ANEMIA

Macrocytic or megaloblastic pattern on the CBC is caused by pernicious anemia, B$_{12}$ or folic acid deficiency, HIV/AIDS medications, and some cytotoxic drugs affecting DNA synthesis. B$_{12}$ deficiency anemia is common in older women, ages 55–60. The initial complaint often is **burning** of the tongue. The patient may be labeled as being psychosomatic, because no other symptoms or signs may be present on intraoral examination as a cause for the burning. As the condition progresses, there is depapillation of the tongue, microglossia, beefy red tongue, angular cheilitis, and circumoral and peripheral tingling numbness. All symptoms and signs mentioned above with the **exception** of the **neurological symptoms** also occur with folic acid deficiency anemia. The neurological symptoms are specific for B$_{12}$ deficiency only.

PERNICIOUS ANEMIA

Pernicious anemia is associated with an autoimmune destruction of the parietal cells in the stomach. The parietal cells produce the intrinsic factor, which is needed for B$_{12}$ absorption. Pernicious anemia is therefore associated with a poor absorption of vitamin B$_{12}$. The following are other conditions associated with low levels of vitamin B$_{12}$ due to low levels of intrinsic factor:

1. Partial gasterectomy (partial removal of stomach)
2. Inadequate absorption due to bowel disease
3. Bacterial overgrowth in the intestine
4. Pancreatic insufficiency or certain medications

The Schilling's Test

The Shilling's test is performed to evaluate vitamin B$_{12}$ absorption, and it is most commonly used to evaluate patients having pernicious anemia.

Vitamin B$_{12}$ deficiency due to any cause is treated with vitamin B$_{12}$ injections in the gluteus muscle, once or twice per month.

FOLIC ACID DEFICIENCY ANEMIA

Folic acid deficiency anemia has the same symptoms and signs as B$_{12}$ deficiency with the exception of the neurological symptoms, as noted earlier. Folic acid deficiency anemia occurs at any age.

Folic Acid Deficiency Anemia Etiological Factors

Leading etiological factors for folic acid deficiency are chronic alcoholism, phenytoin sodium (Dilantin) intake for grand mal epilepsy, cytotoxic/cancer drugs, or HIV/AIDS medications. Diagnosis is confirmed by evaluating the serum folic acid level.

Folic Acid Deficiency Anemia Treatment

Treatment consists of daily oral intake of folic acid tablets.

DIAGNOSTIC CRITERIA FOR ALL TYPES OF ANEMIAS

It is evident from all the previous discussions that the diagnosis of anemia is best achieved by assessing the medical history, physical examination, and the laboratory tests.

Anemia Symptoms and Signs

The general symptoms associated with anemia can be categorized according to the severity of the anemia.

Symptoms of Mild Anemia

Tiredness, weakness, and fatigue along with shortness of breath **on exertion**. Additionally, the patient experiences general malaise, loss of appetite, palpitations, and chest pain.

Symptoms of Moderate to Severe Anemia

The intensity of the symptoms listed above worsens. The patient experiences the symptoms not only on exertion, but also at rest. History-taking will demonstrate that a patient, who was active in the past, now has decreased level of activity that is well spaced out on purpose. This is a lifestyle modification to minimize the anemia symptoms.

Symptoms of Severe Anemia

Significant worsening of the symptoms and signs described in the previous sections occur, leading to cardiac failure. Thus, hospitalization becomes inevitable as the patient experiences the symptoms and signs associated with congestive heart failure (CHF).

Anemia Signs

The following are signs associated with anemia:

1. **Pallor** of the conjunctiva, oral mucosa, and nail beds. Severe cases will also show pallor of the palmar creases.
2. **Nail changes:** Chronic anemia will show brittle nails and clubbing or convexity of the nails. Koilonychia or spooning or concavity of the nails can occur with chronic iron deficiency anemia.
3. **Tachycardia:** The body tries to compensate for the anemia by increasing the cardiac output and consequently the heart rate.
4. **Severe anemia-associated congestive heart failure (CHF) signs.**
5. **Functional systolic murmur:** Severe anemia is associated with a hyperdynamic circulation and gushing of blood through the pulmonic valve causing a functional systolic murmur. This murmur does not need to be premedicated prior to dentistry.

ANEMIA LABORATORY DIAGNOSIS AND TREATMENTS

The complete blood count, as discussed, is the gold standard test used to assess anemia.

Anemia Patterns

Look for the following specific patterns:

- ↓ **Hemoglobin (Hb)**, ↓ **hematocrit (Hct)**, ↓ **mean corpuscular volume (MCV)**, ↓ **mean corpuscular hemoglobin concentration (MCHC):** associated with iron deficiency anemia and thalassemia.
- ↓ **Hemoglobin (Hb)**, ↓ **hematocrit (Hct)**, ↑ **MCV, normal MCHC:** associated with folic acid/B_{12} deficiency, pernicious anemia, HIV/AIDS medications, and some cytotoxic drugs that affect DNA synthesis.
- ↓ **Hemoglobin (Hb)**, ↓ **hematocrit (Hct), normal MCV, normal MCHC:** associated with anemia of chronic disease, malignancy-related anemia, early iron deficiency anemia, acute blood loss, or chronic renal failure (CRF)–associated anemia.

Anemia Treatments

Treatment is as follows:

1. **Eliminate the cause:** Eliminate the underlying cause.
2. **Provide replacement therapy:** Iron/folate/B_{12}
3. **Blood transfusion:** Do this especially in the presence of acute hemolysis.
4. **Erythropoietin (Epogen):** Epogen is used to treat anemia of chronic disease or chronic renal failure (CRF)–associated anemia.
5. **Corticosteroids:** In the very occasional type of antibody-associated RBC destruction anemia, corticosteroids prove helpful.

SUGGESTED ANESTHETIC, ANALGESIC, ANTIBIOTIC, AND STRESS MANAGEMENT PROTOCOLS FOR ALL ANEMIAS

During dental management of the anemic patient, it is suggested you note the percentage drop in the patient's hemoglobin level and mentally categorize the anemia as mild, moderate, or severe. This helps with the decision of whether or not to treat the patient and what local anesthetics to use. Use the guidelines in the following sections.

Mild Anemia: Hemoglobin Drop up to 25% from Normal

The normal hemoglobin is 13.5–17.5 g/dL in males and 12–16 g/dL in females. A reduction up to 25% would be 10.12–13.13 g/dL in males and 9–12 g/dL in females. 2% lidocaine (Xylocaine) with 1:100,000 epinephrine; 0.5% bupivacaine marcaine or 2% mepivacaine (Carbocaine) with 1:20,000 levonordefrin (NeoCobefrin), maximum 2 carpules, can be used. Vasoconstriction with epinephrine will minimize bleeding, but it will not cause any worsening of anemia symptoms. **Avoid** epinephrine containing LAs with G6PD deficiency anemia.

Moderate Anemia: Hemoglobin Drop of 25–50% from Normal

At this level of anemia use local anesthetics without epinephrine because the palpitations and other associated cardiac symptoms can worsen. It is suggested you use only 3% mepivacaine HCL (Carbocaine). Do not use 4% prilocaine (Citanest Plain) or 4% septocaine (Articaine) because these local anesthetics can precipitate methemoglobinemia in the presence of hypoxia.

Note: In addition to anemia, 4% prilocaine HCL with 1:200,000 epinephrine (Citanest Forte) or 4% prilocaine HCL (Citanest Plain) and 4% septocaine (Articaine) also should not be used in all other conditions causing moderate to severe hypoxia. This is advised to prevent methemoglobinemia from occurring. Other conditions associated with hypoxia are chronic cardiac or respiratory disease, cyanotic congenital cardiac defects, chronic renal failure (CRF) due to a lack of erythropoietin, and COPD. These conditions can all cause moderate to severe hypoxia. Methemoglobinemia is a clinical condition in which greater than the normal 1% level of methemoglobin is present in the circulation. Methemoglobin is an oxidative product of hemoglobin. Cyanosis without respiratory distress occurs when the methemoglobin level reaches 10–20%. Methemoglobin level above 20% is lethal.

Avoid epinephrine containing LAs with G6PD deficiency anemia.

Severe Anemia: Hemoglobin Drop of More than 50% from Normal

Routine dental treatment must be deferred in the presence of severe anemia.

Suggested Local Anesthetic for G6PD Anemia

The only local anesthetic that can be used in a patient with G6PD anemia is 3% mepivacaine HCL (Carbocaine) without epinephrine.

Epinephrine-containing local anesthetics contain bisulfites as preservatives. Bisulfites are oxidant drugs and can cause hemolysis in the G6PD patient.

Suggested Analgesic Protocol for All Anemias Except G6PD Anemia

Aspirin and nonsteroidal antiinflammatory drugs (NSAIDS) should not be used in any anemic patient because these drugs promote gastrointestinal bleeding; cause platelet dysfunction; and, being acidic, promote acidosis.

Acetaminophen (Tylenol) or codeine with acetaminophen (Tylenol #1–4), hydrocodone with acetaminophen (Vicodin), or oxycodone with acetaminophen (Percocet) are safe. Avoid aspirin/NSAIDS because these drugs promote bleeding. Immediate and aggressive pain management in the patient with hemolytic anemia will prevent the occurrence of crisis bouts and consequent hemolysis.

Suggested Analgesic Protocol for G6PD Anemia

Do not use acetaminophen (Tylenol) in patients with G6PD anemia because acetaminophen is an oxidant drug.

If a narcotic analgesic is needed in the G6PD patient, prescribe codeine phosphate (not sulphate) without acetaminophen (Tylenol) or prescribe meperidine (Demerol).

Codeine Phosphate is available as a 30 mg tablet. The dose for codeine phosphate is 15–60 mg/dose q4–6 h, for 2–3 days and the maximum dose per day is 360 mg.

Meperidine (Demerol) is available as a 50 mg tablet and the dose is 50 mg qid for 2–3 days. It is advisable to give pain medications for 2–3 days only to prevent overuse or addiction. If the pain still persists beyond 2–3 days, it is best to have the patient come in so that you can evaluate the cause of the persistent pain.

Suggested Antibiotics Protocol for All Anemias

The following antibiotics are safe to use in the anemic patient: penicillins, cephalosporins, macrolides (avoid with iron deficiency anemia, as discussed previously), clindamycin or doxycycline.

Hypoxia, infection, and acidosis promote crisis bouts in the hemolytic anemia patients. Use antibiotics judiciously and aggressively in these patients to prevent infections, promote healing, or treat infections.

Complete Blood Count with WBC Differential and Platelets

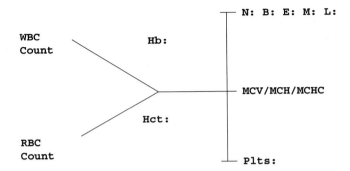

Complete Blood Count Key:
WBC: White Blood Cell; **RBC:** Red Blood Cell; **Hb:** Hemoglobin;
Hct: Hematocrit; **N:** Neutrophils; **B:** Basophils; **E:**
Eosinophils; **M:** Monocytes; **L:** Lymphocytes; **MCV:** Mean
Corpuscular Volume; **MCH:** Mean Corpuscular Hemoglobin; **MCHC:**
Mean Corpuscular Hemoglobin Concentration; **Plts:** Platelets

Figure 12.1. Standardized complete blood count lattice recording.

Anemia and Stress Management

As stated above, hypoxia promotes crisis bouts in the hemolytic anemia patients. These patients benefit when given stress management with O_2 + N_2O. Stress management also decreases stress, which by itself can trigger hemolysis. Provide stress management for all anemic patients using O_2 + N_2O. Do not prescribe the benzodiazepines, diazepam (Valium), or lorazepam (Ativan). Both these drugs depress the respiratory center and worsen the hypoxia.

The CBC recording in medical records is usually indicated as a "lattice" pattern recording in case notes and is often passed on as such when the CBC is requested by the dentist. The lattice pattern is shown in Figure 12.1.

Red Blood Cells Associated Disorder: Polycythemia: Assessment, Analysis, and Associated Dental Management Guidelines

Polycythemia can present as primary or secondary polycythemia. Polycythemia vera is primary polycythemia. It is a myeloproliferative disorder associated with an increased number of circulating RBCs. The white blood cell (WBC) and platelet counts are also increased. The erythropoietin level is low.

Chronic hypoxia causes secondary polycythemia. Chronic obstructive pulmonary disease (COPD), smoking, erythropoietin-producing tumors, and other long-standing heart or lung problems can cause chronic hypoxia (low oxygen level).

The leading physiological cause for erythrocytosis (increased RBC count) or secondary polycythemia is high altitude. The erythropoietin production is always increased in secondary polycythemia.

Polycythemia is mainly a disease of the elderly. Males are affected more than females. An excessive number of RBCs in the circulation causes sluggishness in blood flow, and this increases the incidence of strokes, myocardial infarctions, and deep vein thrombosis (DVTs).

These patients also experience gout and excessive gastrointestinal bleeds. It is not uncommon for these patients to have gout due to the excessive breakdown of RBCs. Increased RBC breakdown increases the serum uric acid level and this in turn precipitates gout. Gout can compromise the kidney status. Always check the CBC and serum creatinine prior to dentistry.

POLYCYTHEMIA SYMPTOMS AND SIGNS

This condition is often asymptomatic initially. When symptoms occur, these patients often experience excessive itching of the skin on exposure to warm water and severe burning of the hands and feet. The patient has a flushed appearance. Physical examination reveals conjunctival engorgement and hepatosplenomegaly.

ABNORMAL LABORATORY VALUES ASSOCIATED WITH POLYCYTHEMIA

The following are abnormal lab values:

1. **Red blood cells (RBCs):** The RBC count is usually elevated to 8–12 million/μL in polycythemia vera. In secondary polycythemia, the RBC count is 6–8 million/μL.

2. **Hemoglobin (Hb):** The hemoglobin is usually increased to 18–24 g/dL.
3. **Hematocrit (Hct):** The Hct is usually increased to 55–60% or 70–80%, depending on the type of polycythemia.
4. **MCV and MCH:** The MCV and MCH are normal or decreased.
5. **Platelets:** The platelets are increased to over $400,000/mm^3$ but they are often dysfunctional.
6. **White blood cell (WBC) count:** The WBC count is elevated to over 12,000 cells/mm^3, and this occurs is in the **absence** of fever.

TREATMENT OF POLYCYTHEMIA

Polycythemia treatment is outlined in the following:

1. Eliminate the precipitating factors
2. Symptomatically treat itching, burning of hands and feet, DVTs, stroke, etc.
3. Give low-dose aspirin to prevent thrombosis.
4. Set up regular phlebotomy, which is the treatment of choice, to decrease the blood volume.

SUGGESTED DENTAL CONSIDERATIONS WITH POLYCYTHEMIA

The following are dental alerts and guidelines for polycythemia:

1. Evaluate the CBC. The patient may need local hemostasis due to poor platelet function.
2. Determine the dose of aspirin or other blood thinners. Always check with the patient's M.D. before you stop the aspirin. In some cases the M.D. may not allow aspirin to be stopped because of the increased threat of thrombosis. In such situations you will use local hemostatic materials. When clearance is obtained for aspirin stoppage, it will need to be stopped 7 days prior to major surgery.
3. Evaluate the status of the affected organ systems: brain, kidney, heart, and deep veins. Assessment of the organ systems will dictate the deviations in the use of stress management, anesthetics, analgesics, and antibiotics in the dental setting.
4. Please review the appropriate sections to determine a final treatment plan for your patient with regard to the use of stress management, anesthetics, analgesics, and antibiotics.

Red Blood Cells Associated Disorder: Hemochromatosis: Assessment, Analysis, and Associated Dental Management Guidelines

Hemochromatosis is a disease state associated with an increased uptake of dietary iron in the presence of excessive iron in the body stores. This causes increased iron deposition in specific tissues (**hemosiderosis**) and organs, particularly the skin, lungs, liver, pancreas, kidney, and heart. Irreversible multiple organ damage ultimately occurs. Lungs and kidneys are particularly affected. Severe pulmonary hemorrhage can deplete the iron levels and cause iron deficiency anemia.

Genetic predisposition is the leading cause of hemochromatosis.

It is common in men age 40 and older and in postmenopausal women.

HEMOCHROMATOSIS SYMPTOMS AND SIGNS

Dark bronze pigmentation of the skin, malaise, abdominal pain, and arthritis are common symptoms. Diabetes type 2, cirrhosis, cardiac arrythmias, cardiomyopathy, congestive heart failure (CHF), Adrenal cortical dysfunction, Pituitary failure, and atrophy of the gonads are common findings associated with hemochromatosis.

HEMOCHROMATOSIS DIAGNOSIS

The following blood tests will establish the diagnosis of hemochromatosis:

1. **Serum iron level:** The serum iron level is markedly increased beyond 200µg/dL.
2. **Complete blood count (CBC):** CBC can indicate the presence of iron deficiency anemia.
3. **Serum ferritin level:** The serum ferritin level is markedly increased. Serum ferritin indicates the total iron stored by the body.
4. **Transferrin level:** The transferrin level is decreased.
5. **Transferrin saturation:** The transferrin saturation is increased beyond 70%. The transferrin saturation indicates the ratio of the serum iron and total iron-binding capacity × (multiplied by) 100.
6. **Liver biopsy:** The liver biopsy confirms the diagnosis of hemochromatosis. The biopsy shows fibrosis or changes due to cirrhosis.

Additional Tests to Evaluate Affected Organ Systems

The following are additional tests for evaluation:

1. The serum creatinine (S.Cr): kidney assessment
2. The liver function tests (LFTs): liver assessment
3. The fasting blood sugar (FBS), postprandial/meal blood sugar (PPBS), and hemoglobinA_1C (HbA$_1$C): diabetes assessment
4. Cortisol levels: adrenal cortical assessment for presence of Addison's disease
5. The electrocardiogram (ECG): cardiac assessment

HEMOCHROMATOSIS MANAGEMENT

Treatment must be started early in the disease process, to minimize organ damage. Treatment consists of the following:

1. **Consultation with the dietician:** The goal is to eliminate foods high in iron and increase the intake of calcium to decrease iron absorption.
2. **Weekly phlebotomy:** Weekly phlebotomy is the treatment of choice when the ferritin level is markedly increased. 500 mL of blood is removed per week by phlebotomy till the iron levels reach baseline and the ferritin level is below 50 ng/L.
3. **Treatment of associated organ problems:** Liver, kidney, pancreas, heart, and pituitary.

Hemochromatosis and Suggested Dental Considerations

The following are considerations for hemochromatosis:

1. Evaluate the status of the affected organ systems: liver, kidney, heart, and adrenal cortex.
2. Assess the PT/INR in the presence of cirrhosis.
3. Coexisting Addison's disease is treated with daily prednisone intake.
4. Determine the daily prednisone dose and provide extra steroids for major dental surgical procedures.
5. Evaluate the presence of diabetes/existing diabetes control.
6. Assessment of items 1–5 will dictate the deviations in the use of stress management, anesthetics, analgesics, and antibiotics in the dental setting.

Please review the appropriate sections for the associated organ system and/or diseases caused by hemochromatosis to determine a final treatment plan for your patient with regard to the use of stress management, anesthetics, analgesics, and antibiotics.

Hemostasis and Associated Bleeding Disorders

Primary and Secondary Hemostasis: Normal Mechanism, Disease States, and Coagulation Tests: Assessment, Analysis, and Associated Dental Management Guidelines

PRIMARY AND SECONDARY HEMOSTASIS OVERVIEW, FACTS, AND ASSOCIATED DISEASE STATES

Hemostasis Introduction

To understand bleeding disorders, one needs a good understanding of the following:

1. The elements of hemostasis
2. The physiology of hemostasis: primary and secondary hemostasis
3. Problems associated with the elements of hemostasis
4. The congenital and acquired bleeding disorders
5. Drugs that potentiate or cause bleeding

The Elements of Hemostasis

The elements of hemostasis are:

1. **Vascular response:** This refers to the vascular contraction or response following injury.
2. **Platelet number:** Bleeding time (BT) is prolonged in the presence of thrombocytopenia (decreased platelet number).
3. **Platelet function:** Bleeding time (BT) is prolonged when platelet function is affected.
4. **Adequate Von Willebrand's Factor (VWF) level:** VWF enhances platelet function.
5. **Adequate Clotting Factor Levels:** PTT and PT/INR assess the functioning status of the intrinsic and extrinsic clotting pathways, respectively.

Physiology of Hemostasis

Primary and secondary hemostasis have to function appropriately for a patient to have a negative bleeding history. The immediate type of bleeding occurs when there are problems associated with the elements involved with primary hemostasis. The delayed type of bleeding occurs when there are problems associated with the elements involved with secondary hemostasis.

151

Elements Associated with Primary Hemostasis

The elements associated with primary hemostasis are:

1. Adequate vascular response
2. Adequate platelet number
3. Adequate platelet function
4. Adequate level of the Von Willebrand's Factor (VWF)

Elements Associated with Secondary Hemostasis

Good secondary hemostasis is dependent on appropriate and adequate Clotting Factor interactions leading to formation of the fibrin clot.

Primary Hemostasis Detailed Discussion

When injury occurs, the blood vessels at the injured site constrict and attract the circulating platelets (out of the circulation) to the site of injury. The platelets aggregate in large number and link with each other to form the platelet plug. Von Willebrand's Factor (VWF) enhances the sticking together, or cohesiveness, of the platelets. This is primary hemostasis. Primary hemostasis defect is associated with excessive oozing at the time of surgery and oozing that continues beyond 24 hr postoperatively. In addition to its effect on the platelets, VWF also helps stabilize and transport Factor VIIIc/Factor VIII clotting, which participates in the clotting cascade. Drugs affecting primary hemostasis are

- Aspirin
- NSAIDS
- Aspirin plus dipyridamole (Aggrenox)
- Adenosine diphosphate inhibitors: clopidogrel (Plavix)
- Ticlopidine (Ticlid)

Note: The immediate type of bleeding can also occur because of increased vascular fragility due to chronic corticosteroid therapy. Chronic steroid use causes thinning of the vascular connective tissue lining and increased fragility of the small blood vessels. The bleeding time (BT) and platelet counts are **normal** and not affected with chronic corticosteroid use. During dentistry these patients respond well to local pressure and local hemostats.

Secondary Hemostasis Detailed Discussion

All Clotting Factors, with the exception of Factor VIII, are manufactured in the liver. Factor VIII and VWF are manufactured in the endothelial cells of the blood vessels. Factors II, VII, IX, and X are vitamin K–dependent clotting factors, and they participate in the intrinsic and extrinsic clotting cascades. The clotting factors are present in the circulation in the inactive form. The intrinsic and extrinsic clotting cascades demonstrate the sequential order in which the clotting factors activate to promote secondary hemostasis. Tissue factor released from the injured vasculature immediately activates Factor VII in the extrinsic clotting pathway and exposure to collagen from the ruptured vessel wall slowly activates Factor XII in the intrinsic pathway. The chain reaction that follows in the intrinsic and extrinsic clotting cascades (Figure 15.1) results in the formation of the fibrin clot that gets deposited on the platelet plug mesh (from primary

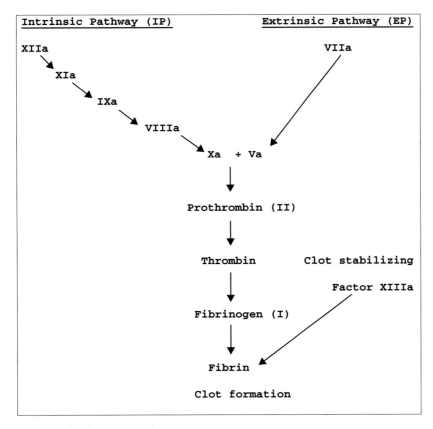

Figure 15.1. The clotting cascade.

hemostasis), and together, the seal the injured site. This is secondary hemostasis. Patients experiencing problems with secondary hemostasis present with deep tissue bleeding 4–10 days postoperatively. Anticoagulants/blood thinners, heparin or warfarin (Coumadin) affect secondary hemostasis.

Clotting Factor Facts

Optimal vitamin K absorption from the gut is needed for the manufacture of Factors II, VII, IX, and X in the liver. Low levels of these factors prolong the PT/INR and the PTT. Liver disease, particularly alcoholic cirrhosis, is the leading cause of Clotting Factor deficiency. Not all patients with cirrhosis will have a prolonged PT/INR. Clotting factor **activity** has to drop by more than **75%** to cause prolongation of the PT/INR.

Note: Platelets are also produced in the liver, and **thrombocytopenia** can be seen with **cirrhosis**. Always determine the PT/INR and the complete blood count (CBC) with platelets prior to probing a cirrhotic patient. Chronic small bowel disease affects vitamin K absorption. Thus Factors II, VII, IX, and X can be low, in the presence of significant vitamin K deficiency. The deficiency can be corrected by injecting 10 mg vitamin K daily, IV for 3 days. Vitamin K IV promotes reversal in 6–12 hr. Oral vitamin K will be ineffective in the presence of chronic malabsorption. IV or oral vitamin K will be ineffective in a cirrhotic patient because the liver is not able to utilize the vitamin K.

$$INR = \left[\frac{Patient's\ PT}{Control\ PT} \right]^{ISI}$$

Key:
PT: Prothrombin Time; **ISI:** International
Sensitivity Index

Figure 15.2. International Normalized Ratio calculation equation.

Clotting Factor Deficiency Causes

The following cause clotting factor deficiency:

1. Hemophilia A (Factor VIII deficiency)
2. Hemophilia B (Factor IX deficiency)
3. Some cases of Von Willebrand's Disease (VWD) can present with Factor VIII deficiency.
4. Anticoagulants heparin (affects the intrinsic pathway) and Coumadin (affects the extrinsic pathway)

CLOTTING FACTOR TESTS PT/INR AND PTT

Prothrombin Time (PT)/International Normalized Ratio (INR)

The PT/INR measures the extrinsic pathway, and the normal range of PT is 10–12 sec.

The International Normalized Ratio (INR)

The INR is a universal test that is used to effectively monitor the effect of warfarin (Coumadin). INR is the prothrombin time (PT) ratio obtained using the international reference thromboplastin reagent (Figure 15.2).

The normal INR range is 0.9–1.2; the average is 1. Only the PT/INR is affected by therapeutic doses of warfarin (Coumadin).

The Partial Thromboplastin Time (PTT)

The PTT measures the intrinsic pathway. The normal PTT range is: 25–38 sec.

PTT is affected by IV heparin and high doses of Coumadin.

When the patient is anticoagulated with IV heparin, the PTT is maintained at 1.5–2.5 times normal. PTT is not affected by low molecular weight heparins (LMWHs).

Platelet Disorders: Thrombocytopenia, Platelet Dysfunction, and Thrombocytosis: Assessment, Analysis, and Associated Dental Management Guidelines

As discussed earlier, platelets play a very important role in primary hemostasis. Platelet deficiency and/or platelet dysfunction can promote excessive oozing during surgery, and the oozing can continue beyond 24 hr postoperatively depending on the extent of the problem.

Common platelet disorders are thrombocytopenia/platelet deficiency, platelet dysfunction, and thrombocytosis.

THROMBOCYTOPENIA/PLATELET DEFICIENCY

The average platelet count is 150,000–400,000/mm^3. The patient is said to have thrombocytopenia if the platelet count is under 150,000/mm^3. Spontaneous bleeding can occur when the platelet count is below 20,000/mm^3.

Thrombocytopenia Causes

The following are causes of thrombocytopenia:

- Drugs such as heparin, chemotherapeutic agents, alcohol
- Leukemia, lymphoma, or bone marrow tumors
- HIV, mumps, rubella, or parvovirus infections
- Sequestration of the platelets by an enlarged spleen. Acute or chronic liver disease is the leading cause for an enlarged spleen.
- Autoimmune destruction of the platelets by IgG antibodies, causing Idiopathic Thrombocytopenia Purpura (ITP). ITP is more common in children and young adults.

Thrombocytopenia Symptoms and Signs

Thrombocytopenia and platelet dysfunction causes easy bruising and easy bleeding. Small, superficial bruises; petechiae; and bleeding mucus membranes are common findings. Petechiae are pinpoint hemmorrhagic flat lesions that occur in clusters. They can be seen on the oral mucosa and on the skin of the extremities.

155

Thrombocytopenia Laboratory Tests

Thrombocytopenia due to any cause is associated with a **prolonged** bleeding time (BT) and a **decreased** platelet count.

Thrombocytopenia Treatment (Except ITP)

Thrombocytopenia (except ITP) can be treated with the following:

1. Platelet Rich Plasma (PRP) or Platelet Rich Concentrate (PRC) transfusion
2. Desmopressin/Stimate/DDAVP. DDAVP elevates the Von Willebrand's Factor level in the blood and stimulates platelet release.

Platelet transfusion when required is given 20 min prior to the planned procedure. One platelet concentrate transfusion increases the platelet count by 10,000/μL.

Thrombocytopenia Dental Alerts

Spontaneous bleeding occurs when the platelet count is below 20,000/mm³. Routine dental treatment is contraindicated if the platelet count is below 50,000/mm³.

In the presence of significant thrombocytopenia, the CBC with platelet count should be assessed prior to dentistry. The test obtained should have been done **within the past 7 days**. For outpatient oral surgery or periodontal surgery procedures the platelet count must be above 75,000/mm³, and for major dental surgical procedures done in the operating room (OR) it is best to have the platelet count above 100,000/mm³.

IDIOPATHIC THROMBOCYTOPENIC PURPURA (ITP)

Thrombocytopenia due to ITP is treated with corticosteroids, immune-globulins, or splenectomy. ITP cannot be treated with platelet replacement therapy because the antibodies will destroy the new platelets.

The steroid protocol for each ITP patient is designed by the patient's M.D. The dose and duration of steroids given will depend on the extent of thrombocytopenia, the gravity of the bleeding, and how affected the patient is with thrombocytopenia.

ITP Steroid Treatment Protocol

Initial Steroid Treatment Protocol for ITP

Initial steroid treatment protocol for ITP is 1 mg/kg/day prednisone, P.O for 2–6 weeks

Subsequent Steroid Treatment Protocol for ITP

Prednisone dose is individualized for every patient. Usually the dose of prednisone is tapered to less than 10 mg per day for 3 months and then withdrawn. Splenectomy is done if discontinuation of prednisone causes a relapse.

Suggested Dental Guidelines for ITP

Always consult with the patient's physician when corticosteroids have been used to treat ITP. If the platelet counts are lower than the required cutoff for dental surgery, the patient could receive additional steroids, per physician's advice. You need to follow the "rule of twos" for major dental treatment and provide extra steroids prior to surgery if the patient is currently on steroids or has used steroids for 2 weeks or longer within the past 2 years.

PLATELET DYSFUNCTION

Platelet function is assessed by the capacity of the platelets to adhere/stick to each other. Antiplatelet drugs minimize platelet aggregation and promote thinning of the blood.

Drugs Associated with Platelet Dysfunction

Drugs associated with platelet dysfunction are NSAIDS, aspirin, dipyridamole (Persanthin), clopidogrel (Plavix), and ticlopidine (Ticlid). All these drugs with the exception of the NSAIDS, irreversibly and permanently affect the entire life span of the platelets which is about 7–10 days (average 7 days). The affect of NSAIDS is temporary and lasts until the drug clears the system, which is about 24 hr. The platelet count is not affected by any one of these drugs.

Platelet dysfunction is confirmed with a prolonged bleeding time (BT). The normal BT is 2.4–8 min.

Platelet Dysfunction and Von Willebrand's Disease (VWD)

Platelet dysfunction can also be associated with deficiency of the Von Willebrand's Factor (VWF). VWF promotes the sticking of the platelets to the injured vascular endothelium and also sticking to each other to form a mesh on which fibrin gets deposited. The platelet count is normal in all types of Von Willebrand's Disease (VWD), except Type 2B (VWD discussion follows).

Antiplatelet Drug Therapy

Conditions Associated with High Risk for Thrombosis

Conditions associated with high risk for thrombosis are transient ischemic attacks (TIAs), cardiovascular accidents (CVA/stroke), unstable angina, myocardial infarction (MI), angioplasty, medicated or bare-metal stents, atrial fibrillation, and peripheral vascular disease. The antiplatelet drugs are given to patients with a high risk for thrombosis.

Suggested Dental Guidelines for Patients on Antiplatelet Drugs

The following are dental guidelines for patients on antiplatelet drugs:

1. Minor procedures like amalgams, composites, and cleanings can be done without stopping any one of these drugs.
2. Always consult with the patient's M.D. before you plan to stop any of these drugs prior to dentistry. If allowed by the M.D., all drugs except NSAIDS, are stopped **7 days prior** to surgery and restarted **1–2 days postop**. NSAIDS are stopped 24 hr prior to surgery and restarted in the evening, once bleeding has stopped, or the next day.

3. Combination therapy with one daily 81 mg/325 mg aspirin and one of the other antiplatelet drugs—Plavix, Persanthin, or Ticlid—is often given to patients with a higher than normal risk for thrombosis. The general trend today is to treat these patients in the dental setting **without** interrupting the intake of any of these medications. The risk of thrombosis far outweighs the bleeding associated with dentistry.

4. For major or minor surgery, sustained pressure and/or local hemostats will control any excessive bleeding. You can serve this population best by providing regular checkups and treating any oral problem immediately.

THROMBOCYTOSIS

Thrombocytosis is a condition associated with platelet counts greater than 450,000/mm³. Thrombocytosis can be due to reactive bone marrow stimulation due to the need for more RBCs, as seen in iron deficiency anemia. It can also occur in the presence of significant inflammation or certain malignancies.

Thrombocytosis-Associated Symptoms

Thrombocytosis-associated symptoms experienced are thrombosis, strokes, and bleeds.

Suggested Dental Guidelines for Thrombocytosis

The following are dental guidelines for thrombocytosis:

1. Assess the cause.
2. Evaluate the medications: antiplatelet or anticoagulants.
3. Incorporate guidelines discussed for antiplatelet activity or anticoagulants.

Von Willebrand's Disease: Assessment, Analysis, and Associated Dental Management Guidelines

Von Willebrand's Disease (VWD), hemophilia A, and hemophilia B are the three leading inherited bleeding disorders, and VWD is the most common of the three. Von Willebrand's Disease (VWD) affects both males and females.

As discussed earlier, when injury occurs the blood vessels at the injured site constrict. This attracts the circulating platelets to the site of injury. The platelets link with each other and form the platelet plug. Von Willebrand's Factor (VWF) thus plays a very important role in primary hemostasis because it enhances platelet cohesiveness. Von Willebrand's Factor also helps transport and stabilize Factor VIIIc (VIII clotting) in the circulation. Factor VIIIc participates in the clotting cascade.

In patients with VWD, depending on the severity of the disease, the half-life and activity of Factor VIIIc is decreased. The PTT will be prolonged in such cases.

Patients with Von Willebrand's disease can therefore present with problems associated with either primary or secondary hemostasis or both.

TYPES OF VON WILLEBRAND'S DISEASE (VWD)

Type 1 VWD

Type 1 VWD is the most common and mildest form of the disease; 85% of patients diagnosed with VWD have Type 1 VWD.

The quality of the VWF is normal. The amount of Von Willebrand's Factor (VWF) in the blood is reduced, but adequate amounts exist in the endothelial stores. These patients are usually asymptomatic but can have the immediate type of bleeding and significant oozing beyond 24 hr following an extraction.

Type 2 VWD

The quality of the VWF is affected, both in the blood and at the storage sites. There are two subtypes of Type 2 VWD: VWD 2A and VWD 2B. Type 2B is additionally associated with a decreased platelet count or thrombocytopenia.

Type 3 VWD

The quality of the VWF is normal, but the amount of VWF is severely depleted in the blood and in the endothelial stores. All Type 3 VWD patients and some cases of Type

2 VWD are not able to transport Factor VIIIc in the blood. In addition to problems with primary hemostasis, these patients have problems with secondary hemostasis when the Factor VIIIc level drops by more than 75%.

Symptoms and Signs of VWD

Excessive bruising at unusual sites, mucous membrane bleeding, heavy nose bleeds, heavy menstrual cycles, and prolonged oozing following extraction(s) are some of the common symptoms experienced with VWD. All these symptoms relate to problems with primary hemostasis.The patients with associated low levels of Factor VIIIc will complain of deep tissue bleeding in the muscles and bleeding in the joints (hemarthrosis).

Diagnosis of VWD

VWD diagnosis is confirmed by the following:

1. **The platelet count:** The platelet count is normal in all types of VWD except, Type 2B VWD. Type 2B VWD is associated with thrombocytopenia.
2. **The bleeding time (BT):** The BT is prolonged in all types of VWD.
3. **The Ristocetin Induced Platelet Aggregation (RIPA) test:** The RIPA test shows decreased platelet aggregation in all types, except Type IIB where the aggregation is increased.
4. **The Ristocetin cofactor activity test:** This test measures the amount of VWF activity. The test shows reduced cofactor activity.
5. **Factor VIII activity:** The Factor VIII activity can be normal or decreased depending on the type of VWD.
6. **The PT/INR:** The PT/INR is normal.
7. **The PTT:** The PTT can be normal or prolonged, depending on the Factor VIIIc activity level. The test will be normal if there is more than 25% Factor VIIIc activity.

VWD TREATMENT

Treatment of Type 1 and Type 2A VWD

Primary Therapy

Primary therapy consists of giving Desmopressin/Vasopressin/DDAVP, IV, intranasal or PO (oral).

Secondary Therapy

Secondary therapy is provided with factor concentrate or cryoprecipitate. Cryoprecipitate contains Factor VIII, VWF, and fibrinogen.

Treatment of Type 2B and Type 3 VWD

Primary Therapy

Primary therapy is provided with factor concentrate.

Secondary Therapy

Secondary therapy for Type 2B VWD is provided with cryoprecipitate.

Secondary Therapy for Type 3 VWD

Secondary Therapy for Type 3 VWD is provided with cryoprecipitate or platelet transfusions.

DDAVP is contraindicated in the Type 2B VWD patient because more of the abnormal VWF will get released causing aggregation of the dysfunctional platelets and thrombosis. DDAVP is of no use in Type 3 VWD because the factor levels are depleted in the blood and in the endothelial stores.

Suggested Dental Guidelines for VWD

The following are dental guidelines for VWD:

1. Consult with the patient's M.D. and determine the type and extent of VWD in the patient.
2. Relay to the M.D. the type of procedures planned, both major and minor dentistry.
3. Confirm with the M.D. the DDAVP or Factor concentrate or cryoprecipitate or platelet transfusion protocol.
4. With IV DDAVP, the surgery can begin in 30–60 min.
5. With oral or intranasal DDAVP, the surgery can begin 60–90 min later.
6. With platelet transfusion, the surgery can begin in 20 min.
7. Surgery can begin immediately after cryoprecipitate (CPP) transfusion. Cryoprecipitate contains 10 times the amount of Factor VIII compared to FFP. One bag of cryoprecipitate contains 100 units of Factor VIII. Cryoprecipitate has the highest concentration of VWF. Ten bags of CPP when given immediately before the procedure shortens the bleeding time for up to 12 hr.
8. The local VWD anesthetic, analgesic, and antibiotic (AAAs) guidelines are similar to the hemophilia guidelines.

Coagulation Disorders: Common Clotting Factor Deficiency Disease States, Associated Systemic and/or Local Hemostasis Adjuncts, and Dental Management Guidelines

HEMOPHILIA A AND HEMOPHILIA B OVERVIEW, FACTS, AND MANAGEMENT

Hemophilia A and Hemophilia B Facts

Hemophilia A, hemophilia B, and Von Willebrand's Disease (VWD) are the three most common inherited bleeding disorders. Hemophilia A and hemophilia B (Christmas disease) affects males only. Females are carriers. Hemophilia A is associated with Factor VIII deficiency and hemophilia B is associated with Factor IX deficiency. Factor VIII has a half-life activity of 8–12 hr. Factor IX has a half-life activity of 12–24 hr. Patients with hemophilia A and B are categorized as having mild, moderate, or severe disease depending on the blood levels of Factor VIII or IX, respectively.

Hemophilia Severity Classification

Hemophilia can be of mild, moderate or severe intensity:

1. **Mild hemophilia:** The specific Factor (VIII or IX) level is 5–30% of normal. The mild hemophiliac bleeds minimally. Bleeding is usually associated with surgery, and the past history may reveal bleeding after a dental extraction.
2. **Moderate hemophilia:** The specific Factor (VIII or IX) level is 1–5% of normal. A moderate hemophiliac bleeds after minor injury and requires immediate attention.
3. **Severe hemophilia:** The specific Factor (VIII or IX) level is less than 1% of normal. A severe hemophiliac bleeds very often, with or without provocation.

Hemophilia A and B Treatment

Factor replacement therapy replacing the specific clotting factor is the treatment of choice for both hemophilia A and B. Most patients with mild hemophilia A can be treated with Desmopressin/DDAVP/Stimate. DDAVP/Stimate is a synthetic analogue of Vasopressin. It stimulates the release of Factor VIIIc, Von Willebrand's Factor (VWF), and tissue plasminogen activator from the endothelial storage sites. There is a two- to threefold increase of Factor VIII from baseline level. At least a 25–30% Factor VIII activity is needed for adequate hemostasis.

DDAVP/Stimate Therapy for Hemophilia A

DDAVP/Stimate is given orally, intravenously, or intranasally, prior to a planned dental procedure, to prevent bleeding. DDAVP should not be used too frequently because it can deplete the storage pools. Do not use DDAVP more than twice or three times over a 48-hr period.

DDAVP Prescriptions

1. **DDAVP IV Dose:**
   Rx: Give 0.3 µg/kg of DDAVP in 50 cc saline IV slowly over 15–30 min. With IV DDAVP Factor VIII and Von Willebrand's Factor (VWF), levels peak in 30–60 min.
2. **DDAVP Intranasal Dose:**
   Rx: Desmopressin/DDAVP, 1.5 mg/mL
   0.1 mL is pumped with each spray, giving a 150 µg dose.
   Adult dose: 300 µg
   Child's dose: 150 µg The intranasal absorption is slow and the effect lasts for 5–21 hr.
   With intranasal DDAVP Factor VIII and Von Willebrand's Factor levels peak in 60–90 min.
3. **DDAVP Oral Dose:**
   Rx: DDAVP, 0.1 or 0.2 mg/tablet
   Sig: 0.05 mg twice daily.
   Total Daily Oral Dose: 0.1–1.2 mg. Onset of action occurs in 0.9–1.5 hr following oral intake.

Note: DDAVP is not used in the management of hemophilia B because it does not stimulate the release of Factor IX.

Hemophilia A and B Clotting Factor Replacement Therapy

The moderate and severe hemophilia A or B patient will always need specific factor replacement prior to any major or minor dental procedure and this includes probing or local anesthesia injection. One unit Factor VIII/kg provides a 2% rise in Factor VIII level. One unit Factor IX/kg provides a 1% rise in Factor IX level. The clotting Factor dose prior to surgery will depend on the severity of bleeding expected and is decided by the patient's physician; **50%** Factor **activity** is a must for block anesthesia.

The commercial factors are powders that need to be dissolved in sterile water, prior to use. Often it is the patient who injects the factor intravenously (IV), just about 15 min prior to a planned procedure.

Repeat infusions every 8–12 hr for Factor VIII and every 12–24 hr for Factor IX; this will depend on the planned dental procedure, postop bleeding, and additional use of antifibrinolytic drugs tranexamic acid (Cyklokapron) or epsilon aminocaproic acid (Amicar). The antifibrinolytic drugs prevent fibrinolysis/clot breakdown, by inhibiting the activation of plasminogen to plasmin.

Factors VIII and IX Sources

Factors VIII and IX are obtained from two sources:

1. Clotting Factor concentrate from plasma
2. Commercially produced Recombinant Factor

Factor VIII Products for Hemophilia A

The Factor VIII products available for hemophilia A are:

1. **Recombinant Products:** Bioclate, Helixate , Kogenate, and Recombinate
2. **Plasma-Derived Product:** Pork plasma-derived hyate

Factor IX Products for Hemophilia B

The Factor IX products available for hemophilia B are:

1. **Recombinant Product:** BeneFIX
2. **Plasma-Derived Products:** AlphaNine SD, Konyne 80, Mononine, Proplex T, and Profilnine

Note: Inhibitors or antibodies to clotting factors can develop in some cases of hemophilia A and hemophilia B. In such situations the patient is infused with the antiinhibitor and the specific clotting factor.

ANTIFIBRINOLYTIC DRUGS EPSILON AMINOCAPROIC ACID (AMICAR) AND TRANEXAMIC ACID (CYKLOKAPRON)

Before you prescribe these drugs always confirm that the patient has no prior history of moderate to severe headaches, acute vision problems, transient ischemic attacks (TIAs), cardiovascular accidents (CVAs/strokes), blood clots, or any other indicators for thrombosis. Confirm that the liver and kidneys are optimally functioning.

The antifibrinolytic drugs can be ingested by mouth (PO), used as a mouth rinse, or injected IV.

Always advise the patient to discontinue the oral or IV antifibrinolytic drug and proceed to the nearest emergency room, should symptoms and signs of thrombosis develop. Sudden, severe headaches; acute vision loss; sudden severe pains in the chest, calves, or abdomen; or sudden motor/sensory deficits in the extremities should be cause for immediate action and attention.

Epsilon Aminocaproic Acid (Amicar) Oral (PO) and Mouthwash Prescriptions

1. **Rx:** Epsilon aminocaproic acid **(Amicar)**, 500 mg/tablet
   Sig: First dose: 5 g (10 tablets) orally, 1 hour postsurgery, followed by 2 g (4 tablets) q6h, postoperatively till the bleeding stops, or prescribe for 5–7 days. **Maximum dose:** 30 g/day
2. **Rx: Amicar syrup**, 250 mg/mL or 1.25 g/tsp (5 ml)
   Sig: 5–10 mL qid × 5–7 days, starting 6 hr prior to surgery, if needed. Use as **mouthwash** for 2 min and **expectorate**.
   The mouthwash decreases recurrent bleeding and the need for factor replacement after surgery. Amicar prevents clot breakdown by the enzymes in the saliva. This allows healing of the tissues beneath the clot.
   Disp: 240 mL/480 mL bottle

Tranexamic Acid/Cyklokapron Oral (PO) and Mouthwash Prescriptions

1. **Rx:** Tranexamic acid **(Cyklokapron)**, 500 mg/tablet
   Sig: 25 mg/kg orally tid/qid × 2–8 days, starting one day prior to surgery

2. **Rx:** 4.8% **Cyklokapron** oral rinse solution
   Sig: Use 10 mL as **mouthwash** for 2 min and **expectorate**, qid × 5–7 days.
   Disp: 280 ml

Cyklokapron is 10 times more potent than Amicar and it has a longer half-life. The Cyklokapron oral rinse is not FDA-approved. It is important to remember that the saliva and the oral mucosa contain plasminogen activators that can trigger fibrinolysis. Use of Amicar or Cyklokapron mouthwash is therefore very beneficial to prevent clot lysis.

Excessive postsurgical oozing can additionally be controlled by sustained pressure and the use of local hemostatic materials. Review Table 18.1 for a summary of hemostatic adjuncts.

Table 18.1. Hemostatic adjuncts: DDAVP, amicar, and tranexamic acid

Therapy	Prescription
Desmopressin or Vasopressin or DDAVP or Stimate therapy: Therapy for Hemophilia A or Von Willebrand's Disease Type 1; 2A	1. **DDAVP IV Dose:** Give 0.3 µg/kg DDAVP in 50cc saline IV slowly over 15–30 min. Levels peak in 30–60 min. 2. **DDAVP Intranasal Dose:** Available as 1.5 mg/mL spray. Each spray pumps 0.1 mL, giving a 150 µg dose. Levels peak in 60–90 mins. Dose lasts for 5–21 h. **Adult Intranasal Dose:** 300 µg **Child Intranasal Dose:** 150 µg 3. **DDAVP Oral Dose:** Rx: DDAVP, 0.1 or 0.2 mg/tablet Sig: 0.05 mg twice daily Total Daily Dose: 0.1–1.2 mg
Antifibrinolytic drug: Epsilon Aminocaproic acid (Amicar)	1. **Oral Amicar Prescription:** Rx: Amicar, 500 mg/tablet Sig: Start dose 5 g (10 tabs) PO 1 h postsurgery, **then** 2 g (4 tabs) q6h till the bleeding stops **or** for 5–7 days. Maximum Oral Dose: 30 g/day 2. **Amicar Mouthwash:** Rx: Amicar syrup, 250 mg/ml or 1.25 g/tsp (5 ml) Sig: 5–10 ml qid × 5–7 days, starting 6 h prior to surgery, if needed. Use as mouthwash for 2 min and **expectorate**. Disp: 240 ml/480 ml bottle
Antifibrinolytic drug: Tranexamic acid (Cyklokapron)	1. **Oral Cyklokapron:** Rx: Cyklokapron, 500 mg/tablet Sig: 25 mg/kg PO tid/qid × 2–8 days, starting one day prior to surgery. 2. **Cyklokapron Mouthwash:** Not FDA approved. Has a longer half-life than Amicar and is also 10 times more potent. Rx: 4.8% Cyklokapron rinse Sig: Use 10 ml as mouthwash for 2 min and **expectorate**, qid × 5–7 days. Disp: 280 ml

LOCAL HEMOSTATIC AGENTS

Microfibrillar Collagen (Avitene or Helistat)

Avitene or Helistat is a meshlike hemostat that attracts and triggers platelet aggregation plus fibrin formation. It can be applied to the bleeding site to control moderate to severe bleeding in 2–5 min. It does not inhibit healing. It can be used in patients taking aspirin or heparin.

Gelfoam

Gelfoam is an absorbable gelatin sponge that is made from purified gelatin solution. It stimulates thromboplastin release and thrombin formation. It gets absorbed in 3–5 days and works best in patients on blood thinners.

Thrombostat

Thrombostat is topical thrombin and it directly converts fibrinogen to fibrin. It works extremely well for severe bleeding.

Fibrin Glues

Fibrin glues contain fibrinogen and thrombin. Rapid hemostasis occurs when used at the bleeding surgical site.

Surgicel

Surgicel is oxidized regenerated cellulose. It swells immediately on contact with blood and forms a sticky mass. On doing so, it presses down on the bleeding site causing hemostasis. It can be kept in place indefinitely or removed after bleeding has stopped. Surgicel works when all other local hemostats have failed.

Amicar or Cyklokapron Mouthwashes

These mouthwashes prevent the conversion of plasminogen to plasmin. Gauze soaked with either mouthwash can be held in place for about 10–30 min, to stop the bleed. Additionally, you can prescribe the mouthwash for 5–7 days, postsurgery.

Calcium Sulfate

An absorbable biocompatible hemostatic agent, calcium sulfate gets resorbed in 2–4 weeks.

Moist Tea Bag

Some literature shows that biting down on a moist tea bag for 10–30 min can decrease bleeding because of the tannic acid present in the tea bag.

SUGGESTED DENTAL GUIDELINES FOR HEMOPHILIA A AND B

The following are dental guidelines for hemophilia:

1. Consult with the M.D. and understand the type and extent of the hemophilia.
2. Inform the patient's M.D. of the dental procedures planned and categorize them as major or minor surgical procedures.
3. Confirm with the M.D. if preoperative DDAVP (Stimate) use will suffice. Confirm route and time of administration for preoperative use. Surgery will begin in 30–60 min with IV use, in 60–90 min with intranasal use, and in 0.9–1.5 hr with oral use. DDAVP can minimize Factor VIII use in some patients.
4. Confirm with the M.D. when the factor replacement should be done. It is usually done 15 min prior to most surgical procedures.
5. Factor VIII levels must be raised to 50% of normal for block anesthesia.
6. Plan on doing more than one procedure at a given time, to optimize the factor transfusion.
7. Keep a 2-week interval if several procedures are planned for the patient. This will ensure optimal postoperative hemostasis and healing.
8. Assess the CBC with platelets and WBC differential to confirm the level of tissue oxygenation (per RBC count), primary hemostasis and immediate bleeding (per platelet count), and healing status (per WBC total and differential count).
9. **Anesthetics:** There is no contraindication to any local anesthetics, but make appropriate changes per anemia guidelines, if the patient has associated anemia. Also, any other existing systemic condition status will need to be factored in when deciding on the local anesthetic.
10. Use local hemostats, when needed.
11. Use reabsorbable sutures because they retain less plaque and therefore cause less inflammation at the surgical site.
12. **Analgesics:** Provide adequate pain management for 2–3 days with acetaminophen (Tylenol), acetaminophen with codeine; acetaminophen with oxycodone (Percocet), or hydrocodone (Vicodin). Do **not** prescribe aspirin or NSAIDS.
13. **Antibiotics:** Provide antibiotic coverage postoperatively with penicillin VK 250–500 mg qid or clindamycin 150–300 mg tid/qid (in the presence of penicillin allergy) for 5 days. This will promote the healing process and prevent infection and inflammation. Local infection and/or inflammation can cause secondary hemorrhage.
14. Advise the patient to consume cold liquids and soft foods until the bleeding stops and avoid using a straw because it promotes sucking and consequent clot displacement.
15. Depending on the procedures done and the gravity of the hemophilia, postsurgical factor replacement should be planned and the protocol communicated to the patient. Factor VIII is given q12h and Factor IX is given q24h.
16. Prescribe Amicar or Cyklokapron orally or as mouthwash, to minimize postoperative factor transfusion.
17. Communicate with the patient for the next 2–3 days to confirm excellent recovery.
18. Last but not least, maintain a good oral status with 4–6 month checkups to prevent major dental problems from developing.

OTHER FACTOR DEFICIENCIES

Factor XII Deficiency

The patient with Factor XII deficiency does not bleed in the presence of a very prolonged PTT.

Factor XIII Deficiency

Factor XIII deficiency can be associated with excessive bleeding in the presence of normal PT/INR and PTT.

19

Anticoagulants Warfarin (Coumadin), Standard Heparin, and Low Molecular Weight Heparin (LMWH): Assessment, Analysis, and Associated Dental Management Guidelines

ANTICOAGULATION THERAPY OVERVIEW

Anticoagulation therapy is indicated in the presence of thrombosis or when there is a risk of thrombosis. Because of its immediate action, IV heparin (standard heparin/unfractionated heparin) is the anticoagulant of choice, used in a hospitalized setting to stabilize a patient experiencing an acute thrombotic episode. Once the acute state is brought under control, warfarin (Coumadin) is started orally. Coumadin cannot be used at the start of an acute thrombotic episode because its onset of action and achievement of optimal action is slow. IV heparin is withdrawn when the therapeutic level of Coumadin is reached and the blood-thinning can be completely maintained by Coumadin. At the time of discharge, the patient is sent home taking only warfarin (Coumadin) to continue maintaining the blood thinning process.

Common Indications for Anticoagulation

Common indications for anticoagulation are transient ischemic attacks (TIAs) or strokes; atrial fibrillation; low ejection fraction causing stasis/pooling of blood; pulmonary embolism; deep vein thrombosis (DVT); and hypercoagulation states: protein C/S deficiency, Factor V Lieden mutation, lupus anticoagulant, antiphospholipid antibody syndrome, and antithrombin III deficiency.

WARFARIN (COUMADIN)

Warfarin (Coumadin) antagonizes the synthesis of the vitamin K–dependent clotting factors II, VII, IX, and X. Deficiency of vitamin K will thus affect the intrinsic and the extrinsic clotting pathways. This will in turn cause a prolongation of the activated partial thromboplastin time (APTT) and the prothrombin time (PT), respectively.

Coumadin is given PO (oral) and it peaks in 60–90 min after oral administration. Once ingested, Coumadin gets bound to albumin. It takes 9–16 hr for Coumadin to be effective and 36–48 hr for therapeutic levels to be established. The plasma half-life of warfarin (Coumadin) is about 37 hr and it is metabolized by the cytochrome P4503A4 enzyme system in the liver.

At the therapeutic level, Coumadin affects only Factor VII, which is associated with the extrinsic pathway. This accounts for why PT/INR is the only test monitored to assess Coumadin response. The half-life of Factor VII is **8 hr**, so when the Coumadin intake is temporarily stopped prior to major dental surgery, it takes **48 hr** (**6 half-lives**) for the PT/INR to normalize.

The Coumadin level is affected by certain dietary foods that are high in vitamin K. Dark green leafy vegetables, avocados, turnips, beets, and liver are the food items that **decrease** the effectiveness of warfarin (Coumadin), thus promoting the risk for thrombosis.

Coumadin Reversal

During dire situations when emergency dental surgery is needed in a patient on Coumadin, the effect of Coumadin can immediately be reversed with Fresh Frozen Plasma (FFP). The PT/INR is always checked post–FFP transfusion to confirm the reversal. Postsurgery, FFP transfusion does not negatively affect the future doses of Coumadin. Vitamin K can also be used to reverse the effects of Coumadin. However, a significantly large dose of vitamin K is needed for the reversal process to be quick. Large doses of vitamin K (oral or IV), used for reversal, have a negative impact on the future doses of Coumadin. Higher doses of Coumadin will be needed, post–emergency surgery. As a preventive measure, only low-dose vitamin K is used to reverse the effects of Coumadin in semiurgent situations. It can take almost 24 hr for Coumadin action reversal to occur. Low-dose vitamin K, as stated above, does not affect the future doses of Coumadin. In most patients with a history of Coumadin intake, the INR is maintained at a therapeutic range of 2.0–3.0. Patients maintained at this range can tolerate a physician-approved, temporary interruption of Coumadin for major surgical procedures. It is always best to communicate with the patient's M.D. for advice when the patient is on Coumadin. Indicate the type of major and/or minor procedures planned and the amount of bleeding expected.

Patients with a high risk for thrombosis need higher doses of Coumadin. **The PT/INR in such cases is maintained between 3.0–4.5 or greater**. In the presence of higher Coumadin doses, the PTT will also be affected. Nevertheless, the PT/INR is the only test evaluated when monitoring even the high-risk patients.

Conditions Associated with Increased Risk of Thrombosis

The following are conditions associated with increased risk of thrombosis:

1. Mechanical prosthetic heart valves
2. Recent deep vein thrombosis (DVT)
3. Recent massive myocardial infarction (MI)
4. Atrial fibrillation (AF) associated with stroke/MI
5. Recent or multiple episodes of pulmonary embolism (PE)

Presence of any documented end-organ thrombosis-associated condition with AF places the patient at high risk for thrombosis. The end-organ conditions can be TIA/CVA/MI.

High-risk patients thus cannot afford to have their blood-thinning process stopped at any time, and for all surgical procedures these patients will have to be switched from Coumadin to heparin.

Depending on the dental procedure planned, the patient's M.D. could switch the patient to either low molecular weight heparin (LMWH) or standard/unfractionated/ IV heparin.

The PT/INR is monitored every 4–6 weeks when the patient is on Coumadin. The dentist must always request and evaluate the latest PT/INR from the physician's office before starting any dental treatment.

In a patient who has always been in the therapeutic range, a PT/INR done no earlier than 1 week prior is most reliable and helpful.

STANDARD AND LOW MOLECULAR WEIGHT HEPARINS (LMWHS)

Mechanism of Action of IV and Low Molecular Weight Heparins

Unfractionated or IV heparin potentiates the action of anti–thrombin III, and this inactivates active factor IIa or prothrombin. IV heparin also inactivates Factors IX, X, XI, XII, and plasmin. IV heparin additionally inhibits the conversion of fibrinogen to fibrin. LMWHs have less anti–factor IIa activity and more factor Xa activity. LMWHs bind to anti–thrombin III and this instantly inactivates factor Xa and factor II (prothrombin)

IV or standard heparin **inhibits** thrombin-induced platelet activation, thus causing IV heparin-induced thrombocytopenia. This effect is more pronounced if the patient has had several past exposures to IV heparin. This accounts for why it is important to check the platelet count at 1, 3, and 7 days postoperatively after the use of IV heparin. LMWHs have decreased platelet activation action and affinity and are less likely to cause thrombocytopenia.

IV heparin is extensively bound to plasma proteins and has a short half-life. LMWHs have a longer plasma half-life. LMWHs are minimally bound to plasma proteins and the proteins released from activated platelets and endothelial cells. Thus the anticoagulation action of LMWH is more consistent and predictable.

IV heparin does not cross the placental barrier so it can be safely given to pregnant patients, when needed. Heparin clearance from the plasma is **reduced** in patients with cirrhosis or severe kidney disease.

The plasma half-life of IV heparin or unfractionated heparin is approximately 1 hr. It is injected intravenously (IV).

The onset of action is immediate following an IV injection and the total clearance time is 6 hr.

Standard heparin effectiveness is judged by monitoring the PTT. Standard heparin is *the* drug used in the hospitalized setting when any acute thromboembolic state needs immediate attention. Once stable, warfarin (Coumadin) is added orally. When the anticoagulation is completely supported by Coumadin in about 2–4 days, standard heparin is then totally withdrawn.

Massive myocardial infarction (MI), stroke, atrial fibrillation (AF) associated with stroke/MI (end-organ problems), heart valve surgery, deep vein thrombosis (DVT), or pulmonary embolism (PE) are examples of acute thromboembolic states. LMWHs are prepared by depolymerization of unfractionated heparin chains. They are injected subcutaneously (SC) by the patient. This is a huge advantage because the patient can be ambulatory and needs no hospitalization.

The onset of action of LMWH occurs in 30 min–1 hr. The plasma half-life of LMWHs is 2–4 hr. The amount of LMWH given is determined by the patient's height and weight. LMWH is usually given q12h.

LMWHs, as discussed earlier, have better bioavailability, longer half-lives, more predictable dose response, and less negative effect on the platelets, compared to standard heparin. LMWHs are the preferred choice in the dental setting when blood thinning has to be continued for high-risk patients (after Coumadin withdrawal) for major procedures.

LMWH Preparations

The LMWHs preparations available are enoxaparine (Lovenox), ardeparin (Normiflo), dalteparin (Fragmin), nadroparin (Fraxiparine), reviparin (Clivarin), and tinzaparin (Innohep). Enoxaparin (Lovenox) is the most commonly prescribed LMWH.

Drug-Drug Interactions Associated with Heparin

The following drugs enhance heparin action and should not be prescribed in the dental setting: aspirin, NSAIDS, cephalosporins, tetracyclines, and antihistamines.

Heparin Antidote

Excessive bleeding associated with heparin can be reversed by protamine sulphate: 1 mg protamine sulphate neutralizes 100 units of heparin, dose for dose.

WARFARIN (COUMADIN), HEPARIN PROTOCOLS, AND SUGGESTED DENTAL GUIDELINES

The following are protocols and dental guidelines:

1. Always consult with the patient's M.D. to determine whether warfarin (Coumadin) can be stopped prior to the surgical procedure.
2. Most physicians will feel comfortable advising when you let them know the extent of surgery planned. State whether you plan on doing a major or minor dental procedure or both.
3. Amalgams, composites, cleanings, and endodontic or prosthodontic procedures are considered "minor procedures" because the bleeding is minimal or easy to control.
4. Gum surgery, extractions, sinus lifts, etc., are considered "major procedures" because of the increased risk for bleeding, tissue trauma, local inflammation, and/or infection.
5. In most patients when the PT/INR is in the therapeutic range, amalgams, composites, cleanings, and endodontic and prosthodontic procedures can be done without stopping the Coumadin. The bleeding is minimal and can be controlled by adequate pressure or local hemostats.
6. For some of the planned major procedures, when Coumadin can be temporarily stopped without a risk to thrombosis per M.D., it is usually stopped 48 hr (2 days) prior to the surgical procedure. Occasionally, some physicians may want you to stop the Coumadin 5 days prior to the planned surgical procedure. The Coumadin in such cases is restarted the evening of the surgical procedure or the next day, depending on when the patient typically takes the Coumadin.

7. If the patient's PT/INR has always been in the therapeutic range in the past, you can proceed without confirming the PT/INR prior to surgery. You will, however, need to confirm the PT/INR prior to major surgery for those patients with a pre-treatment PT/INR above the therapeutic range.

8. Trauma should be kept to a minimum in all cases, and the INR should ideally be checked on the day of the treatment.

9. Follow the sutures and local hemostat use guidelines discussed in Chapter 18, "Coagulation Disorders: Common Clotting Factor Deficiency Disease States, Associated Systemic and/or Local Hemostasis Adjuncts, and Dental Management Guidelines."

10. For patients with an increased risk for thrombosis, heparin is the bridging blood-thinning medication used during the period prior to and immediately following the dental procedure. You need to let the M.D. know whether you plan on doing major or minor dentistry. The M.D. will then decide whether IV heparin or low molecular weight heparin (LMWH) is to be used. For anticoagulation conversion from Coumadin to IV heparin, the patient is hospitalized. On the day of admission the Coumadin intake is stopped and the PT/INR plus APTT are constantly monitored. IV heparin is started q6h (every 6 hr) when the INR drops below 2. The IV heparin dose is progressively increased to compensate for the Coumadin washout. Heparin ultimately takes over the anticoagulation process from Coumadin. When complete Coumadin washout has been achieved the PT/INR attains baseline level (1.0). At this point, IV heparin is the only anticoagulant that provides the blood thinning. Always confirm that the PT/INR is normal before you begin the surgical procedure. The major surgical procedure is done **6 hr after** the last IV heparin dose. Once adequate hemostasis is achieved postsurgery, IV heparin is restarted. The APTT is monitored to regulate the IV heparin dose.

    When the patient is stable postoperatively, Coumadin is restarted by mouth on the evening of the procedure or the next day. The PT/INR and the APTT are now monitored. As the PT/INR rises, the IV Heparin dose is progressively decreased. The dropping APTT will reflect the heparin washout. The entire process from start to finish takes approximately 7 days.

11. For anticoagulation conversion to LMWH, no hospitalization is needed. The patient injects the LMWH, subcutaneously (SC). The APTT is **not** monitored with LMWH use. The M.D. will decide the Coumadin washout and LMWH protocols, prior to the surgery.

12. Lovenox is the most common LMWH preparation prescribed. Planned major surgical procedures in patients on Lovenox should be done 18–24 hr (6 half-lives) **after the last intake** of the drug. The patient usually **skips** the Lovenox injection on the evening prior to **and** the morning of the surgery.

    Lovenox is restarted the **evening of or the next day**, depending on the thrombosis risk status of the patient.

    Patients with a higher risk will restart the Lovenox on the evening following the procedure, once hemostasis has occurred.

    Once the patient is stable with the LMWH, Coumadin is restarted by mouth and then the PT/INR is monitored. When the PT/INR is in the therapeutic range of 2–3, the LMWH is withdrawn.

13. Aspirin, NSAIDS, alcohol, liver disease, kidney disease, and other bleeding disorders can increase the risk of bleeding in patients on Coumadin and heparin.

14. Uncomplicated oral surgical procedures can be performed without altering the Coumadin dose in patients with an INR less than 3.0. Minimal trauma during surgery, absorbable sutures, and local hemostats will additionally help. Amicar or Tranexamic acid mouthwash can also provide hemostatic support.

15. For emergency dental surgery it is best to rely on an INR test no more than 1 week old.

16. Intrapapillary and intraligamentary injections are far safer than regional block anesthesia in patients with an INR above the therapeutic range. Regional block anesthesia can cause bleeding into the facial spaces, which can precipitate airway obstruction.

17. Intramuscular injections are contraindicated in the following patients: patients on anticoagulants, cirrhosis patients, and patients with Crohn's or Celiac disease–associated malabsorption of vitamin K.

Drug-Drug Interactions (DDIs) with Warfarin (Coumadin)
Antibiotics

The more potent antibiotics such as amoxicillin plus clavulanic acid (Augmentin), cephalexin (Keflex), cephadroxyl (Duricef), doxycycline (Vibramycin), and metronidazole (Flagyl) should be **avoided** because they deplete the intestinal flora bacteria and thus promote bleeding by increasing the INR. Penicillin VK and clindamycin are **safe** to use with Coumadin.

Analgesics

Recent studies have shown that excessive use of acetaminophen (Tylenol), particularly Extra-Strength Tylenol with Coumadin, can cause a 4–9 times increase in the INR within 18–48 hr. It is best to use regular-strength Tylenol, Tylenol with codeine, Tylenol with hydrocodone (Vicodin), or oxycodone (Percocet) for 2–3 days only. Stress adequate hydration (6–8 glasses of water/day) and no alcohol use while on the pain medications. Avoid using morphine analogues, dihydrocodeine, acetaminophen-propoxyphene (Darvocet), and Pethidine because they raise the INR. Excessive pain may prevent the patient from eating, so start the pain medication just prior to major surgery or soon after. Fasting raises the INR, so prompt and proper analgesic use will prevent this from happening.

Antifungals

The **systemic** azole antifungals, fluconazole (Diflucan), ketoconazole (Nizoral), and griseofulvin (Fulvicin) **promote** bleeding, in the presence of Coumadin. Use the topical antifungals, clotrimazole (Mycelex) or nystatin (Mycostatin) instead, when needed.

VI

Cardiology

Rheumatic Fever (RF): Assessment, Analysis, and Associated Dental Management Guidelines

RHEUMATIC FEVER FACTS AND OVERVIEW

Rheumatic fever (RF) is a nonsuppurative acute inflammatory response to a previously untreated or partially treated Group A, β hemolytic streptococcus infection.

Patients with a diagnosis of RF will give a history of having had strep throat or scarlet fever a few weeks prior to the start of the symptoms and signs associated with RF. RF can occur within 3 to 4 weeks of an infection with β hemolytic streptococcus. The prevalence rate of RF following an untreated or incompletely treated β hemolytic infection is 3%.

RF is thought to be an abnormal immune system response to the streptoccal antigens, streptolysin O and streptolysin S.

Streptolysin O is strongly antigenic and triggers the production of antistreptolysin-O antibody (ASLO). The presence of high levels of ASLO during the acute phase of RF confirms the likelihood of the condition.

The RF-triggered antigen-antibody cross-reactivity affects the periarteriolar connective tissue, targeting the heart, joints, skin, and neurological tissues.

Note: Acute RF is associated with a negative throat culture because it occurs a few weeks **after** a β hemolytic streptococcus infection.

The Major and Minor Jones Criteria

The Major and Minor Jones Criteria, established in 1944, help with the diagnosis of RF.

Major Jones Criteria

The Major Criteria for RF are polyarthritis, carditis, rheumatic chorea, erythema marginatum, and erythema nodosum.

Arthritis

Major joints, when affected, are involved bilaterally and it is an aseptic arthritis. The joints swell and become extremely painful. Recovery of one set of joints is associated with involvement of another set of joints. Once recovery occurs, there is no residual joint deformity.

This type of arthritis is called *fleeting polyarthritis* because of the moving pattern of joint involvement. The polyarthritis is aggressively treated with pain medications, until resolution occurs within a few weeks. Rheumatic arthritis is seen commonly in children.

Carditis

All three layers of the heart can get involved with RF. The endocardium is the most frequently affected layer of the heart. Fibrosis of the valves can lead to stenosis (narrowing) or incompetence (widening).

When the blood passes through a stenosed valve it causes turbulence in blood flow, resulting in a heart murmur. With valvular incompetence the blood regurgitates back into the heart chamber above and this also causes turbulance and a heart murmur.

Mitral stenosis (MS) and mitral incompetence (MI) are common RF-associated valvular lesions, in children. Aortic stenosis (AS) and aortic incompetence (AI) are common lesions seen in adults. The most affected heart valve is the mitral valve and the least affected heart valve is the pulmonic valve. As per the **new 2007** American Heart Association (AHA) guidelines, RF-associated heart valve damage/lesions **no longer** need premedication with antibiotics prior to dentistry. Premedication is, however, **needed** if any of the damaged heart valves are replaced with **prosthetic valves**.

Involvement of the myocardium is rare, but if it occurs it presents as cardiomyopathy. Patients with cardiomyopathy also do not need to be premedicated any more, per the new 2007 AHA guidelines.

Pericardial involvement occurs more frequently in children than adults, and pericardial effusion (fluid collection in the pericardial sac) is the most common form of presentation. Pericardial involvement also no longer needs premedication prior to invasive dental treatments, per the 2007 AHA guidelines.

Rheumatic Chorea/Sydenham's Chorea/St. Vitus' Dance

Rheumatic chorea occurs exclusively in children. It causes involuntary, jerky movements involving the face and the upper extremities. These movements are absent when the child sleeps but are exacerbated with emotional disturbance. Rheumatic chorea affects females more frequently and the condition improves as the child grows. **Stress management** during dentistry is extremely **helpful** for these patients.

Erythema Marginatum

Erythema Marginatum is a rash that occurs in only 10% of patients affected with RF. Erythema Marginatum is characterized by a doughnut-shaped (pale center, dark margins) serpegineous rash that occurs on the trunk and upper limbs. As the rash migrates upward from the lower trunk area, the lower rash starts to disappear. This rash, which is more frequently seen on light-skinned than dark-skinned individuals, is diagnostic of RF when present.

Erythema Nodosum/Subcutaneous Nodules/Aschoff's Bodies

Erythema Nodosum/subcutaneous nodules are pea-sized, painless nodules. They recur periodically on bony areas of the elbows, wrist, and shins.

Minor Jones Criteria

Minor Jones Criteria are presented in the following sections.

Fever

Moderately high fever is common.

Arthralgia

Patients experience recurrent joint pains but there is no joint swelling or deformity.

Pain in the Right Upper Quadrant (RUQ) of the Abdomen

Liver enlargement/engorgement occurs when RF precipitates congestive heart failure (CHF). This causes pain in the RUQ of the abdomen.

Elevated ESR

Elevated erythrocyte sedimentation rate (ESR) is seen commonly with RF and it indicates acute inflammation. ESR measures the levels of globulin and fibrinogen in the blood. A decreasing ESR during the management phase indicates that the patient is responding to the treatment and that the inflammation is resolving.

Increased WBC Count

Leukocytosis occurs in response to the acute inflammation associated with RF.

Increased C-Reactive Protein

Increased C-reactive protein titer is a marker that identifies a recent β hemolytic streptococcal infection.

Elevated Anti-Streptolysin O (ALSO) Titer

Rising ASLO titer is a strong marker for RF.

EKG Changes

RF-associated myocardial involvement is associated with EKG changes. Cardiac conduction can be affected with RF.

RHEUMATIC FEVER (RF) DIAGNOSIS

To confirm the diagnosis of RF, the patient must have at least two Major or one Major plus two Minor Jones criteria present.

Rheumatic Fever (RF) Treatment

RF treatment is a two-phased treatment.

RF Acute Phase Treatment

Pain medications and steroids are aggressively used to counteract the intense pain and inflammation associated with acute RF.

Rheumatic Fever (RF) Secondary Prevention Treatment

Once the primary RF attack has resolved, future attacks of RF are prevented by maintaining uninterrupted low-dose antibiotic levels in the patient for the next 5 years. This prevents invasion of the β hemolytic streptococcus. The nonpenicillin allergic patient gets 1.2 million units benzathine penicillin G IM (intramuscularly), once per month for 5 years. Each injection provides a low concentration of the antibiotic for 4 weeks. Penicillin-allergic patients are given erythromycin or azythromycin (Zithromax), 250 mg/day × 5 years.

Infective Endocarditis and Current Premedication Prophylaxis Guidelines

INFECTIVE ENDOCARDITIS

Overview

Infective endocarditis is a condition associated with microbial infection of the endocardial surface of the heart. The valves are particularly affected with vegetation that contains bacteria, platelets, and inflammatory cells. Infective endocarditis can present as acute bacterial endocarditis (ABE) or subacute bacterial endocarditis (SBE).

Infective endocarditis is prevented by premedicating the patient prior to dentistry, when premedication is called for or required. Premedication provides a high level of antibiotic in the blood **prior** to the dental procedure and helps destroy any bacteria that enter the bloodstream during invasive dentistry.

Acute Bacterial Endocarditis (ABE)

ABE is an aggressive type of endocarditis with galloping symptoms. It occurs within about 7 days of an invasive dental procedure done without premedication, when premedication is required. ABE is common in the elderly and in IV drug users. Staphylococcus aureus, viruses, and fungii are the most common offending organisms causing ABE.

Subacute Bacterial Endocarditis (SBE)

SBE is the most common form of infective endocarditis, and streptococcus viridans is the most common offending organism. Symptoms and signs usually present insidiously within 2–3 weeks after an invasive dental procedure done without premedication, when premedication is required. SBE presentation can also occur 2–3 months later.

Infective Endocarditis Clinical Features

It is quite common for patients to experience "flulike" symptoms, at the start of the endocarditis. The symptoms with ABE are rapidly progressive; those associated with SBE are gradual in onset. Fever, anorexia, malaise, weight loss, night sweats, salmon-colored urine or hematuria, conduction abnormalities, new valvular regurgitation, and CHF are common findings associated with infective endocarditis.

Splinter hemorrhage of the fingernails, Roth's spots (retinal hemorrhages), Osler's nodes (painful red bumps on the fingertips), and Janeway lesions (nontender hemorrhagic nodules on the palms and soles) are common peripheral signs associated with infective endocarditis.

Infective Endocarditis Treatment

Any patient presenting with ABE or SBE is immediately hospitalized for treatment of the systemic infection and associated vital organ involvements. A maximum of three blood cultures are obtained to determine the offending organism (bacterial/viral/fungus), and the specific infection is aggressively treated for 2–3 weeks with IV antibiotics (penicillin plus gentamycin or vancomycin in the penicillin-allergic patient); antivirals; or antifungals, dependent on the outcome of the blood cultures.

Symptomatic care is additionally provided for the associated symptoms and vital organ involvements (heart and kidneys). Postrecovery, all patients with a past history of infective endocarditis (ABE or SBE) must be premedicated prior to all invasive dental procedures, per the 2007 American Heart Association (AHA) guidelines. Any antibiotic listed in the AHA premedication guideline protocol can be used, depending on the patient's allergy status (Table 21.1).

PREMEDICATION PROPHYLAXIS

Conditions That Require AHA Premedication Prophylaxis

- Prosthetic heart valves
- Past history of infective endocarditis
- Unrepaired or incompletely repaired cyanotic congenital heart disease, including those with palliative shunts or conduits
- A completely repaired congenital heart defect with prosthetic material or device, during the first 6 months after the procedure. Epithelial overgrowth of the graft material usually occurs within the first 6 months of repair.
- Any repaired congenital heart defect with persistent residual defect at the site or adjacent to the site of a prosthetic patch or a prosthetic device
- Cardiac transplant patients who develop heart valve–associated problems.
- Systemic intracranial hydrocephalic shunt: ventriculoatrial (VA) or ventriculovenous (VV).
- Systemic hemodialysis shunts (arteriovenous catheter or arteriovenous synthetic graft shunt): Do not monitor the blood pressure or draw blood from the arm with the shunt.
- Peritoneal dialysis: Only patients with an indwelling catheter.
- Synthetic graft materials (Dacron, Teflon, etc.) when used for **extracardiac** vascular repairs. Epithelial overgrowth of the graft material is never 100%, and some areas may stay denuded and promote infective endocarditis.
- Patients receiving cancer drugs through an infuse port or a Hickman catheter line
- Patients with a history of cirrhosis and associated **ascites** need to be premedicated as per AHA guidelines. The ascitic fluid can promote bacterial growth and increase the risk for infective endocarditis.
- **Prosthetic Joints:** Premedication is required for the first 2 years following joint replacement. Premedication **beyond** the first 2 years of joint replacement is needed for patients with the following:

Table 21.1. 2007 American Heart Association (AHA) recommended antibiotic prophylaxis regimen

Recommended Regimens for Dental Procedures

Standard Regimen:
Amoxicillin (Amoxil, Trimox, Wymox, etc.):
Adults: 2.0 g PO (oral), 1 h before the procedure
Children*: 50 mg/kg PO, 1 h before the procedure

Patients Unable to Take Oral Medications:
Ampicillin:
Adults: 2.0 g intramuscular (IM) or intravenous (IV) 30 min before the procedure
Children: 50 mg/kg IM or IV 30 min before the procedure
OR
Cefazolin (Ancef) or Ceftriaxone (Rocephin):
Adults: 1 g IM or IV 30 min before the procedure
Children: 50 mg/kg IM or IV 30 min before the procedure

Amoxicillin/Penicillin–Allergic Patients:
Clindamycin (Cleocin):
Adults: 600 mg PO (oral), 1 h before the procedure
Children: 20 mg/kg PO 1 h before the procedure
Cephalexin (Keflex)**
Adults: 2.0 g oral 1 h before the procedure
Children: 50 mg/kg oral 1 h before the procedure
Azithromycin (Zithromax) or Clarithromycin (Biaxin):
Adults: 500 mg oral 1 h before the procedure
Children: 15 mg/kg oral 1 h before the procedure

Penicillin-Allergic Patient Unable to Take Oral Medications:
Cefazolin (Ancef) or Ceftiaxone (Rocephin)**
Adults: 1.0 g IV or IM 30 min before the procedure
Children: 50 mg/kg IM or IV 30 min before the procedure
Systemic Clindamycin:
Adults: 600 mg IV 30 min before the procedure
Children: 20 mg/kg IV 30 min before the procedure

*Total children's dose should **not** exceed adult dose.
**Avoid Cephalosporins in patients with immediate-type hypersensitivity/acute anaphylaxis reaction to Penicillin.

1. Congenital or acquired immunocompromised states: diabetes, HIV/AIDS, chemotherapy or radiotherapy, malignancy
2. Chronic joint diseases: rheumatoid arthritis, lupus arthritis, or osteoarthritis
3. Multiple joint prosthesis history
4. Past history of joint prosthesis infection
5. Congenital bleeding disorders: hemophilias, VWD
6. Chronic skin conditions associated with open sores (psoriasis/eczema: distant source of infection propogation)
7. Severe periodontal disease: local source of infection propagation

Conditions That Do Not Require AHA Premedication Prophylaxis

- All types of atrial septal defects: primum or secundum atrial septal defect (ASD)
- Ventricular septal defect (VSD)
- Hypertrophic cardiomyopathy
- Mitral valve prolapse, with or without regurgitation
- Rheumatic heart disease
- Bicuspid valve disease
- Calcified aortic stenosis
- No premedication is required **after** the first 6 months for atrial septal defect (ASD), ventricular septal defect (VSD), or patent ductus arteriosus (PDA) repairs.
- Coronary artery bypass surgery
- Extracranial hydrocephalic shunt: ventriculoperitoneal (VP) shunt
- Severe anemia, hyperthyroidism, or multiple pregnancies–associated functional systolic murmur
- Cardiac pacemakers or defibrillators
- Phen-fen–associated heart valve damage
- Arteriovenous fistula for hemodialysis

As is evident from the 2007 AHA guidelines, many patients who were previously premedicated **now do not** need the antibiotic coverage. It is suggested you always confirm the cessation of premedication with the patient's physician prior to initiation of dentistry without antibiotic coverage.

Note: There will still be an occasional patient for whom the physician may want to continue with the premedication to prevent infective endocarditis, in spite of the new guidelines.

PROSTHETIC CARDIAC VALVES

There are two types of prosthetic/artificial valves: bioprosthetic valves and mechanical/metal valves. Both of these valves require endocarditis prophylaxis prior to invasive dentistry as per the 2007 AHA guidelines.

Bioprosthetic Valves

Bioprosthetic valves come from three sources: pig, bovine, or human cryopreserved heart valves. The pig valves have a shorter lifespan compared to the bovine valves and, in comparison, the human cryopreserved heart valves have the longest lifespan. The bioprosthetic valves in general have a low risk for clot formation.

Calcium deposition and consequent calcification and hardening of the valves accounts for the decreased longevity of the bioprosthetic valves compared to the mechanical valves. The average life-span of the pig and bovine bioprosthetic valves is approximately 10 years; it is longer than 10 years for the human valves. All bioprosthetic valves require **uninterrupted** blood thinning with warfarin (Coumadin) in the initial 3–6 months and then the patient with pig or bovine valve prosthesis is switched to daily aspirin. The human prosthetic valves **do not** require any blood thinning with aspirin beyond the initial 3–6-month postoperative period.

It is best to **delay** routine dental treatment for the time the patient has to be on the **uninterrupted** anticoagulation. When treatment has to be done during the first 3–6 months, either be conservative or consult with the patient's physician, who may then decide to switch the patient to IV or low molecular weight heparin. Premedication is needed prior to invasive dentistry for **all types** of bioprosthetic valves.

Mechanical Valves

Mechanical valves last about 20 years and have a high risk for clot formation. Lifetime anticoagulation with warfarin (Coumadin) is standard with the mechanical valves. Accordingly, when major or minor surgery is needed, the patient will have to be switched from Coumadin to heparin. It is best to plan one or two procedures at a given time to minimize the need for frequent switches.

JOINT PROSTHESIS

Joint Prosthesis Overview and Facts

The American Dental Association (ADA) and the American Academy of Orthopedic Surgeons (AAOS) advisory statement "Antibiotic prophylaxis for dental patients with total joint replacements," clearly states that **all** patients must be premedicated during the **first two years** of getting a joint prosthesis, and premedication can be discontinued for the healthy patient beyond the initial 2 years. Premedication beyond the initial 2 years of the prosthesis, for invasive procedures, should be continued for patients with systemic diseases associated with decreased immunity due to HIV/AIDS, diabetes, radiotherapy, or chemotherapy; chronic joint diseases associated with rheumatoid arthritis, osteoarthritis, or systemic lupus erythematosus; past history of prosthetic joint infection; history of hemophilia A/B, VWD, and other congenital bleeding disorders; malnourishment; or malignancy. It is suggested that patients with a peripheral site of chronic skin infection (oozing eczema/bleeding dermatitis) or patients with poor dental status and moderate to severe periodontal disease also be premedicated beyond the standard 2 years to prevent joint prosthesis infection. Bacteremias can infect the artificial joint and cause rejection. The consequence of joint prostheses infection far outweigh the risk for antibiotic prophylaxis. Always consult with the orthopedic surgeon regarding prophylaxis so you can optimally protect your patient. According to the advisory statement mentioned above, extractions, periodontal surgery, implants, endodontic surgery beyond the apex, cleaning, placement of orthodontic bands, and intraligamentary and intraosseous injections are dental procedures linked to a high risk of bacteremia.

The taking of impressions in a partially edentulous patient should also be added to this list because the impression material can often lodge between the teeth and cause mucosal tears as the impression is removed.

Joint Prosthesis Premedication Antibiotic Selection Criteria

Studies have shown staphylococcus aureus to be the most common offending organism involved with infections of the prosthetic joint. Streptococci have been isolated on occasion. Staphylococcus aureus is often resistant to penicillin. Amoxicillin is **not** as efficient at providing prophylaxis against staphylococcus aureus compared to the oral penicillinase-resistent penicillin (Dicloxacillin), Augmentin, cephalosporins (Cephalexin/Keflex, Cephadroxyl/Duricef or Cephazolin/Ancef), the newer macrolides (Azithromycin, Clarithromycin) or clindamycin. The AHA recommended dose of cephalosporins, macrolides, and clindamycin should be used for premedication of patients with joint prostheses. Some orthopedic surgeons occasionally recommend the use of Augmentin or Dicloxacillin or Keflex/Cephalexin for an extended 2–3 days period of prophylaxis, before and after the procedure. Communicate with the surgeon in such cases to understand why this altered guideline is needed for the patient. The patient may have multiple joint prostheses or may have some additional underlying factors known to the surgeon that make such a patient a high risk requiring an altered regimen.

Patients with pins and plates do not need to be premedicated. Some orthopedic surgeons, however, premedicate a patient with multiple pins and plates and here, too, confirm the need by directly communicating with the surgeon to understand the need.

SUGGESTED DENTAL GUIDELINES IN THE PRESENCE OF PREMEDICATION PROPHYLAXIS

The following are dental guidelines for premedication prophylaxis:

1. When successive appointments are planned for a patient needing premedication with one specific antibiotic for all visits, the appointments must be spaced **7 days apart** to allow for the regrowth of antibiotic-susceptible flora and prevent any bacterial resistance to the premedication antibiotic. The streptococcus viridans can get resistant when the same antibiotic is given more frequently or when given less than 7 days apart.
2. Plan more than one procedure to minimize antibiotic use.
3. Patients who need SBE prophylaxis should have good oral hygiene. Have the patient **gently rinse for 30 sec** with any mouthwash or use chlorhexidine. Rinsing the mouth prior to treatment will degerm the oral cavity and minimize the bacteremia.
4. Avoid aggressive gingival irritation and repeat prolonged use of chlorhexidine during visits, because this will increase the population of resistant bacteria.
5. Acutely infected teeth must be extracted 10–14 days prior to any planned cardiac/ major surgery to prevent SBE. The 10–14 days provides adequate time for healing to occur.
6. Use amoxicillin/azithromycin/clindamycin alternatively if appointments are necessary at intervals shorter than 7 days. Always make certain that the required gap of 7 days is maintained for each class of antibiotic. As an example, use amoxicillin on day 1, switch to azithromycin on day 3, switch to clindamycin on day 6, and go back to amoxicillin again on day 9. This protocol will effectively maintain the required interval. Use this protocol **only** when you think you really need it.

    Try scheduling the patient no more than twice per week because there is always the risk of intestinal flora washout with the high premedication dosages.
7. Recommend simultaneous use of probiotics or acidophilus/yogurt drinks when prescribing antibiotics because this will definitely help maintain the intestinal flora.
8. For patients who want to come in once per week for dental care and do not mind longer appointments for the day, you can schedule such a patient using the following protocol:

a. In a dental school setting you can have the patient for a morning 9:00am and an afternoon 1:00pm appointment. If you schedule a procedure associated with bleeding in the morning and a supragingival procedure in the afternoon, you need to premedicate the patient only **once**, 1 hr prior to the start of the first appointment. If both the procedures are going to be associated with bleeding, you need to give an additional **half-dose** of the premedication antibiotic prior to the 1:00pm appointment and proceed without waiting for an hour. There is no need to wait after the second dose because the second dose provides merely a boost for the morning dose of the antibiotic.

b. In a private practice setting, one single dose of premedication can provide sufficient antibiotic coverage for 5–6 hr and that would be sufficient time for more than one procedure!

9. Coinfection in a premedicated patient can be treated in one of two ways:

a. Use the **same antibiotic** for premedication and the treatment of infection.

   Using the same antibiotic is much preferred and less confusing to the patient.

   Example: Give amoxicillin as premedication, 2.0 g PO 1 hr prior to treatment **followed** by amoxicillin 250/500 mg tid × 5 days, **starting** 6 hr after the 2.0 g amoxicillin intake. With this protocol you have to **change** the premedication antibiotic for the visits planned in the next 2–3 weeks because the streptococcus viridans will become resistant with the 5-day intake of amoxicillin. It takes about 2–3 weeks for a responsive oral flora to be reestablished and become sensitive to the same antibiotic. Thus amoxicillin can be used again for premedication in 2–3 weeks. It is important to remember that this protocol, using amoxicillin for treatment of infection can be implemented only if the patient has been symptomatic with the infection for **less** than 3 days. If the symptoms have lasted longer than 3 days, clindamycin is **the** antibiotic of choice for treatment of the infection.

b. Another option is available using a different antibiotic for premedication and treatment of infection:

   Example: Give amoxicillin for premedication and clindamycin for treatment of the infection; 6 hr after the intake of 2.0 g amoxicillin, start clindamycin 300 mg tid/qid for 5 days to treat the infection. No change in the premedication antibiotic is needed for subsequent dental visits with this protocol.

10. Before starting any dental treatment, always confirm with the patient that he/she has taken the premedication antibiotic. Occasionally the patient forgets to take the antibiotic. You might also forget to ask the patient whether the antibiotic was taken. You could complete a procedure associated with bleeding and realize this error subsequently. Giving the premedication antibiotic **within 2 hr** after the procedure will provide effective prophylaxis. Any prophylaxis after 2 hr will not be beneficial.

11. As discussed earlier in Chapter 20, "Rheumatic Fever (RF): Assessment, Analysis, and Associated Dental Management Guidelines," immediately after recovering from an acute RF attack the patient is given **secondary prevention treatment** with penicillin, erythromycin, or azithromycin.

   The streptococcus viridans or α-hemolytic streptococcus is constantly exposed to the antibiotic during this secondary prevention treatment phase and thus becomes resistant to the specific antibiotic. If premedication is needed during dentistry in this phase for reasons specified under conditions that call for premedication, always select an antibiotic that belongs to **another** family.

Because penicillin is bactericidal you will need to select a bactericidal premedication antibiotic. Due to the possibility of cross-resistance with the cephalosporins, it is best to select 600 mg clindamycin (bactericidal dose) for premedication. In the patient getting erythromycin/azithromycin for secondary prevention treatment, the only premedication antibiotic that can be used is 600 mg clindamycin. Always keep an interval of **6 hr** between the bacteriostatic erythromycin/azithromycin and the bactericidal dosed 600 mg clindamycin, because cidal and static drugs cannot be combined.

22

Hypertension and Target Organ Disease States: Assessment, Analysis, and Associated Dental Management Guidelines

HYPERTENSION

Hypertension Classification

Hypertension (Htn) is classified as primary/essential and secondary.

Primary/Essential Hypertension

Primary/essential hypertension is the most common type of hypertension and accounts for 95% of all cases presenting with high blood pressure. This type of hypertension has a genetic link and is often associated with cardiovascular risk factors, smoking, obesity, lipid problems, and diabetes. It is insidious in onset and is often asymptomatic in the early stages.

Secondary Hypertension

Secondary hypertension is always due to an underlying cause. Renovascular disease, renal artery stenosis, coarctation of the aorta, pheochromocytoma, Cushing's syndrome, thyroid or parathyroid disease, heavy alcohol consumption, chronic corticosteroid therapy, chronic NSAIDS therapy, or long-term oral contraceptive use can lead to secondary hypertension. The secondary hypertension patient experiences symptoms quite early on compared to the primary/essential hypertension patient, and the symptoms are more severe.

2003 VII JOINT NATIONAL COMMISSION'S HIGH BLOOD PRESSURE GUIDELINES FOR ADULTS AGED 18 YEARS AND OLDER

The following are high blood pressure guidelines from the 2003 VII Joint National Commission (see also Table 22.1).

1. Classification of Blood Pressure for Adults Aged 18 Years and Older
2. List of Major Risk Factors for Hypertension
3. List of Target Organ Damage/Clinical Cardiovascular Disease
4. Recommendations for Follow-Up Based on Initial Set of BP Readings for Adults

Table 22.1.   VII Joint National Commission (JNC-2003) blood pressure classification for adults aged 18 years and older*

Category/BP Staging	Blood Pressure Classification	
	Systolic, mmHg	Diastolic, mmHg
Normal	<120	<80
Pre-Hypertension	120–139	80–89
Stage I	140–159	90–99
Stage II	≥160	≥100
Stage III: DEFER DENTAL TREATMENT	≥180	≥110

*Based on the average of 2 or more readings taken at **each** of 2 or more visits after an initial screening, not taking BP medications and not acutely ill. When systolic and diastolic pressures fall into different categories, the higher category should be selected to classify the individual's blood pressure status. For instance, 154/82 mmHg should be classified as Stage 1, and 164/95 mmHg should be classified as Stage 2. Isolated systolic hypertension is defined as a systolic blood pressure of 140 mmHg or more and a diastolic blood pressure of less than 90 mmHg plus it is staged appropriately (e.g., 154/82 mmHg is defined as Stage 1 isolated systolic hypertension). In addition to staging hypertension on the basis of average blood pressure levels, the clinician should specify presence or absence of target-organ disease and additional risk factors. This specificity is important for risk classification and treatment.

* Smoking
* Dyslipidemia
* Diabetes mellitus
* Age >60 y
* Sex: Men and postmenopausal women
* Family history of cardiovascular disease: women <65 y or men <55 y

Figure 22.1.   Major risk factors for hypertension.

* Heart diseases
* Left ventricular hypertrophy
* Angina or prior myocardial infarction
* Prior coronary revascularization
* Heart failure
* Stroke or transient ischemic attack
* Nephropathy
* Peripheral arterial disease
* Retinopathy

Figure 22.2.   List of target organ damage/clinical cardiovascular diseases.

MAJOR RISK FACTORS FOR HYPERTENSION

Major risk factors for hypertension are listed in Figure 22.1.

Target Organ Damage/Clinical Cardiovascular Diseases

The target organ damage or clinical cardiovascular diseases that result from hypertension are listed in Figure 22.2.

Table 22.2. Blood pressure monitoring follow-up guidelines

Systolic	Diastolic	BP Monitoring Follow-Up Guidelines
<120 mmHg	**<80 mmHg**	Recheck in 2 years
120–139	80–89	Recheck in 1 year
140–159	90–99	Confirm within 2 months
≥160	≥100	Assess or refer to MD in 1 month.
≥180	≥110	Refer symptomatic patient to MD/ER immediately. Refer asymptomatic patient to MD within 1 week.

Blood Pressure Measurement Follow-Up Guidelines

Recommendations for follow-up based on the initial set of BP readings for adults is listed in Table 22.2.

Blood Pressure (BP) Monitoring and Hypertension-Related Facts

When monitoring the BP make sure that the patient has not smoked or had a caffeinated drink 30 min prior to measuring the BP, because this will erroneously **raise** the BP. If the patient has just consumed a heavy meal, it will erroneously record a **lower** BP reading.

Use an appropriate-sized cuff when recording the patient's BP. Use a pediatric/adult/thigh cuff to match the patient's arm size. When monitoring the BP, the patient's arm should be relaxed and supported over your arm or should be resting on the arm of the dental chair. The arm should be positioned such that the cuff is at the cardiac level. Allow a 5-min interval between BP measurements. Take an average of 2–4 readings to diagnose hypertension.

Elevated systolic blood pressure (SBP) and widened pulse pressure are associated with greater cardiovascular risk compared to the diastolic blood pressure (DBP). The pulse pressure (PP) is the difference between the SBP and the DBP. The normal PP is 40 mmHg.

Each increment of 20 mmHg SBP/10 mmHg DBP **doubles** the cardiovascular risk for the patient. More than two-thirds of elderly patients today are hypertensive. The high prevalence of obesity is largely responsible for the increased incidence of hypertension in both children and adults. Hypertension should be suspected during pregnancy if the patient presents with either an elevation of the SBP by 30 mmHg or an elevation of the DBP by 15 mmHg, when compared to the average BP reading obtained prepregnancy or prior to 20 weeks of pregnancy. It should also be suspected when you detect a BP reading **greater** than 140/90 mmHg, when no previous reading for the patient is known. Routine dental treatment **must be deferred** in patients presenting with Stage III hypertension. Refer immediately to the emergency room (ER) if the patient is experiencing new onset target organ damage (TOD): stroke, angina, MI, etc. For the Stage III asymptomatic patient contact the patient's physician and refer for immediate care **within 1 week**.

Postural/Orthostatic Hypotension

Always monitor the BP **prior** to dentistry in the upright and lying-down positions in patients giving a history of postural hypotension, and assist such a patient out of the chair following completion of dental treatment. Refer to Chapter 9, "Management of Medical Emergencies in the Dental Setting: Assessment, Analysis, and Associated Dental Management Guidelines," for discussion of etiology, prevention, and management of orthostatic hypotension.

Hypertension Treatment

Lifestyle modification to eliminate risk factors, weight loss, diet modification, and drugs are the main tools for treatment of hypertension (Table 22.3). The clinician's goal should be always to maintain the BP below 140/90 mmHg in all patients **except** the patient with chronic kidney disease and diabetes. In these patients the goal is to maintain the BP below 130/80 mmHg.

HYPERTENSION AND TARGET ORGAN DISEASE (TOD)

Hypertension can cause target organ disease (TOD) and thus affect the major circulations. Atherosclerosis, thrombosis, or arterial spasm due to long-standing hypertension can affect any one of the following circulations: cerebral, coronary, renal, or peripheral. Transient ischemic attack (TIA) or cerebrovascular accident (CVA) can occur with involvement of cerebral circulation. Involvement of coronary circulation can cause angina (stable, unstable) or myocardial infarction (MI). Involvement of the renal circulation can result in chronic renal failure (CRF). Involvement of the peripheral circulation affecting the medium-sized arteries of legs can cause intermittent claudication, which is associated with severe pain in the calves when walking briskly or walking uphill.

Presence or absence of TOD determines how the patient is faring with hypertension control. The patient's current BP readings and the current status of *each* major circulation must be *collectively* evaluated to ultimately decide **when** to proceed with dentistry and **what** anesthetics, analgesics, and antibiotics (AAAs) to use during dental care.

HYPERTENSION-ASSOCIATED SUGGESTED DENTAL GUIDELINES

Anesthetics and Hypertension

The following are dental guidelines for anesthetics and hypertension:

1. The decision about the type of LA that can be used in the hypertensive patient as stated above depends on the **average BP reading** obtained **and** the presence or absence of **end organ disease**.
2. Use xylocaine with epinephrine or 2% mepivacaine (Carbocaine) with 1:20,000 levonordefrin (NeoCobefrin), maximum 2 carpules if the patient is well controlled, has an ASA status I/II, and there is **no** underlying history of arrhythmias, TIA, CVA, unstable angina, or renal disease. Also, the patient should not be taking digoxin (Lanoxin).
3. As specified under the end organ circulation's discussions in the **subsequent** sections, epinephrine is contraindicated in any patient with a history of arrhythmias, unstable angina, chronic renal failure (CRF), TIA, recent CVA, intermittent claudication, digoxin, and ASA III/IV.
4. 4% Prilocaine HCL with 1:200,000 epinephrine (Citanest Forte) or 0.5% bupivacaine (Marcaine) with 1:200,000 epinephrine should be used in the mild hypertension patient with **no** end organ problems.

Table 22.3. Drug therapy for hypertension

Drug Category	Generic/Trade Name	Side Effects
I. Diuretics	**A:** **Thiazides:** Hydrochlorothiazide (Esidrex) Hydrochlorothiazide (Hydrodiuril) **B:** **Loop Diuretics:** Bumetanide (Bumex) Ethacrynic Acid (Edecrin) Furosemide (Lasix) **C:** **Potassium-Sparing Agents:** Spironolactone (Aldactone) Triamterene (Dyrenium) Amiloride (Midamor) **D:** **Combination Acting Agents:** Spironolactone + Hydrochlorothiazide/HCTZ Triamterene + HCTZ Amiloride + HCTZ	Hypokalemia Hypercholesterolemia Glucose intolerance or hyperglycemia Hyperuricemia Muscle spasm Hypomagnesemia
II. Adrenergic Inhibitors	**A:** **Peripheral Acting Agents:** Reserpine (Serpasil) Guanethidine (Ismelin) **B:** **Central Alpha Agonists:** Methyldopa (Aldomet) Clonidine (Catapres) **C:** **Alpha Blockers:** Prazosin (Minipress) Tetrazosin (Hytrin) Doxazosin (Cardura) **D:** **Beta Blockers**: **D-I:** **Selective beta blockers** Acebutolol (Sectral) Atenolol (Tenormin) Metoprolol (Lopressor) **D-II:** **Nonselective Beta Blockers** Propranolol (Inderal) Timolol (Biocadren) Pindolol (Viskenm) **E:** **Combined Alpha and Beta Blockers:** Labetalol (Normodyne) Labetelol (Trandate) Carvedilol (Coreg)	**A:** **Side effects** Sedation Nasal congestion Depression Orthostatic hypotension Diarrhea **B:** **Side effects:** Sedation Liver dysfunction Fever Autoimmune disorders Sedation Dry mouth Withdrawal hypertension **C:** **Side effects:** Postural hypotension mainly with first dose * Lassitude **D:** **Side effects:** Serious side effects: * Brochospasm: more with the nonselective drugs * Congestive heart failure * Masking of insulin-induced hypoglycemia * Depression Less serious SE: * Poor peripheral circulation * Insomnia * Bradycardia * Fatigue * Increased triglycerides * Decreased HDL-cholesterol **E:** **Side effects:** * Postural hypotension * Upset stomach * Beta-blocking side effects and masking of hypoglycemic symptoms

Table 22.3.   *Continued*

Drug Category	Generic/Trade Name	Side Effects
III. Vasodilators	**A: Direct Vasodilators:** Hydralazine (Apresoline) **B: Calcium Channel Blockers (CCBs):** Nifedipine (Procardia) Nifedipine (Procardia XL) Nifedipine (Adalat CC) Verapamil (Isoptin or Calan) Diltiazem (Cardizem) Diltiazem (Dilacor XR) Felodipine (Plendil) Nicardipine (Cardene) Nicardipine (Cardene SR) Isradipine (DynaCirc) **C: Angiotensin Converting Enzyme(ACE) Inhibitors:** Captopril (Capoten) Enalapril (Vasotec) Lisinopril (Zestril) Lisinopril (Prinivil) Fosinopril (Monopril) Ramipril (Altase) Moexipril (Univasc) Quinapril (Accupril)	**A: Side effects** Fluid retention Tachycardia Headaches **B: Side effects** Flushing Headache Gingival hyperplasia: most with Nifedipine Constipation Upset stomach Conduction defects **C: Side effects** Rash Loss of taste or metallic taste Dry hacking cough with all ACE-I **Rare side effects:** Leukopenia Proteinuria Angioneurotic edema **ACE-I Alert:** ACE inhibitors are contraindicated in pregnancy
IV **Angiotensin-II** **Receptor** **Blockers** **(ARBs)**	Losartan (Cozaar) Valsartan (Diovan) Irbesartan (Avapro) Candesartan (Atacand) Olmesartan (Benicar) Telmisartan (Micardis) Eprosartan (Teveten)	**ARB side effects:** No metallic taste or the dry hacking cough with ARBs May cause upset stomach, dizziness Contraindicated in pregnancy

5. 3% Mepivacaine HCL (Carbocaine) with no epinephrine should be used in the moderately hypertensive patient with **no** end organ problems.
6. 4% Prilocaine HCL (Citanest Plain) should be the **ONLY LA** used in the hypertensive pregnant patient.
7. Routine dental treatment is deferred if the patient has severe hypertension.

Cerebral Circulation Diseases TIAs and CVAs: Assessment, Analysis, and Associated Dental Management Guidelines

TRANSIENT ISCHEMIC ATTACKS (TIAs)

TIA is associated with temporary cerebral ischemia due to cerebral vascular spasm. No permanent brain damage occurs. Once the spasm is released the symptoms disappear. The symptoms last for a few seconds to a few minutes but occasionally they can last for a few hours. Resolution of symptoms occurs within 24 hr. Patients with a history of TIA have a 50–60% chance of progressing to CVA/stroke.

Acute TIA Attack Management

Please refer to Chapter 9, "Management of Medical Emergencies in the Dental Setting: Assessment, Analysis, and Associated Dental Management Guidelines," for a discussion on the etiology, clinical features, and management of an acute TIA attack.

TIA-Associated Suggested Dental Management Guidelines

The following are dental guidelines for TIA:

1. TIA patients could be on any one of the following blood thinners: aspirin, dipyridamole (Persantine), clopidogrel (Plavix), or Coumadin. Always consult with the M.D. to determine whether the drug or drugs can be temporarily discontinued prior to major surgery. When possible, Coumadin is usually stopped 48 hr prior to treatment and restarted the evening of surgery or the next day. The restart time depends on when the patient typically takes the warfarin (Coumadin). Aspirin, dipyridamole (Persantine), and clopidogrel (Plavix), when approved for stopping, can be stopped 7 days prior to treatment and restarted 1–2 days postoperatively.
2. **TIAs and Local Anesthetics (LAs):** 3% mepivacaine HCL (Carbocaine) or 4% prilocaine HCL (Citanest Plain) are the only LAs that can be used. No epinephrine containing LAs should be used at any time during dentistry because epinephrine promotes vasoconstriction and this in turn can trigger TIAs and consequent cerebral hypoxia.
3. **TIAs and Analgesics:** Regular or extra-strength acetaminophen (Tylenol) is safe. Tylenol with codeine, Tylenol with hydrocodone (Vicodin), or Tylenol with

oxycodone (Percocet) can also be used as long as you use them judiciously and dispense them for 2–3 days only.

4. **TIAs and Antibiotics:** No antibiotics are contraindicated with TIAs.

5. **TIAs and Stress Management:** The benzodiazepines—lorazepam (Ativan) or diazepam (Valium)—should be avoided because these drugs depress the respiratory center and can promote TIAs.

STROKE/CEREBROVASCULAR ACCIDENTS (CVA)

Obstruction of the cerebral circulation by a thrombus, embolus, or ruptured intracranial aneurysm can precipitate stroke. Stroke causes permanent neurological damage, usually affecting the contralateral side of the body.

Acute CVA Attack Management

Please refer to Chapter 9, "Management of Medical Emergencies in the Dental Setting: Assessment, Analysis, and Associated Dental Management Guidelines," for discussion of etiology, clinical features, and management of CVA.

CVA-Associated Suggested Dental Management Guidelines

The following are dental guidelines for CVA:

1. Stroke patients could be on blood thinners, such as aspirin, dipyradamole (Persantine), clopidogrol (Plavix), or Coumadin, postrecovery. Prior to major surgery, always consult with the patient's physician to determine whether and when the blood thinners can be stopped and subsequently restarted.

2. Following a CVA that required significant hospitalization, routine dental treatment must be **delayed by 6 months**.

3. Routine dental treatment should be **delayed by 3 months** if the post-CVA recovery was uneventful and the patient was admitted overnight just for observation.

4. **CVA and Local Anesthetics:** Avoid epinephrine containing LAs during the **first 6 months** of dental treatment. Subsequent use of epinephrine depends on the patient's prognosis. Epinephrine containing LAs can be used starting 1 year after the stroke, when the patient demonstrates progressive improvement of the CVA and absence of TIAs.

5. **CVA analgesics, antibiotics, and stress management:** The guidelines are the same as those with TIAs.

Coronary Circulation Diseases, Classic Angina and Myocardial Infarction: Assessment, Analysis, and Associated Dental Management Guidelines

24

Angina and myocardial infarction (MI) can occur with involvement of the coronary circulation. Hypertension causes narrowing of the coronary arteries and when the patient is involved in an activity these narrowed arteries are unable to supply adequate nutrition and oxygenation to the heart, thus leading to angina. Hypertension-associated angina is classic angina and it can be stable or unstable.

ANGINA

Stable Angina

Stable angina is always brought on by activity; it happens infrequently and it is always controlled immediately with 1–3 nitroglycerine (NTG) pills.

Unstable Angina

Progressive worsening of stable angina over time can lead to the development of unstable angina. A change occurs in the ASA status from ASA II to ASA III. The patient does not need much activity at this stage to trigger an attack. The coronary arteries are narrowed quite significantly. The patient is on daily isosorbide (Isordil) or the patient uses a daily nitroglycerine patch to control the unstable angina. NTG pills are additionally used during an attack. Isosorbide (Isordil) is a long-acting nitrate and a very potent vasodilator.

Acute Angina Attack

Please refer to Chapter 9, "Management of Medical Emergencies in the Dental Setting: Assessment, Analysis, and Associated Dental Management Guidelines," for discussion of etiology, clinical features, and management of stable and unstable angina attacks.

Angina Pectoris–Associated Suggested Dental Guidelines

Anesthetics for Stable Angina

Local anesthetics with or without epinephrine can be used. Use maximum 2 carpules of 2% lidocaine (Xylocaine), 0.5% bupivacaine (Marcaine), 4% prilocaine HCL (Citanest Forte), 3% mepivacaine (Carbocaine), 4% prilocaine HCL (Citanest Plain), 4% septocaine

(Articaine), or 2% mepivacaine (Carbocaine) with 1:20,000 levonordefrin (NeoCobefrin).

Anesthetics for Unstable Angina

Avoid LAs with epinephrine.

Analgesics and Antibiotics for Angina Pectoris

There are no analgesics or antibiotics contraindicated per se with stable or unstable angina; however, be discreet in prescribing narcotic analgesics in the unstable angina patient.

Angina Stress Management

Benzodiazepines or $O_2 + N_2O$ can be used for stress management in the stable angina patient. Benzodiazepines are contraindicated in the unstable angina patient, and you should use only $O_2 + N_2O$ in these patients. Prophylactic use of NTG/Isordil is advised in anticipation of stress for the unstable angina patient.

Prinzmetal's Angina

Prinzmetal's angina is due to coronary artery spasm. This angina is more common in females, often affecting the type A personality woman. Prinzmetal's angina occurs mostly at rest and is often cyclical. It can occur continuously for a period of time and then disappear.

Prinzmetal's Angina Symptoms and Signs

Symptoms and signs are similar to stable angina.

Prinzmetal's Angina Medical Management

Nifedipine (Procardia), a Ca^{+2} channel blocker is the treatment of choice; 10 or 20 mg Procardia SL (sublingual) helps relieve the spasm.

Prinzmetal's Angina Anesthetics, Analgesics, Antibiotics, and Stress Management Suggested Dental Guidelines

Determine the severity of Prinzmetal's angina along with the ASA status of the patient, and then follow the guidelines as outlined for classic angina.

MYOCARDIAL INFARCTION

Myocardial infarction (MI) is a consequence of complete obstruction in the coronary artery blood supply to the heart resulting in death of the myocardium beyond the obstruction.

Acute Myocardial Infarction Attack

Please refer to Chapter 9, "Management of Medical Emergencies in the Dental Setting: Assessment, Analysis, and Associated Dental Management Guidelines," for discussion of etiology, clinical features, and management of myocardial infarction (MI) attack.

MI Diagnosis Confirmation in a Hospital Setting

In the hospital setting the diagnosis of a suspect case of MI is confirmed with analyses of the clinical presentation, specific EKG findings (most commonly ST segment elevation, T wave inversion, new bundle-branch blocks), and specific laboratory test results indicating myocardial injury—elevated SGOT, LDH, creatine kinase (CK), Troponin I and T.

In-Hospital MI Reperfusion Management

The confirmed MI cases are immediately triaged for reperfusion with thrombolytic drugs and/or surgical reperfusion options.

MI Management with Thrombolytic Drugs

Thrombolytic drugs, streptokinase, or recombinant tissue plasminogen activator (rTPA) are most effective when given in the first 2 hr of the MI. IV heparin, LMWH, aspirin, and clopidogrel (Plavix) are additional blood thinners used for the care of MI.

Surgical Reperfusion Options Post-MI

Percutaneous coronary interventions (PCI) via cardiac catheterization (formerly called *angioplasty, percutaneous transluminal coronary angioplasty* [*PTCA*], or *balloon angioplasty*), laser angioplasty, stents, or coronary artery bypass graft (CABG) surgery are invasive surgical treatment options commonly used to reperfuse the myocardium.

Stents Post-MI

Two kinds of stents are used during angioplasty: bare metal stents and drug-eluting stents (DES). Bare metal stents require **uninterrupted** antiplatelet activity with aspirin and Plavix for a minimum period of **6 weeks** and drug-eluting stents (DES) require Plavix and aspirin **uninterrupted** for a minimum period of **6 months**.

Coronary Artery Bypass Post-MI

Bypass rates have gone down because of the high success rates of PCI. The internal mammary artery or the long saphenous vein grafts are used for bypass surgery. Bypass surgery patients do not need premedication prior to dentistry.

MI Management Post–Acute Phase Recovery

Once recovered, the MI patient is maintained on aspirin and/or clopidogrel (Plavix), beta blockers, ACE inhibitors, and cholesterol-lowering drugs to prevent future myocardial infarction attacks.

Myocardial Infarction–Associated Complication: CHF and Cardiac Arrythmias

Complications associated with MI are congestive heart failure (CHF) and cardiac arrythmias. MI causes structural changes that affect the proper filling and pumping of the heart, leading to CHF. CHF can also be due to worsening severe anemia, anorexia, or thyrotoxicosis where the failure occurs because of a hyperdynamic circulation caused by the underlying disease state. Worsening cardiac disease or worsening pulmonary disease can also lead to CHF.

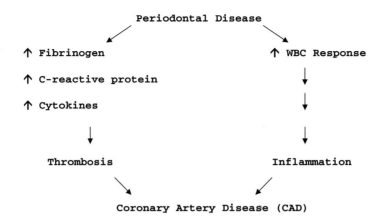

Figure 24.1. Periodontal disease and coronary artery disease link.

Dental Disease and Myocardial Infarction (MI) Link

Periodontal inflammation is associated with increased levels of fibrinogen, C-reactive protein (CRP), and cytokines. Extensive research has shown that inflammation is an important step in the formation of atherosclerotic plaques. The link between periodontal disease and coronary artery disease (CAD) has been extensively discussed in the literature; this link is schematically illustrated in Figure 24.1.

MYOCARDIAL INFARCTION (MI)–ASSOCIATED SUGGESTED DENTAL GUIDELINES

The following are dental guidelines for MI:

1. It is worth scheduling frequent hygiene recalls every 3–4 months for patients with severe periodontal disease and/or coronary artery disease.
2. In patients with significant cardiac disease (ASA III/IV or patients on lanoxin/ digoxin, isosorbide/isordil, or nitroglycerine patch), minimize stress and avoid the use of vasoconstrictors in the local anesthetics.
3. Delay routine dental treatment post-MI, by **6 months** if the patient has had a massive MI that required significant hospitalization.
4. Delay dental treatment post-MI, by **3 months** for a patient with minimal MI that might have needed overnight or short-term hospitalization for observation.
5. After stent placement, angioplasty, or CABG, the patient can be scheduled for routine dental procedure once daily activities have begun. This resumption of activity usually occurs within 2–4 weeks of the procedure.
6. As indicated earlier, bare metal stents require **uninterrupted** antiplatelet activity with aspirin and Plavix for a minimum period of **6 weeks** and drug-eluting stents (DES) require Plavix and aspirin **uninterrupted** for a minimum period of **6 months**. Planned dentistry has to accommodate the uninterrupted antiplatelet activity period.

   One way is to schedule minor procedures (amalgams, composites, or cleanings) causing minimal/no bleeding during the uninterrupted antiplatelet activity period; this care will not be affected with the aspirin and Plavix.

For major procedures you can incorporate one of two options. One is to schedule major procedures that can be done with the use of local hemostats to control the bleeding in the presence of aspirin and Plavix. Another way is to delay the major dental treatment needing the temporary interruption of aspirin and/or Plavix for a time **beyond** the above specified time periods.

7. Drug-eluting stents (DES) lately have been associated with an increased risk of thrombosis, compared to the bare metal stents. The drug-eluding stents have been found to prevent the regrowth of normal arterial tissue lining in immediate or close proximity to the stents, thus causing an increased incidence of thrombosis. Many cardiologists, for this reason, prefer using aspirin and Plavix for 1–2 years or indefinitely, depending on the patient's current medical status and bleeding history.

8. It's quite evident, therefore, for a dental practitioner always to consult with the patient's M.D. to determine whether the antiplatelet medications can be temporarily interrupted and **when**, in relation to the time of angioplasty or stents.

   Dependent on the patient's current cardiac status and risk for thrombosis, the M.D. could **extend** the above specified time lines for **uninterrupted** aspirin and Plavix intake. In such situations, when major surgery is needed, local hemostats and appropriate suturing should be utilized to minimize bleeding.

9. Stents do not require premedication. However, with the recent focus on the higher threat for thrombosis with stents, some cardiologists want their patients to receive premedication prior to dentistry.

10. During the early recovery period, patients with MI do best with shorter appointments scheduled in the morning.

11. **Anesthetics and MI:** Use 3% mepivacaine HCL (Carbocaine) without epinephrine or 4% prilocaine HCL (Citanest Plain) during the first 6 months of dental care. 0.5% bupivacaine (Marcaine) or 4% prilocaine HCL (Citanest Forte), both with 1:200,000 epinephrine, can be used subsequently, if the patient has been stable during the first 6 months of dental care. Remember, however, that this switch to local anesthetics with epinephrine is moot if the patient is on lanoxin (digoxin) following recovery from MI. According to the suggested guidelines set for digoxin, epinephrine is contraindicated.

12. High-risk patients should have questionable teeth extracted and removable prosthetic management provided.

13. Advanced periodontal surgery and complex fixed prosthetics are generally contraindicated.

Congestive Heart Failure (CHF): Assessment, Analysis, and Associated Dental Management Guidelines

CONGESTIVE HEART FAILURE (CHF) SYMPTOMS AND SIGNS

CHF Symptoms

The following are CHF symptoms:

1. **Orthopnea:** Orthopnea is the shortness of breath experienced on lying down. The patient therefore is always propped up in bed.
2. **Paroxysmal nocturnal dyspnea or "cardiac asthma":** Shortness of breath is experienced hours or minutes after lying in bed.
3. **Cough with frothy sputum:** Severe CHF compromises cardiac output and this leads to pulmonary congestion or edema. Significant pulmonary congestion causes cough with a frothy sputum expectoration.

CHF Signs

The following are CHF signs:

1. **Distended neck veins:** The forward flow of blood is compromised with CHF, causing a backup and consequent distention of the neck veins.
2. **Rales on auscultation:** Rales or coarse crackles on auscultation are heard in the base of both lungs and indicate the presence of fluid in the lungs.
3. **Functional systolic murmur:** CHF can be associated with a functional systolic murmur, and this murmur is corrected following treatment and recovery. This murmur is heard in the second left intercostal or pulmonic space on physical examination of the chest.
4. **Ankle edema** The compromised cardiac status causes a fluid collection in the peripheral tissues and **pitting** edema. Pitting edema can be confirmed by applying transient pressure with your thumb on the patient's edematous tissue on the feet. Transcient pressure leaves a dent, indicating fluid collection.

CONGESTIVE HEART FAILURE (CHF) MEDICAL MANAGEMENT

The type of CHF treatment implemented is dictated by the cause of CHF. The common drugs used in the management of CHF are diuretics, vasodilators, ACE inhibitors, beta blockers, and digoxin. CHF drug facts of importance to the dentist are outlined in the following sections.

Diuretics

Diuretics help deplete the excess fluid collection and correct the peripheral and pulmonary edema associated with CHF. Hypokalemia, hypocalcemia (muscle spasm), hypomagnesemia, hyperglycemia, hyperuricemia, and hypercholesterolemia are major side effects associated with the thiazide diuretics.

Vasodilators

ACE inhibitors and angiotensin II receptor blockers are used for the management of CHF. Dry cough and metallic taste in the mouth are frequent side effects associated with the ACE inhibitors. Hydralazine/Apresoline is another vasodilator that is used to treat moderate to severe CHF. Orthostatic hypotension, dizziness, light-headedness, or fainting spells may occur with the vasodilators.

Lanoxin (Digoxin)

Digoxin is a cardiac glycoside that helps a diseased heart function well. Digoxin is used to treat CHF; atrial fibrillation (AF), or supraventricular arrhythmias. Lanoxin (digoxin) has significant DDIs with the anesthetics, analgesics, and antibiotics (AAAs) used in dentistry. To determine what AAAs are safe to use with lanoxin (digoxin), it is important to know the drug's mechanism of action and the specific AAAs that negatively interact with it.

Please refer to Chapter 2, "History and Physical Assessment of the Medically Compromised Dental Patient (MCP)," plus Table 2.1 for information on digoxin and associated DDIs with the AAAs.

Digoxin and Hypokalemia

In addition to the medications listed in Table 2.1, digoxin toxicity can also be precipitated by hypokalemia. Always look for the symptoms and signs of hypokalemia in patients taking digoxin or thiazide diuretics. Hypokalemia may also be seen with prolonged vomiting or diarrhea or with laxative abuse. The normal Serum K^+ level is 3.5–5.5 mEq/L.

Hypokalemia Symptoms

Hypokalemia can be associated with muscle weakness, muscle fatigue, severe muscle pain, muscle cramps, and irregular heartbeat due to abnormal cardiac contraction.

Hypokalemia Treatment

A symptomatic hypokalemia patient can feel better drinking a cup of orange juice or eating a banana. If this does not prove to be effective the patient must seek medical care. Avoid dental treatment in the presence of symptomatic hypokalemia and refer the patient to the M.D.

Digoxin Toxicity

Digoxin overdose can cause nausea, vomiting, anorexia, blurring of vision, green or yellow halos, or green/yellow tinting of images and arrhythmias. Hypokalemia markedly increases the incidence of arrhythmias during digoxin toxicity.

Cardiac Arrhythmias: Assessment, Analysis, and Associated Dental Management Guidelines

CARDIAC ARRHYTHMIAS OVERVIEW

Cardiac arrhythmias can be an increase in heart rate, a decrease in heart rate, or an irregularity in heart rate. An increased heart rate can be associated with sinus tachycardia, atrial or supraventricular arrythmias, and ventricular arrythmias. When the heart rate is decreased the patient is said to have bradycardia.

Sinus Tachycardia

Sinus tachycardia is associated with a pulse rate above 100 beats/min and it occurs in response to stress, anxiety, excitement, or exercise. The patient experiences no prolonged symptoms and no treatment is required.

Atrial or Supraventricular Arrhythmias (AF)

Atrial arrythmias are seldom life threatening. The symptoms experienced with AF will depend on the severity of the arrhythmia. Common symptoms experienced are palpitations, light-headedness, dizziness, chest pain, shortness of breath (SOB), hypotension, CHF, syncope, or thrombosis-associated TIAs or CVAs. Thrombosis is often a complication of AF due to the chaotic beating of the heart. Drugs like warfarin (Coumadin), aspirin, or clopidogrel (Plavix) are often included in the management of AF for this reason, to prevent complications from emboli.

AF is frequently treated with cardiac glycosides (digoxin), calcium channel blockers (Diltiazam/Cardizam), or beta blockers (Metaprolol or Propranolol) that help slow down the heart rate. Quinidine or Amiodarone are used to treat refractory cases of atrial fibrillation (AF).

Atrial Fibrillation (AF) and Ablation Therapy

The most recent advances in the management of atrial fibrillation is ablation therapy of the ectopic foci in the atrial wall around the pulmonary vein or ablation of the AV node. The patient is up and about within a few days following the ablation therapy, which corrects the arrhythmia and allows for the discontinuation of the arrhythmia medications. Routine dental treatment can continue once the patient resumes normal activity.

Ventricular Arrhythmias

Ventricular arrhythmia and ventricular tachycardia (VT) are potentially life-threatening complications of MI. Electrical cardioversion, defibrillators, quinidine, procainamide, lidocaine, propranolol are often used to manage ventricular arrhythmias. Patients on procainamide may occasionally develop a lupus-like syndrome. An implantable defibrillator is often the choice to help restore normal sinus rhythm in patients with a high risk for ventricular fibrillation.

SUGGESTED DENTAL GUIDELINES FOR ARRHYTHMIAS

Suggested Dental Guidelines for Tachyarrhythmias

Consult with the M.D. and understand the nature of the arrhythmia. Provide stress management because it helps reduce the occurrence of exacerbation of arrhythmias. These patients do best with shorter appointments. Avoid epinephrine because it can precipitate life-threatening arrhythmias.

Bradycardia

Bradycardia is associated with a pulse rate <60 beats/min. A pulse rate <60 beats/min at rest can be physiological or pathological. Physically active individuals can have a slow heart rate or physiological sinus bradycardia due to daily exercise. Certain medications with increased parasympathetic effects like phenothiazines or digoxin can cause bradycardia. Beta blockers like propranolol and metaprolol decrease cardiac excitability and also cause bradycardia. Pathologically, cardiac conduction problems can be associated with bradycardia, and this is treated with an implanted pacemaker.

Bradycardia Symptoms

With significant bradycardia the patient can experience lightheadedness, dizziness, and fainting spells due to poor blood flow in the cerebral circulation. Diagnosis is confirmed with a Holter monitor.

Suggested Dental Guidelines for Patients with Bradycardia

The following are dental guidelines for bradycardia:

1. Consult with the M.D. and understand the severity of the bradycardia.
2. Provide stress management and have the patient in for shorter appointments.
3. Do not use a pulp tester, cavitron, or any other electrical device on patients with pacemakers. Electrical devices, when used in an adjacent operatory, must be at a distance beyond the pacemaker patient's outstretched arm span.

Peripheral Circulation Disease

Long-standing hypertension-associated involvement of the peripheral vascular circulation causes narrowing of the medium-sized arteries of the leg due to severe atherosclerosis.

PERIPHERAL CIRCULATION DISEASE–ASSOCIATED-SYMPTOMS

The patient experiences intermittent claudication or pain in the legs, calves, or feet while walking a few blocks or uphill. The narrowed vessels are not able to meet the tissue oxygen demand with activity, prompting the patient to stop. The patient often experiences relief of symptoms with rest.

PERIPHERAL CIRCULATION DISEASE–ASSOCIATED SIGNS

The patient's skin on the lower extremities will be shiny and show hair loss.

PERIPHERAL CIRCULATION DISEASE–ASSOCIATED SUGGESTED DENTAL GUIDELINE

The atherosclerosis is significant, causing a narrowing of the medium-sized arteries, and it is best to avoid epinephrine containing local anesthetics.

Renal Function Tests, Renal Disease, and Dialysis: Assessment, Analysis, and Associated Dental Management Guidelines

KIDNEY FUNCTION TESTS

Tests evaluated to assess kidney function are:

1. The serum creatinine
2. The creatinine clearance
3. The extent of proteinurea
4. The blood urea nitrogen (BUN)
5. The glomerular filtration rate (GFR)
6. Renal imaging

Serum Creatinine (S. Cr)

Creatinine is a waste product generated from muscle cell breakdown, and it is filtered out in the urine by the kidneys. As kidney function decreases, the serum creatinine levels rise. Diet can affect serum creatinine values, so it is best to estimate renal function by calculating the GFR. The normal s. creatinine in most labs is 0.4–1.2 mg/dL. In general, a patient is said to have a 50% **reduction** of kidney function when the serum creatinine is ≥1.7 mg/dL in men and ≥1.4 mg/dL in women.

It is safe to say that individuals with a serum creatinine of 2.0 mg/dL have moderate to severe decrease in GFR, regardless of the equation used to estimate GFR.

Creatinine Clearance (CrCl)

The creatinine clearance shows how well the kidneys are functioning. This test indicates **how efficiently** the kidneys can remove creatinine from the blood and pass it into the urine. The test compares the amount of urine creatinine in a 24-hr collection with the level of serum creatinine.

Creatinine Clearance Equation

$$\text{Cr. } Cl = \frac{\text{Urine Creatinine} \times \text{24-hr Urine Volume}}{\text{Plasma or Serum Creatinine}}$$

Creatinine clearance is measured as mL/min. The normal creatinine clearance is 80–130 mL/min.

Proteinurea

Another marker of kidney function is the presence of protein in the urine. Protein normally **does not** filter out of the kidneys. Healthy kidneys remove all wastes from the blood but do not remove protein. Diseased kidneys may fail to separate albumin from the wastes. Initially, only small amounts of albumin leak into the urine. This *micro-albuminuria* is an indication of deteriorating kidney function. As kidney function worsens, the amount of albumin and other proteins in the urine increases, resulting in proteinuria. A 24-hr urine collection measures the total amount of protein lost in the urine.

Blood Urea Nitrogen (BUN)

Urea is formed in the liver as a waste product when protein is broken down in the body. The urea is then eliminated in the urine. Blood urea nitrogen (BUN) measures the amount of **nitrogen** in the blood. The nitrogen comes from urea. BUN thus gives an estimate of how effectively the kidneys are removing urea from the blood. The normal BUN in most labs is 7–20 mg/dL.

Glomerular Filtration Rate (GFR)

The GFR shows how efficiently the kidneys are filtering wastes from the blood in normal and diseased patients. GFR is estimated by using the modification of diet in renal disease study group (MDRD) equation, which is based on the patient's age, weight, gender, race, and serum creatinine. Use the following site to calculate your patient's GFR:www.kidney.org/professionals/kdoqi/gfr_calculator.cfm

Serum creatinine-based estimation of GFR provides a basis for the classification of chronic kidney disease.

Glomerular Filtration Rate (GFR) and Staging of Chronic Renal Disease

The GFR is used to determine the severity of kidney disease and the five levels of severity or stages are:

Stage 1:	GFR $\geq$90 mL/min/1.73 m^2
Stage 2 (Mild):	GFR 60–89 mL/min/1.73 m^2
Stage 3 (Moderate):	GFR 30–59 mL/min/1.73 m^2
Stage 4 (Severe):	GFR 15–29 mL/min/1.73 m^2
Stage 5 (Kidney Failure):	GFR <15 mL/min/1.73 m^2

A patient is said to have chronic kidney disease when the GFR is <60 mL/min/1.73 m^2 for 3 months. As a conscientious provider, you must help prevent the progression of kidney disease by **using the appropriate AAAs** and insist that the patient control the associated diseases such as hypertension/diabetes that commonly cause chronic kidney disease.

Renal Imaging

Ultrasound, computed tomography (CT scan), and magnetic resonance imaging (MRI) are tools to detect unusual changes in the kidney structure or impairment in urinary flow.

DECREASED RENAL FUNCTION AND ASSOCIATED HEMATOLOGICAL CHANGES SIGNIFICANT FOR DENTISTRY

Every dental provider must be aware of the following hematological changes associated with decreased renal function:

1. **Anemia:** Anemia is caused by decreased erythropoietin production associated with kidney disease.
2. **Increased Potassium:** Decreased renal function is associated with an increase in the serum potassium level.
3. **Sodium:** The serum sodium level is **unchanged** with kidney disease but it could get altered with volume fluctuation.
4. **Increased Phosphate:** Increased phosphate level is a consequence of low level of 1,25 dihydroxy-D (active Vitamin D).
5. **Decreased Calcium:** Low calcium level is caused by low levels of 1,25 dihydroxy-D.
6. **Decreased Magnesium:** Kidney disease can decrease the magnesium level, and low magnesium often causes skeletal muscle soreness, tingling, and TMJ dysfunction.
7. **Prolonged Bleeding Time (BT):** Uremia causes decreased platelet cohesiveness and a prolongation of the bleeding time (BT).

HEMODIALYSIS AND PERITONEAL DIALYSIS

Dialysis Overview

Dialysis is a means to remove waste products and excess fluid from the blood on a regular basis when the patient's kidneys have failed and are nonfunctional. There are two main types of dialysis: hemodialysis and peritoneal. Patients with chronic renal failure may be on peritoneal dialysis or hemodialysis.

Hemodialysis

Hemodialysis treatments are typically done at a dialysis center through a **hemodialysis access** created in the patient's arm, leg, or neck. It is important that every provider know some important facts about the various forms of hemodialysis access to treat optimally and correctly these patients in the dental setting.

Hemodialysis Accesses

Hemodialysis access can be attained through an intravenous catheter, an arteriovenous (AV) fistula, or a synthetic graft. These accesses help connect the patient to the dialysis machine. These accesses are **not removed** when the kidney failure patient gets a renal transplant. Thus, the premedication requirements indicated for specific accesses pre-transplant, **must be followed** posttransplant also.

Intravenous Catheter Access

Intravenous catheter access is a **short-term access** and is typically reserved for immediate or sudden onset need for dialysis. This form of access is associated with catheter-induced infection and stenosis of the vasculature with the indwelling IV catheter. A patient with an **indwelling catheter** should always be **premedicated** prior to invasive dentistry.

Arteriovenous (AV) Fistula or Arteriovenous Synthetic Graft

The AV fistula and the synthetic graft are the **more permanent** forms of hemodialysis accesses. Both forms, however, have to **mature** before becoming available for hemodialysis.

The Arteriovenous (AV) Fistula

The arteriovenous (AV) fistula is the **most opted** mode of access. An artery and a vein are joined together through an anastomosis using the patient's own vasculature, and it takes an average of about 4–6 weeks for the fistula to mature. Fistulas are usually created in the arm and it is extremely important for the provider **not** to use that arm for BP monitoring or IV/IM injections. The AV fistula infection rate is low compared to the synthetic graft or the intravenous catheter, since no foreign material is used in its formation. The potential for thrombosis is also low with the AV fistulas. A patient with an AV fistula **does not** require premedication for invasive dental procedures. However, always confirm this fact with the patient's physician before you proceed with dentistry without premedication. Occasionally, the M.D. may want premedication with a "young" or newly forming fistula if the patient has severe periodontal infection.

Arteriovenous Synthetic Graft

An arteriovenous graft is almost like a fistula, except that synthetic material is used to join or link the artery and vein. An AV graft is created when the patient's blood vessels are not optimal and so do not allow the creation of a fistula. An AV graft matures faster than a fistula and it can be placed in the thigh or even in the neck. Grafts are associated with a higher risk for thrombosis and infection because of the use of synthetic material. The patient with an **AV graft** should always be **premedicated** prior to dentistry.

The patient gets dialyzed three times per week, and each dialysis session lasts 4 hr. IV heparin is administered during the first 3 hr of hemodialysis and 50% of the IV heparin is cleared at the end of the 4th hr of hemodialysis. Total heparin clearance occurs 5 hr after the **end** of the hemodialysis. You need to thus wait 5 hr posthemodialysis, if you plan on treating the patient on the day of hemodialysis. It is always best to treat these patients on the "off days" of dialysis.

Peritoneal Dialysis

Peritoneal dialysis is less efficient than hemodialysis and it is carried out at home by the patient using the portable peritoneal dialysis machine. This accounts for the peritoneal dialysis patient being a lot more mobile compared to the patient undergoing hemodialysis. The hemodialysis patient has to visit a dialysis center for dialysis to occur.

In peritoneal dialysis, the peritoneal membrane acts as a semipermeable membrane through which dialysis or exchange occurs. Premedication prophylaxis per se is not needed with peritoneal dialysis. However, in some cases the patient will need to be premedicated prior to invasive dentistry if there is an **indwelling catheter** for peritoneal dialysis.

The dialysate consists of a sterile solution of minerals and glucose. It is run through a tube into the peritoneal cavity where it is left for some time so the waste products can be absorbed. This waste product–containing fluid is then drained out through the tube and discarded. This exchange cycle is repeated 4–5 times during the day and/or overnight with an automated dialysis machine.

ANESTHETICS, ANALGESICS, ANTIBIOTICS, AND KIDNEY DISEASE

Longstanding daily use of painkillers composed of two or more analgesics (particularly acetaminophen and aspirin together) with caffeine or codeine are most likely to damage the kidneys (Table 28.1).

NSAIDS block prostaglandin (PG) formation. Vasodilator PG inhibition can impair glomerular filtration, especially in volume-depleted states. Acetaminophen has reactive metabolites that are neutralized by glutathione. Significant nephrotoxicity can occur when the neutralizing capacity of glutathione is taxed. Long-term use of NSAIDS and acetaminophen has been linked with an increased risk of end-stage renal disease (ESRD).

Table 28.1. Renal disease and dental drugs guidelines

Drugs: Generic/Trade	Suggestion(s)
ANESTHETICS	
2% Lidocaine (Xylocaine)	Use maximum 2 carpules. Use with Serum Creatinine <2.0 mg/dL.
2% Mepivacaine (Carbocaine) with 1:20,000 Levonordefrin (NeoCobefrin)	Use maximum 2 carpules. Use with Serum (S) Creatinine (Cr) <2.0 mg/dL.
3% Mepivacaine HCL (Carbocaine)	*The* LA with S. Cr. >2.0 mg/dL
4% Prilocaine HCL (Citanest Forte or Citanest Plain)	**Avoid Citanest** in the presence of **hypoxia** due to low Erythropoeitin.
4% Septocaine (Articaine)	**Avoid Articaine** in the presence of **hypoxia** due to low Erythropoeitin.
ANALGESICS	
Aspirin	**Predialysis:** Use normal dose. **Dialysis:** Avoid. **Best to avoid.**
NSAIDS **Acetaminophen (Tylenol)**	**Avoid NSAIDS.** 1. **CrCl >50 mL/min or S.Cr <2 mg/dL:** Dose normally: 325–650 mg q4–6h OR 1000 mg 3–4 times/day 2. **CrCl 10–50 mL/min or S.Cr >2 mg/dL to Predialysis:** Give 325–650 mg **q6h.** 3. **CrCl <10 mL/min or Dialysis:** Use 325–650 mg **q8h.** **Avoid extra strength Tylenol with S.Cr >2 mg/dL.**

Table 28.1. *Continued*

Drugs: Generic/Trade	Suggestion(s)
Codeine + Acetaminophen: (Tylenol #1–4)	1. **CrCl >50 mL/min or S.Cr <2 mg/dL:** Normal Codeine dose, 30–60 mg. Give 1–2 Tylenol #3 **q4h** PRN. 2. **CrCl 10–50 mL/min or S.Cr >2 mg/dL to Predialysis:** Use 50% dose of Codeine (15–30 mg). Dispense 1–2 Tylenol #2 **q6h** PRN. 3. **CrCl <10 mL/min or Dialysis:** Use 75% dose of Codeine (7.5–15 mg): 1–2 Tylenol #1 **q8h** PRN.
Propoxyphene (Darvon)	**Contraindicated.** Metabolites accumulate in ESRD (end-stage renal disease)
Meperidine (Demerol)	**Contraindicated** because metabolites accumulate in ESRD
Hydrocodone + Acetaminophen: (Vicodin)	**Predialysis:** Vicodin, 1 tab **q6h** PRN **Dialysis:** Vicodin, 1 tab **q8h** PRN
Oxycodone + Acetaminophen: (Percocet)	**Predialysis:** One 2.5/325 tab **q6h** PRN **Dialysis:** One 2.5/325 tab **q8h** PRN
ANTIBIOTICS	
Penicillin VK	1. **S. Cr <2.0 mg/dL:** Normal dose 2. **S. Cr >2.0 mg/dL to Predialysis:** Pen VK 250–500 mg **q8–12h** 3. **Dialysis:** Pen VK 250–500 **q12–16h**
Amoxicillin	1. **S.Cr <3.3 mg/dL:** Normal dose 2. **S.Cr >3.3 mg/dL to Predialysis:** 250–500 mg **q12h** 3. **Dialysis:** 250–500 **q24h**
Other Penicillins	Decrease dose by 50%.
Cephalosporins	Decrease dose by 50%.
Erythromycin	Safe but no longer used in dentistry.
Azithromycin (Zithromax)	Safe to use.
Clarithromycin (Biaxin): Best to **avoid**, but if needed, use the scripts listed.	1. **S. Cr. <3.3 mg/dL:** 250 mg **q12h.** 2. **S. Cr. >3.3 mg/dL to predialysis:** Give 125 mg **q12h.** 3. **Dialysis:** 125 mg **q24h**
Clindamycin (Cleocin)	No dose adjustment for renal failure.
Tetracycline HCl: Best to **avoid** with kidney disease. If absolutely needed *then* use the listed scripts	1. **S.Cr 1.25–2 mg/dL:** 250–500 mg **q8–12h** 2. **S.Cr 2 mg/dL to Predialysis:** 250–500 mg **q12–24h** 3. **Dialysis:** 250–500 mg **q24h**
Doxycycline (Vibramycin)	No dose change.
Diazepam (Valium) **Lorazepam (Ativan)**	Safe to use if the patient is on Erythropoeitin replacement therapy.

VII

Pulmonary Diseases

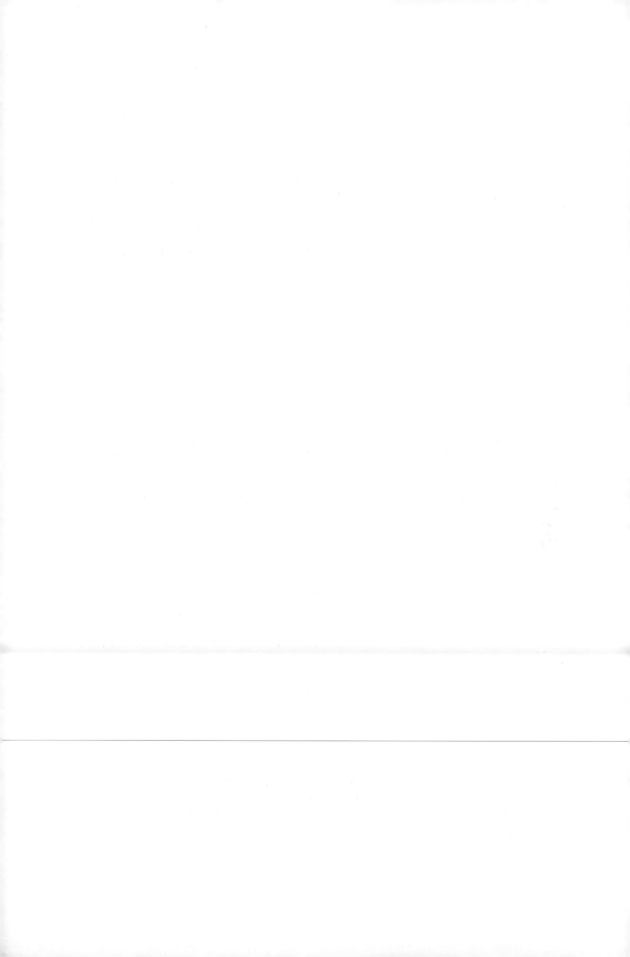

Pulmonary Function Tests and Sedation with Pulmonary Diseases: Assessment, Analysis, and Associated Dental Management Guidelines

Pulmonary disease can involve the upper airway or the lower airway. Rhinitis, sinusitis, and pharyngitis are common upper airway diseases. Asthma, bronchitis, emphysema, and chronic obstructive pulmonary disease (COPD) are conditions that affect the lower airways.

The dentist should not only be familiar with the disease states but should also be knowledgeable about the diagnostic tools to detect and assess pulmonary disease. This becomes particularly important with the conditions causing significant changes in the ASA status of the patient.

THE DIAGNOSTIC TOOLS TO DETECT PULMONARY DISEASE

The diagnostic tools to detect pulmonary disease are presented in the following sections.

History and Physical Examination

History can reveal the presence of symptoms and/or the etiological factors such as smoking, specific allergens, or genetic predisposition, that are responsible for the pulmonary disease(s). Sinus congestion, headaches, cough, dyspnea, wheezing, hemoptysis (coughing up blood), sleepiness, snoring, and morning headaches are some of the more common symptoms experienced with pulmonary disease. Physical examination can show nasal congestion, nasal inflammation, cobblestoning of the pharynx, macroglossia, nasal polyps, cervical lymphadenopathy plus classic inspection, palpation, percussion, and auscultation findings in the lungs.

Laboratory Tests

Pulmonary Function Tests (PFTs)

Pulmonary function is measured by spirometry. The tests detect how efficiently the oxygen from the lungs is transferred into the blood and how well the carbon dioxide is removed from the blood. The specific measurements obtained by spirometry are:

- **Forced Vital Capacity (FVC):** FVC is the amount of air exhaled with force, after inhaling completely.

- **Forced Expiratory Volume in 1 Second (FEV$_1$):** FEV$_1$ is the amount of air exhaled with force in 1 sec of expiration.

Spirometry/Pulmonary Function Tests and Disease Evaluation

- **Obstructive lung diseases:** asthma, chronic bronchitis, emphysema, bronchiectasis, bronchiolitis, and chronic obstructive pulmonary disease (COPD) are listed as obstructive lung diseases. Asthma, chronic bronchitis, emphysema, and chronic obstructive pulmonary disease (COPD) are the most common obstructive lung diseases encountered. The narrowed airways in these states are associated with increased airway resistance.

- The FEV$_1$ and FVC tests are used to evaluate these disease states, and a low FEV$_1$/FVC ratio found on spirometry indicates obstruction. The severity of obstruction is defined as the absolute value of the FEV$_1$. The lower the FEV$_1$ the worse is the obstruction.

- **Restrictive lung diseases:** restrictive lung diseases are associated with decreased distensibility of the lungs, pleura, or chest wall during inhalation; thus, increased pressure is required to distend the lungs.

A diseased thickened interstitium can be associated with diffusion problems. Therefore, scarring of lung tissues, chest wall deformity, or problems with the chest wall muscles can also cause inability to inhale a normal volume. Restrictive lung disease can be due to

- Lung parenchymal disease: pulmonary fibrosis, sarcoidosis
- Pleural disease: pleural effusion, pneumothorax
- Inadequate filling from acute lung disease: pneumonia or CHF
- Neuromuscular conditions: muscular dystrophy, myasthenia gravis
- Chest wall anomalies: obesity-related chest deformity, kyphosis, or scoliosis

Restrictive lung diseases are best assessed by measuring the lung volume. A normal FEV$_1$/FVC ratio occurs in a normal patient or a patient with restrictive lung disease. The difference is that the FVC is low in the patient with restrictive lung disease and normal in a healthy patient.

Arterial Blood Gases (ABGs)

Arterial blood gases detect the amount of oxygen and carbon dioxide in the blood. The PaO$_2$ indicates how efficiently the oxygen is able to move from the lungs into the blood. The PaCO$_2$ indicates how efficiently the carbon dioxide is able to move from the blood into the lungs and then out of the lungs. The normal partial pressure of oxygen (PaO$_2$) is 75–100 mmHg. Values below 60 mmHg require immediate action to correct the hypoxia. The normal partial pressure of carbon dioxide (PaCO$_2$) is 35–45 mmHg. A high PCO$_2$ indicates respiratory acidosis and poor ventilation. A low PCO$_2$ indicates respiratory alkalosis and hyperventilation.

With asthma there is no reduction in lung volumes and there is no impairment in the gas transportation from the alveoli to the blood. Therefore, the PFTs in asthma show a low FEV$_1$/FVC ratio, normal total lung capacity (TLC), and normal gases diffusion. The obstruction typically improves with a bronchodilator challenge.

Emphysema is associated with obstruction, hyperinflation, air trapping, and impairment in gas transportation from the air to the blood. Therefore, the PFTs in emphysema show a low FEV_1/FVC ratio, an elevated total lung capacity (TLC) and a reduced diffusion of gases. The obstruction is not reversible in emphysema.

In interstitial lung disease the lungs progressively develop smaller lung volumes and impairment to gas exchange. The PFTs show a normal FEV_1/FVC ratio, a low TLC, and a low diffusion of gases.

GENERAL ANESTHESIA OR CONSCIOUS SEDATION CONSIDERATIONS WITH PULMONARY DISEASES

An increase in adverse outcomes can occur with outpatient general anesthesia; conscious sedation in patients with pulmonary disease and complications are more common in the ASA III/IV patient. Hypoxemia and drug overdose are the most frequent problems encountered. When conscious sedation or general anesthesia is used it is best to increase the dose slowly, especially in the elderly patient.

Conscious Sedation

Benzodiazepines and opioids suppress the respiratory drive and this is a significant problem in obstructive sleep apnea (OSA).

Oxygen Plus Nitrous Oxide

Oxygen plus nitrous oxide has the advantage of rapid onset and recovery. The disadvantage is that it can expand and rupture the bullae. Thus it is contraindicated if the patient cannot tolerate an increase in the PO_2.

Upper Airway Disease: Assessment, Analysis, and Associated Dental Management Guidelines

ALLERGIC RHINITIS

Allergic rhinitis can be seasonal or constant. Most patients have associated allergies of some sort.

Allergic Rhinitis Symptoms

Nasal discharge, sneezing, and itchy eyes are the most common symptoms experienced.

Allergic Rhinitis Treatment

The patient should avoid exposure to allergens. Additionally, the patient should be evaluated for underlying allergies and receive appropriate allergy shots when possible. Nasal or oral antihistamines are often prescribed along with nasal or systemic steroids to gain relief.

SINUSITIS

Sinusitis could be bacterial or viral in origin. Streptococcus pneumonea and staphylococcus aureus are the leading organisms associated with bacterial sinusitis. Hemophyllus influenza is the virus associated with viral sinusitis. Patients can sometimes present with unilateral sinusitis, and in such cases it is always important to rule out a dentally related or underlying neoplasm cause.

Sinusitis Symptoms

The patient experiences mild, moderate, or severe pain over the sinuses affecting the cheeks, forehead, eyes, and top and back of the head. Additionally, the patient experiences malaise, nasal obstruction, headaches, purulent rhinorrhea, and sometimes thick nasal discharge.

Sinusitis Treatment

Medical Management

Treatment often consists of antibiotics for 3 weeks and decongestants such as Afrin spray for *less than* 4 days. Afrin spray, when used for more than 4 days, will cause rebound congestion and consequent worsening of symptoms.

Surgical Intervention

Surgery becomes necessary sometimes in refractory cases.

STREPTOCOCCAL THROAT INFECTION/BACTERIAL PHARYNGITIS

The normal oral flora contains α-hemolytic streptococcus, also called *streptococcus viridans*. Group A β-hemolytic streptococcus, an invading bacterium is the organism associated with causing streptococcal infection of the throat or streptococcal pharyngitis.

Symptoms and Signs of Streptococcal Throat Infection

Symptoms and signs of streptococcal throat infection include fever, muscle aches and pains (myalgia), dysphagia (difficulty swallowing), lack of cough, swollen and painful anterior cervical lymph nodes in the neck, and tonsillar exudates. The watery eyes and runny nose that typically occur with viral pharyngitis do not occur with bacterial pharyngitis.

Streptococcal Pharyngitis Diagnosis

Streptococcal pharyngitis diagnosis is confirmed with a rapid antigen detection test (RADT) and/or a throat culture.

The Rapid Antigen Detection Test (RADT)

The RADT detects the presence of group A streptococcal carbohydrate on a throat swab, and the result is obtained in 5–10 mins. A positive RADT confirms the presence of streptococcal pharyngitis. The validity of a negative RADT must be confirmed with a follow-up throat culture when there is a high suspicion of streptococcal pharyngitis, because the RADT is less sensitive than the throat culture test.

Throat Culture Test

The culture of a throat swab on a sheep-blood agar plate is the standard test to document the presence of acute streptococcal pharyngitis. The throat culture provides results in 24–48 hr, and it is 90–95% sensitive.

Streptococcal Pharyngitis Treatment

Treatment is as follows:

1. **Non-penicillin Sensitive Patients:**
   1a. **Pen VK or Amoxicillin** Adult dose: 500 mg bid × 10 days
      Adolescent dose: 250 mg tid/qid × 10 days
      Child dose: 250 mg bid/tid × 10 days Treatment with Pen VK or Amoxicillin must be given for **10 days.**
   1b. **Amoxicillin Extended-Release Tablets (Moxatag)**
      Adult dose: 775 mg Moxatag, once daily × 10 days with meal. Do not chew or crush the tablet.
      Note: Moxatag contains three components, one immediate-release and two delayed-release amoxicillin formulations.
2. **Penicillin Allergy Patients:** Azithromycin (Zithromax), 500 mg on the first day, followed by 250 mg per day for the next 4 days
   Treatment with azithromycin is provided for **5 days** only.

Asthma and Airway Emergencies: Assessment, Analysis, and Associated Dental Management Guidelines

ASTHMA

Asthma is a condition that is a consequence of an immune response. The airways become sensitive to allergens causing bronchial hyperresponsiveness and narrowing. Increased inflammation and increased mucus production during an asthma attack causes further narrowing of the airways. Wheezing, coughing, shortness of breath, chest tightness, and increased respiratory rate are the hallmark features of asthma. Patients with allergies and eczema have a higher predilection for asthma. IgE is produced in excess in these patients and IgE blocks the β_2 receptors, causing asthma.

Extrinsic Asthma

Allergy-associated asthma is labeled as *extrinsic asthma*. This type of asthma is more common in childhood and improves with age or disappears in adulthood. Extrinsic asthma could, however, persist in adulthood but it rarely progresses to COPD. COPD is less often associated with familial allergies or eczema and is more often associated with intrinsic asthma and smoking.

Intrinsic Asthma

Intrinsic asthma occurs in adulthood and is often triggered by pulmonary infections. As stated above, intrinsic asthma often leads to COPD and COPD in general is less responsive to brochodilators compared to asthma.

Asthma Symptoms and Signs

Patients are usually symptomatic with asthma at night or during the early morning hours. During an asthma attack the respiratory rate is increased, the expiration is prolonged, and the patient experiences tachycardia. Ronchi and wheezing are primarily heard on expiration initially, but with progressive worsening of the asthma the ronchi and wheezing can occur, in both the inspiration and expiration phases. The patient uses the accessory muscles of respiration and the sternocleidomastoid and scalene muscles of the neck to assist with the breathing and oxygenation. Asthma is also associated with a paradoxical pulse, wherein the pulse increases during expiration and decreases during inspiration.

Asthma can be intermittent or it can result in chronic respiratory impairment. The range of severity of asthma is determined by the frequency of asthma attacks and the number of attacks that occur at night or in the early hours of the morning.

Asthma Classification per the U.S. National Heart, Lung and Blood Institute (US NHLBI)

The four categories of asthma identified by the US NHLBI are mild intermittent, mild persistent, moderate persistent, and severe persistent. A severe asthma attack is a true emergency needing immediate attention because it can be associated with near closure of the airways and decreased oxygen supply to the vital organs. This is of particular concern in the patient with severe persistent asthma where the FEV_1 is <60%.

Asthma Etiological Factors

Common etiological factors causing asthma are

- Viral infections, which are the leading cause for asthma attacks in children
- Irritants such as cigarette smoke and cold air
- Allergens such as dust and pollen
- Exercise
- Medications such as β blockers, aspirin, sulfites, penicillin, glaucoma medications, and NSAIDS

Asthmatic patients often have allergies, and allergy-associated asthma most often begins in childhood.

ASTHMA DIAGNOSIS

Diagnosis of asthma is made with the following:

1. **History of Asthma Attack Presentation:** Presenting symptoms of asthma attacks are adequate in many cases where the presenting features are classic.
2. **Spirometry:** Spirometry, as stated earlier, demonstrates the amount of air that the patient's lungs can take in and the rapidity with which the inhaled air can be thrown out by the patient. Narrowed inflamed airways will show lower results. Spirometry can also be used to determine the extent of improvement in the airway status with medications, once treatment is instituted.
3. **Allergy Testing:** Because allergens frequently cause asthma, patients are often subjected to allergy testing to determine the cause of asthma.
4. **Chest X-Ray:** The chest x-rays determine whether there is any other associated lung disease.

ASTHMA TREATMENT

The goal of asthma management should be for the patient to have good exercise capacity, have fewer attacks, and be less dependent on immediate-relief drugs, as much as possible. Asthma management is best achieved by the following:

- Elimination of the precipitating factors where possible, especially with allergens
- Implementation of care by the patient immediately on recognizing the signs and symptoms of asthma
- Medications

Asthma Medications

The medications for the management of asthma can be categorized as presented in the following sections.

Immediate-Relief Medications

Short-acting inhaled β_2 agonist bronchodilators (Metaproterenol, Albuterol, Terbutaline, Pirbutrol) are the preferred quick relief medications that open up the airways and bring relief within minutes of using the inhaler.

Patients should always carry their bronchodilator with them and use it immediately on becoming symptomatic. An early addition of corticosteroid inhalants with the β_2 agonist can often show an arrest in the progression of asthma.

Occasionally, the β_2 agonist bronchodilators can cause an increased heart rate or an increased BP at higher doses. When this happens, Ipratropium bromide, an anticholinergic medication, can be used instead because the drug has no cardiac side effects. The disadvantage, however, is that Ipratropium bromide is not immediate in action and is not as effective as the β_2 agonist.

Medications for Long-Term Control and Prevention of Asthma Attacks

Medications for long-term control and prevention of asthma are taken daily (Table 31.1). To become optimally effective they need to be taken for weeks.

Be aware that the long-acting inhalers are slow in action, so the short-acting inhalers may have to be used during an asthma attack.

Inhaled glucocorticoids (Beclomethasone, Triamcinolone), long-acting β_2 agonist (Salmeterol, Albuteral SR), mast-cell stabilizers (Cromolyn), leukotreine modifiers (Zafirlukast), anticholinergics (Ipratropium bromide), and methylxanthines (Theophylline, Aminophylline) provide long-term control and prevention of asthma attacks. Methylxanthines are often added when inhaled steroids and the other long-acting β agonists have not provided adequate control.

Asthma Emergency Treatment Drugs

When the patient's own medications are not as effective during an asthma attack, other medications or measures such as short-acting β_2 agonists, systemic steroids, methylxanthines, and oxygen are used.

Asthma Facts

Patients having mild persistent asthma with more than two attacks per week are often treated with inhaled corticosteroids as the first drug of choice and mast-cell stabilizers, leukotreine modifiers, or theophylline as alternates.

Moderate persistent asthma patients are given higher doses of glucocorticoids plus long-acting β_2 agonists primarily. The long-acting β_2 agonists are bronchodilators or muscle relaxants, and they do not have antiinflamatory action. Glucocorticoids plus leukotriene modifier or theophylline are used as alternates.

Along with the inhalants used by the moderate persistent asthma patient, oral glucocorticoids are frequently added to enhance recovery in the severe persistent asthma patients.

Inhaled corticosteroids are the most common long-term control medications that decrease inflammation and airway swelling, especially in the mild, moderate, or severe

Table 31.1. Asthma medications

Drug Class	Drug Name: Generic (Trade)	Comments
Inhaled Selective β_2 Adrenergic Agonists	Metaproterenol (Alupent) Albuterol (Ventolin or Proventil) Terbutaline (Brethaire) Pirbutrol (Maxair) Salmeterol (Serevent)	Serevent is a much better β_2 selective agent. It is a long-acting drug that has a slow onset of action. Serevent, however, is **not** advised for the management of an acute asthma attack.
Antiinflammatory Drugs: Corticosteroids	**Inhaled steroids:** Triamcinolone (Azmacort) Beclomethasone (Beclovent or Vanceril) Flunisolide (Aerobid or Nasalide) Budesonide (Rhinocort) Fluticasone (Flonase)	Inhaled steroids are not systemically absorbed and you do **not** need to follow "the rule of twos" with inhaled steroids. Inhaled steroids can cause candida infection affecting the palate.
Oral Steroids	Prednisone Prednisolone Dexamethasone	Prednisone is most often used. Dexamethasone is the longest-acting steroid with frequent systemic side effects.
Injectable Steroids	Hydrocortisone sodium succinate (Solucortef)	Reserved for very severe attacks.
Methyl-Xanthines	Theophylline (Theodur/Theobid) Aminophylline Oxtriphylline (Choledyl)	Theodur has a very narrow therapeutic index. Toxicity occurs with caffeine, chocolate, epinephrine, macrolides, quinolones, or cimetidine. Signs and symptoms of Theophylline toxicity: The patient is agitated and the pulse becomes very rapid and fluttery. Aminophylline is the injectable form of Theophylline.
Mast Cell Stabilizers	Cromolyn sodium (Intal) Nidocromil (Tilade)	Prevent allergic rhinitis and asthma by decreasing histamine release from mast cells. **Not** used for acute asthma attack.
Leukotriene Receptor Antagonists	Zafirlucast (Accolate) Monteleukast sodium (Singulair)	Prevent Leukotriene release from mast cells, eosinophils, and basophils. Leukotrienes cause bronchial smooth muscle contraction. Avoid Macrolides because they decrease drug bioavailability.
Lipoxygenase Inhibitors	Zileuton (Zyflo)	These drugs inhibit Leukotriene formation. Used for asthma prevention, **not** to treat an acute attack.
Muscarinic Antagonists	Ipratropium bromide (Atrovent) Tiotropium (Spireva)	They inhibit acetylcholine released from parasympathetic nerve terminals. Acetylcholine causes bronchial smooth muscle contraction
Combination Drugs	Salbutamol + Beclomethasone (Aerocort) A steroid, Fluticasone + Salmeterol, a selective β_2 Agonist (Advair)	

persistent asthma patients. They are generally safe when used as directed but can cause **oral candidiasis** in the roof of the mouth. This can be prevented by asking the patient to **rinse** the mouth after inhaler use.

Leukotriene modifiers treat mild persistent asthma when used alone, and when combined with steroid inhalants they treat moderate or severe asthma. Cromolyn sodium is used to treat mild persistent asthma. Theophylline, when used alone, treats mild persistent asthma. When combined with inhaled steroids, it treats moderate persistent asthma. Short-acting inhalants **are needed** to control an attack in patients using the long-acting inhalers.

Patients suffering from severe asthma often use handheld peak flow meters to estimate the effectiveness of their medications.

Combinations of inhaled steroids and the long-acting β_2 agonists (Fluticasone + Salmeterol/Advair) have recently become available and are often being prescribed.

ASTHMA-ASSOCIATED SUGGESTED DENTAL GUIDELINES

The following are dental guidelines for asthma:

1. Question the patient about what triggers the asthma attacks and be aware that 95% of attacks are stress-related. Provide stress management if needed.
2. Have the patient use a puff of their bronchodilator prior to treatment as an alternate to stress management, particularly in the ASA III and IV patient.
3. Confirm the medications used for asthma management and have the patient bring the inhalers to the dental office.
4. Evaluate the severity of the asthma and determine how quickly the medications are effective during an attack.
5. Avoid using antihistamines **during** an asthma attack because antihistamines cause mucus thickening, worsening the asthma attack.
6. Aspirin, Indocin, NSAIDs (ibuprofen, Anaprox), penicillin, codeine, and morphine can frequently precipitate allergies and/or asthma attacks. Check whether the patient has used these medications before without any adverse reactions. Use these drugs **only** if they have caused no reactions.
7. Determine whether the patient has used oral or injectable corticosteroids for 2 weeks or longer in the past 2 years. You will have to follow "the rule of twos" for major dental surgery in such patients.
8. Treat the ASA III and IV patient in a semi-sitting position.

Local Anesthetics and Asthma

The following are local anesthetics used with asthma:

- **A well-controlled asthmatic (ASA I/II):** Use 2% Lidocaine with epinephrine (Xylocaine) or 2% mepivacaine (Carbocaine) with 1:20,000 levonordefrin (NeoCobefrin), but use no more than 2 carpules.
- **Severe asthma (ASA III/IV):** Use 3% mepivacaine (Carbocaine) or 4% prilocaine HCL (Citanest plain) because epinephrine is contraindicated.

Analgesics and Asthma

Avoid narcotic analgesics in the ASA III and IV patient.

Oral Antibiotics and Asthma

Macrolides are contraindicated with the following:

1. **The β$_2$ Adrenergic Agonists:** Alupent, Proventil, Brethaire, Maxair, and Serevent
2. **The Methylxanthines:** Theophylline, Amminophylline
3. **The Leukotreine Receptor Antagonists:** Accolate and Singulair

Acute Airway Emergencies

Please refer to Chapter 9, "Management of Medical Emergencies in the Dental Setting: Assessment, Analysis, and Associated Dental Management Guidelines," for discussions on clinical features and management of acute asthma, hyperventilation syndrome, and foreign body obstruction.

Chronic Bronchitis: Assessment, Analysis, and Associated Dental Management Guidelines

Chronic bronchitis is a disease state where the patient has had cough with expectoration for **2–3 months** of the year for **2** successive years at least. This patient will give a history of using bronchodilators, antibiotics during flare-ups, and oral or injectible corticosteroids during exacerbation of the chronic bronchitis.

Chronic Bronchitis Treatment

Chronic bronchitis management consists of quitting smoking, using bronchodilators, and using corticosteroids to control or attenuate a flare-up.

Chronic Bronchitis Suggested Dental Guidelines

The following are dental guidelines for chronic bronchitis:

1. Follow the suggested dental and AAA guidelines as outlined for asthma focusing on the specific bronchodilators used by the patient.
2. Follow "the rule of twos" if steroids were used for 2 weeks or longer within the past 2 years.

Emphysema: Assessment, Analysis, and Associated Dental Management Guidelines

EMPHYSEMA FACTS

Emphysema is associated with abnormal and permanent enlargement of the airspaces distal to the terminal bronchioles. There is destruction of the walls with or without fibrosis and loss of elastic recoil of the lungs.

The long-standing history of smoking, cough with expectoration, and progressive dyspnea are quite suggestive of emphysema, and spirometry clinches the diagnosis. Emphysema and chronic bronchitis, when present together, constitute COPD.

EMPHYSEMA TREATMENT

Treatment options for emphysema are:

- Quit smoking.
- Use bronchodilators.
- Oxygen therapy: Intermittent or continuous low-flow oxygen is prescribed. Bronchodilators, oxygen, and theophylline form the mainstay of treatment for emphysema.
- Antibiotics are used to control and treat pulmonary infection.
- Pulmonary rehabilitation is used to improve breathing and oxygenation.
- Lung reduction surgery provides relief to some patients.
- Lung transplant is the ultimate choice when all else fails.

Note: Inhaled corticosteroids do not work well in emphysema but they work extremely well in asthmatics.

EMPHYSEMA-ASSOCIATED SUGGESTED DENTAL GUIDELINES

The following are dental guidelines for emphysema:

1. Evaluate the PFTs to determine the severity of the disease and treat the patient in a semi-sitting position.
2. Follow the suggested dental and AAA guidelines as outlined for asthma, focusing on the specific bronchodilators used by the patient.
3. Follow "the rule of twos" if steroids were used for 2 weeks or longer within the past 2 years.

Chronic Obstructive Pulmonary Disease (COPD): Assessment, Analysis, and Associated Dental Management Guidelines

COPD is a disease state associated with irreversible pulmonary damage, progressive airflow limitation, partially obstructed airways, breathing difficulty, and an abnormal inflammatory response. In COPD the alveoli lose their elasticity resulting in some areas of collapsed airways and some areas of hyperinflated airways. Alveolar damage causes poor air exchange. Additionally, excess mucus production by the mucus-producing cells causes thickening of the airways and airway blockade. COPD is most prevalent in the elderly.

COPD is a disease state associated with emphysema and chronic bronchitis. Emphysema is associated with hyperinflated alveoli interspersed with alveoli that have been destroyed. Chronic bronchitis is associated with thickened inflamed airways. Frequent lung infections therefore result in rapid progression toward COPD in such patients.

COPD ETIOLOGY

The etiological factors associated with COPD are:

1. Smoking: Smoking is the leading cause for COPD.
2. Inhaled irritants
3. Genetic predisposition: Familial COPD is often associated with α_1 antitrypsin deficiency. Alpha-1 antitrypsin inactivates destructive proteins, so lack of α_1 antitrypsin leads to destruction of the lungs and COPD.

COPD SYMPTOMS AND SIGNS

COPD patients frequently experience shortness of breath on exertion and at rest plus persistent cough with excessive expectoration, wheezing, and chest tightness.

COPD DIAGNOSIS

Diagnosis of COPD is made with the following:

1. History: Typical history of presentation helps with the diagnosis.
2. Spirometry breathing tests: The spirometry test demonstrates the amount of air that the patient's lungs can take in and the rapidity with which the inhaled air can be thrown out by the patient. The FEV_1 is markedly decreased in these patients.

3. Chest X-Ray: The chest x-ray shows the classic changes associated with chronic bronchitis and emphysema.
4. Arterial blood gases: Arterial blood gases show a decreased PO_2 and a normal/ increased PCO_2.

COPD CLASSIFICATION

COPD can be classified as

-   Mild COPD
-   Moderate COPD
-   Severe COPD

Mild COPD

The patient may not yet be aware of the airway limitation; and it is detected only by spirometry, which shows mild airflow limitation. The PO_2 is close to 75 mmHg and the PCO_2 is normal at 35–45 mmHg.

Moderate COPD

Symptoms occur on exertion and this prompts the patient to seek help. Spirometry shows worsening of airflow. A Moderate COPD patient has a PO_2 close to 60 mmHg and the PCO_2 is normal.

Severe COPD

Symptoms and signs associated with COPD are present at rest. Spirometry shows severe airflow limitation, and heart or respiratory failure can occur in these patients. In severe COPD the PO_2 is ≤ 50 mmHg and the PCO_2 is ≥ 50 mmHg.

COPD TREATMENT GOALS

Relief of the symptoms and signs, improvement in exercise tolerance and slowing of the progression of the disease are the prime treatment goals. Treatment options include the following:

-   **Smoking cessation**
-   **Bronchodilators:** The short-acting bronchodilators are used for immediate effect that lasts for 4–6 hr and is implemented PRN (as and when needed). The long-acting bronchodilators are used daily and their effects last for 12 hr.
-   The short-acting bronchodilators may be the only inhalants used for mild COPD. The moderate COPD patient may be prescribed just a long-acting bronchodilator or a combination of short- and long-acting bronchodilators.
-   **Inhaled steroids:** Inhaled steroids are often prescribed for moderate to severe COPD. Steroids work by decreasing the airway inflammation.
-   **Oral or injectable steroids:** These steroids provide additional support to decrease airway inflammation.
-   **Oxygen:** Oxygen is used as adjunctive management in the severe COPD patient to correct the shortness of breath (SOB) caused by decreased oxygenation of the blood. Oxygen may be given intermittently or continuously.
-   **Pulmonary Rehabilitation**

Table 34.1. COPD staging, tests, symptoms, and treatment

COPD Severity	FEV$_1$ ÷ FVC	FEV$_1$	Symptoms	Treatment
Mild or Stage 1 COPD	<70%	>80%	The patient may or may not be symptomatic.	Stop smoking; short-acting bronchodilators and flu vaccine
Moderate or Stage 2 COPD	<70%	50–80%	The patient may or may not be symptomatic.	Stop smoking; short- and long-acting bronchodilators; rehabilitation and flu vaccine
Severe or Stage 3 COPD	<70%	30–50%	The patient may or may not be symptomatic.	Same as Stage 2 **plus** steroids with frequent infections
Very Severe or Stage 4 COPD	<70%	<30%	Respiratory and right heart failure are common.	Same as Stage 3 **plus** oxygen for respiratory failure

COPD Staging, Tests, Symptoms, and Treatment

The mainstay of COPD staging, tests, symptoms, and treatment are shown in Table 34.1.

COPD Dental Alerts and Suggested Dental Guidelines

The following are dental alerts and guidelines for COPD:

1. The normal FEV$_1$ is 1.5 L. Patients with 50% reduction in FEV$_1$ experience shortness of breath (SOB) on exertion and patients with 75% reduction in FEV$_1$ experience SOB at rest.
2. In the COPD patient hypoxia triggers the respiratory drive by stimulating the carotid chemoreceptors and this helps the patient breathe.
3. If O$_2$ is administered during nonemergency states, one can cause problems in the COPD patient's breathing because this will eliminate the hypoxic drive. Hypoventilation and CO$_2$ retention will occur.
4. During acute respiratory distress (ARD) when the PO$_2$ is further decreased and PCO$_2$ is elevated, O$_2$ should be given at a flow rate of 5–6 L/min to treat the hypoxia. This is a true emergency and the oxygen is supplied until the emergency is corrected.
5. O$_2$ + N$_2$O **cannot** be used for stress management in the COPD patient. If stress management becomes necessary, cautiously give low dose diazepam (Valium) to a mild COPD patient only.
6. **Never** put the patient in a horizontal position.
7. Do **not** use epinephrine or epinephrine cords in the COPD patient.
8. Often the patients are using theophylline, aminophylline, and inhaled and/or oral steroids. Use the guidelines already discussed for these drugs.
9. Avoid aspirin, Indocin, NSAIDS, and penicillin if these drugs have caused allergies.

10. Check whether the patient needs steroid supplementation for major dentistry when oral or injectible steroids have been used in the past 2 years.
11. Codeine, morphine, and other sedatives/hypnotics are contraindicated in the COPD patient because these drugs depress the respiratory center and will worsen the patient's breathing status.
12. Follow the antibiotic guidelines for asthma, depending on which antiasthma drugs are being used in the COPD patient.

Obstructive Sleep Apnea (OSA): Assessment, Analysis, and Associated Dental Management Guidelines

OBSTRUCTIVE SLEEP APNEA (OSA) FACTS

The patient with OSA experiences repetitive episodes of upper airway obstruction associated with a reduction in blood oxygen saturation, arousal from sleep, snoring, sleepiness, morning headaches, excessive daytime sleepiness, and mood swings. OSA is more prevalent in men than women.

OSA RISK FACTORS

Obesity, male patient, snoring, craniofacial abnormalities, nasal obstruction, redundant soft palate, endocrine abnormalities, and family history are some of the common risk factors associated with OSA.

OSA TREATMENT

OSA treatment consists of the following:

- The patient must avoid alcohol or sedating medications and reduce weight.
- A dentally prepared mandibular advancement device can help with the management of OSA.
- Nasal continuous positive airway pressure (CPAP) helps keep the airway open.

Tuberculosis: Assessment, Analysis, and Associated Dental Management Guidelines

TUBERCULOSIS EPIDEMIOLOGY

Mycobacterium tuberculosis (MTB) is an aerobic, acid fast bacillus that usually affects the lungs. There has been an increased incidence of MTB secondary to HIV, homelessness, and emigration. 90% of the adult cases are due to reactivation of a dormant infection.

TB RISK FACTORS

Risk factors for TB are HIV, diabetes, prolonged steroid use, alcoholism, prisoners, nursing home residents, health care workers, immunosuppressive treatment, close contact with infectious patients, underweight patients, and persons from countries with a high TB prevalence.

TB TRANSMISSION

TB is spread from person to person through the air via coughed-infected droplets. Coughed-up, aerosolized particles stay around for a long time and infect susceptible individuals.

TB SYMPTOMS AND SIGNS

Symptoms and signs frequently associated with TB are fever, chest pain, chills, cough, weight loss, hemoptysis, night fever, night sweats, and fatigue.

TB DIAGNOSIS

The diagnosis of TB is made with:

1. **The Tuberculin skin test (TST):** The TST is done using purified protein derivative (PPD) from M. tuberculosis. The PPD skin test is a delayed hypersensitivity reaction that shows response in 48–72 hr. The response is indicated by an induration or thickening at the site of the inoculum that is measured to identify if the reaction is positive or negative (Table 36.1).

Table 36.1. Interpretation of a positive TST PPD reaction

Induration Size	Interpretation
5-mm induration	**A 5-mm reaction is positive in** • An immune-compromised patient • A close contact of a patient with TB
10-mm induration	**A 10-mm reaction is positive in** • Recent migrant to the U.S. • An IV drug user • A patient less than 4 years old
15-mm induration	**A 15-mm reaction is positive in** • One with no known TB risk factors

2. **QuantiFERON TB Gold Test (QFT-G):** The QFT-G is a new test for diagnosing latent Mycobacterium tuberculosis infection. It is an in vitro diagnostic test that measures a component of cell-mediated immune reactivity to M. tuberculosis. The test is based on the quantification of interferon-gamma (IFN-γ) released from sensitized lymphocytes in whole blood incubated overnight with purified protein derivative (PPD) obtained from M. tuberculosis. The QFT-G can be used in place of the TST.
3. **Sputum Smear and Culture:** The bacteria, when cultured, can take 3–6 weeks to grow.
4. **Chest X-Ray:** The chest x-ray can show hilar adenopathy; upper lobe infiltrates; pleural effusion, especially in young patients; and calcifications. The chest x-ray is done if the PPD is positive. If the chest x-ray is abnormal, the patient is evaluated for active TB.

WHEN TO INITIATE TB TREATMENT

Treatment for TB should be initiated with the presence of a positive AFB smear or when there is a high clinical suspicion.

TYPES/FORMS OF TB

The three forms of TB are:

• Latent TB
• Active TB/Pulmonary TB
• Multidrug-Resistant (MDR) and Extensively Drug-Resistant (XDR) TB

Latent TB

With latent TB the patient has a positive skin test; negative chest x-ray; and no symptoms, signs, or physical findings of TB. The patient is treated to prevent future reactivation to the active form of TB.

Active TB/Pulmonary TB

A patient is said to have active/pulmonary TB when the patient has a positive skin test; the chest x-ray may be abnormal; the patient experiences fever, cough, night sweats, hemopytosis, anorexia, weight loss; and the respiratory specimen smear test is positive.

Multidrug Resistant (MDR) and Extensively Drug-Resistant (XDR) TB

The four drug standard regimen—or the first-line, anti-TB drugs—when used correctly can successfully treat TB. When these drugs are used incompletely, incorrectly, or not at all, multidrug-resistant TB (MDR-TB) can develop. Drug-resistant TB is a dangerous form of TB caused by the TB bacillus becoming resistant to at least Isoniazid and Rifampicin, the two most powerful anti-TB drugs. MDR-TB takes longer to treat with second-line drugs and the care is often expensive. Extensively drug-resistant tuberculosis (XDR-TB) develops when the second-line drugs are also incompletely used or inappropriately used such that they become ineffective. Treatment options for XDR-TB are even more restrictive and expensive because the patient has severe resistance to the first **and** second line of TB treatment.

Latent TB Treatment

If the patient is HIV-negative, Isoniazide (INH) is given for 6–9 months. If the patient is HIV-positive and has fibrotic lesions on the chest x-ray, INH is given for 9 months. For all patients with latent TB, Rifampin for 4 months can be another option instead of INH.

Active TB/Pulmonary TB Treatment Regimens

Initial Phase

The initial phase therapy consists of rifampin, isoniazide, pyrazinamide, and ethambutol (RIPE) for 2 months.

Continuation Phase

The continuation phase therapy consists of 4 months INH/Rifampin daily or twice/week of INH/Rifampin for 7 months. The multidrug approach is needed due to the high incidence of resistance.

TB PRECAUTIONS

Transmission of TB can be curtailed by using the following precautions: wash hands, sterilize instruments, surface disinfection, minimize splash/aerosols, and use approved masks.

TUBERCULOSIS TREATMENT GUIDELINES EXPANDED DISCUSSION

Treatment regimens are decided by the United States Public Health Service (USPHS) and the Infectious Diseases Society of America (IDSA).

Directly observed therapy (DOT) involves monitoring ingestion of each antituberculosis dose to maximize the completion of treatment. This is of particular benefit in the homeless or the drug abuse population or in individuals with a poor drug compliance history.

Each antituberculosis regimen has an initial phase of 2 months of treatment followed by a continuation phase of 4 or 7 months. Isoniazide (INH), rifampin (RIF), ethambutol (EMB), and pyrazinamide (PZA) are considered the first-line drugs in the treatment of tuberculosis. The second-line drugs consist of cycloserine, ethionamide, streptomycin, and capromycin.

All *asymptomatic* patients with positive TST/PPD skin reactions (latent TB) should get preventive therapy with INH and pyridoxine (vitamin B$_6$) supplementation for 6–9 months.

BCG vaccine is given to all newborns in developing countries where tuberculosis is endemic. It is given to attenuate an actual attack. A PPD skin test with an induration of ≥15 mm in a vaccinated individual warrants anti-TB treatment.

Without interruption, 6 months is the minimum duration of TB treatment. When interruption occurs because of missed doses or drug toxicity, the treatment should be completed in 9 months.

In the **initial phase** of 2 months, the symptomatic patient (active TB) is treated with all four drugs: isoniazide (INH), rifampin (RIF), ethambutol (EMB), and pyrazinamide (PZA). Once the organism shows susceptibility on testing, EMB is discontinued.The **initial phase** may be given in one of three ways: daily for 2 months, daily for 2 weeks followed by twice weekly for 6 weeks, or thrice weekly for 2 months.

In the **continuation phase** there are three treatment options also: daily, twice weekly, or three times weekly, by DOT. The 4 months continuation phase is used for most patients.

INH and RIF are given for 4 months if the initial chest x-ray was positive *or* the sputum smear was positive at 2 months. If the initial cultures were negative and treatment with the four drugs was initiated for 2 months, resulting in improvement of the symptoms and signs or improvement of the chest x-ray at 2 months, INH and RIF can be given for 2 additional months to complete treatment, as an alternate option. If the initial chest x-ray was positive *along with* a positive smear at 2 months, the patient is given an extended treatment for 7 months. Extended treatment is therefore recommended for patients with drug-susceptible tuberculosis who have cavitation on the chest x-ray and positive sputum cultures after completion of 2 months of treatment.

The 7-month phase treatment *is also used* in those patients where PZA could not be used for the initial treatment because of liver problems or gout.

INH, RIF, and PZA can cause hepatitis. If hepatitis occurs, the drugs are stopped immediately for a short period. The medications are restarted once the hepatitis resolves. The liver, kidney, and platelet function are routinely monitored by the physician during anti-TB treatment. The dental practitioner *must always evaluate* these results *prior* to the start of dental treatment. If the patient has preexisting hepatitis, INH is avoided and the patient is given RIF, EMB, and PZA for 6 months. In the presence of severe liver disease, only one hepatotoxic anti-TB drug is used along with EMB. This patient is given RIF plus EMB for 12 months.

Gastrointestinal upsets are **common in the first few weeks** of treatment and they resolve progressively. The drugs can, however, be taken with food to minimize the gastrointestinal side effects.

Two drug combinations are approved in the U.S.:

1. INH and RIF (Rifamate®)
2. INH, RIF, and PZA (Rifater®)

Isoniazide (INH) Side Effects

Hepatotoxicity

Hepatotoxicity with enzyme elevations occurs in 10–20% of the patients. The hepatotoxicity is the worst in males around 40 years of age.

Peripheral Neuropathy

The neuropathy is dose-related and is uncommon at conventional doses. It is more common in the presence of conditions that predispose to neuropathy—e.g., diabetes, HIV, renal failure, alcoholism, pregnancy, and breast-feeding. Pyridoxine (vitamin B_6) supplementation is given to prevent this neuropathy. It typically causes circumoral tingling numbness and tingling numbness in the hands and feet.

Rifampin (RIF) Side Effects

The following are RIF side effects:

- **Body-fluid discoloration:** Orange discoloration of bodily fluids such as saliva, tears, sweat, and urine occurs.
- **Cutaneous reactions:** Pruritis with or without a rash can occur.
- **Transient hepatotoxicity:** Liver toxicity can occur and monitoring of LFTs is a requirement with anti-TB treatment.

Ethambutol (EMB) Side Effects

The following are EMB side effects:

- **Retrobulbar neuritis:** Retrobulbar neuritis that occurs is irreversible. It is dose-related and the risk is minimal with routine dose.
- **Peripheral neuritis:** Peripheral neuritis with ethambutol and INH are similar in presentation.

Pyrazinamide (PZA) Side Effects

PZA is associated with the following:

- Hepatotoxicity
- Gastrointestinal side effects: nausea and vomiting
- Nongouty polyarthritis

Drug-Drug Interactions (DDIs) Between the Anti-TB Medications and the Anesthetics, Analgesics, and Antibiotics (AAAs) Used in Dentistry

The following are drug-drug interactions between anti-TB medications and the AAAs:

- **Antibiotics:** The concentrations of clarithromycin, erythromycin, and doxycycline are **decreased** (thus becoming ineffective) by RIF because of the effect on the P4503A4 enzyme system.
- **Azole antifungals:** Due to the effect on the P4503A4 enzyme, the concentration of the azole antifungals are also negatively affected. Fluconozole, however, can be used with increased doses.
- **Methadone:** Methadone levels are also negatively affected by the anti-TB medications.

SUGGESTED DENTAL GUIDELINES FOR TUBERCULOSIS

The following are dental guidelines for TB:

1. The nonsymptomatic TST/PPD skin test–positive patient does not transmit the disease. This patient needs preventative anti-TB treatment to prevent any **future reactivation** with decreased immunity or when exposed to a symptomatic coughing patient or "open" case of tuberculosis. This patient can have routine dentistry without any delay as the patient is not infective.

2. The **noncoughing symptomatic patient:** Within 2–4 weeks of the initial phase of anti-TB treatment, the bacterial count is negligible in the sputum *in most of the noncoughing symptomatic cases*. The patient can be treated in the dental setting subsequent to this time period after obtaining a clearance from the patient's physician.

3. **The symptomatic coughing patient:** The *symptomatic coughing patient* must complete the first **2 months** of the initial phase treatment, start the continuation phase treatment, obtain a clearance from the physician, *and then* be scheduled for routine dentistry. Avoid the use of a high-speed hand-piece in the first month of dentistry in such patients to avoid aerosolization of droplets into the environment.

4. Always consult and confirm with the patient's M.D. the type of drug therapy recommended for your patient and the status of the disease.

5. Evaluate the liver function tests (LFTs), serum creatinine, complete blood count (CBC) with platelets, and WBC differential before initiating dental treatment.

6. Always use strict universal precautions when treating **all** patients and not just the TB patient.

7. Avoid all drugs metabolized by the liver to minimize hepatotoxicity.

8. **TB and local anesthetics:** Use no more than 2 carpules of local anesthetics.

9. **TB and analgesics:** Avoid aspirin, NSAIDS, extra-strength acetaminophen (Tylenol), meperidine (Demerol), and propoxyphene (Darvon). Use regular-strength Tylenol or Tylenol #1–3 or Vicodin or Percocet for 2–3 days only.

10. **TB and antibiotics:** Avoid macrolides, ampicillin, tetracycline HCL, and metronidazole. Use penicillins, cephalosporins, and clindamycin when needed. Clindamycin can be used without dose alteration in the presence of a normal liver or hepatitis. Decrease the dose by 50% in the presence of cirrhosis.

11. Mycobacterium avium intracellulare (MAI) and/or Mycobacterium kansassi (MK) occurs only in the HIV patient due to a dramatic reduction in immunity. The T_4 cell count is usually <200 cells/mm^3 when MK occurs. MAI is frequently seen with a T_4 count of 50 cells/mm^3. Anti-TB management protocol for MAI and MK is the same as with MTB, as stated above.

VIII

Clinical Pharmacology

Prescribed and Nonprescribed/ Over-the-Counter Medications: Assessment, Analysis, and Associated Dental Management Guidelines

The following are medications that should be evaluated during patient assessment:

- Prescribed medications
- Over-the-counter (OTC) medications
- Drugs associated with or causing allergic reactions
- Corticosteroids (discussed in Chapter 40, "Adrenal Gland Cortex and Medulla Disease States: Assessment, Analysis, and Associated Dental Management Guidelines"
- Recreational drugs
- Herbal medications

PRESCRIBED MEDICATIONS

As discussed in Chapter 1, "Routine History-Taking and Physical Examination," you must obtain a complete list of medications prescribed by the patient's physician and determine the drug-drug interactions (DDIs) with the anesthetics, analgesics, and antibiotics (AAAs) used in dentistry. The ideal way to assess prescribed medications is presented in Chapter 2, "History and Physical Assessment of the Medically Compromised Dental Patient" (MCP) where lanoxin (Digoxin) and theophylline (TheoDur) are discussed.

OVER-THE-COUNTER (OTC) MEDICATIONS

Review the history and determine what OTC medications the patient is taking.

Aspirin or NSAIDS

Aspirin permanently affects the platelet cyclo-oxygenase system causing decreased platelet cohesiveness. NSAIDS also affect the same system but the effect is temporary. The platelet function returns to normal once the NSAID has cleared the system.

Nasal Decongestants, Cough or Cold Preparations, and Appetite Suppressants

All these preparations contain sympathomimetic agents, epinephrine or neosynephrine. The epinephrine in local anesthetics can synergize with the sympathomimetic agents in these preparations and cause an epinephrine overdose-type reaction resulting in blood pressure elevation. Obviously it is best to avoid dental treatment for the short term if the patient is too sick. If, however, you have to treat the patient for a dental emergency, use 3% mepivacaine (Carbocaine) or 4% prilocaine HCL (Citanest Plain) instead.

Laxatives

Check for laxative use. Laxatives do not interfere with dental treatment when used in therapeutic doses. Do not prescribe codeine or other narcotic analgesics that cause constipation to a patient on laxatives.

Laxative overuse is not uncommon in patients with eating disorders, such as anorexia and bulimia. Laxative overuse or abuse can cause significant hypokalemia or low potassium level.

The normal serum potassium is 3.5–5.5 mEq/dL, and the patient becomes symptomatic in the presence of hypokalemia. Muscle cramps, muscle weakness, tingling numbness in the hands and feet, and irregular pulse can occur with hypokalemia.

Do not give any local anesthetic during hypokalemia because arrhythmias could occur. Be aware that hypokalemia can also occur in a patient with a history of severe vomiting and/or diarrhea.

DRUGS CAUSING OR ASSOCIATED WITH ALLERGIES

Sulfites, bisulfites, aspirin, NSAIDS, penicillins, cephalosporins, codeine, or morphine can cause allergies, and you must determine the presence of an allergy history to these medications before you begin any dental treatment.

Anaphylactic reactions can be mild, moderate, or severe. The longer it takes for reactions to occur, the better the prognosis. Acute reactions occur within the **first hour** of taking the drug. Most frequently however, the reaction occurs within minutes after taking the drug.

Acute Anaphylactic Reaction

Please refer to Chapter 9, "Management of Medical Emergencies in the Dental Setting: Assessment, Analysis, and Associated Dental Management Guidelines," for discussion of the clinical features and management of an acute anaphylactic reaction.

Mild or Moderate Anaphylaxis Reaction Management

When a patient experiences a milder form of anaphylactic reaction, the drug or preparation that caused a reaction is discontinued and the patient is given diphenhydramine (Benadryl), 25–50 mg/tablet PO q6h for 48–72 hr.

25 mg per dose is best for a mild reaction, and 50 mg per dose is best for a moderate reaction. Warn the patient not to drive while on Benadryl as it causes drowsiness.

Write a case note in the record that you have informed the patient about the drowsiness caused by Benadryl. Fexofenatidine (Allegra), loratadine (Claritin), and cetirizine

Table 37.1. Common herbals and their side effects

Herbal Preparation	Side Effects; Drug-Drug Interactions (DDIs) with Anesthetics, Analgesics, Antibiotics (AAAs); and Advice
Chamomile **Garlic** **Ginger** **Gingko**	All these interfere with blood clotting and may cause pre/postop bleeding. Have the patient stop the herbals 7 days prior to surgery.
Echinacea	Inhibits wound healing by interfering with the immune function. Increases the risk of postsurgical infection. Patient using this herbal may need antibiotics postop to promote healing. Can alter the effectiveness of posttransplant immunosuppressant drugs.
Ephedra	Can cause abnormal heartbeat, extreme BP elevation, and coma when combined with some antidepressants and anesthesia. Stop intake 7 days prior to surgery.
Ginseng	Can cause arrhythmias and can interact with epinephrine in the local anesthesia and trigger arrhythmias. Can cause bleeding during and after surgery, but no interference with clotting or local anesthetics with epinephrine, if stopped 7 days prior to surgery.
Kava	Interacts with sedatives, causing excessive drowsiness. Can interfere with anesthesia. Must be stopped 7 days before surgery.
Licorice Herb (not the candy)	Can interfere with BP medications. Stop intake 7 days prior to surgery.
St. John's Wort	Has DDIs with blood thinners and several cardiac and blood pressure medications. Stop 7 days prior to surgery.
Valerian Root	Causes excessive drowsiness with sedatives, can interfere with anesthesia. Stop 7 days prior to surgery.

(Zyrtec) are H_1 blockers that do not cause drowsiness. As an alternate any one of these drugs can be used, and all these drugs are now available OTC.

RECREATIONAL DRUGS

The patient could be using/abusing uppers (stimulants) or downer (depressant) drugs that can interfere with dental treatment. Delay dental treatment in an intoxicated patient because this patient will not be cooperative during dentistry and needle-stick; percutaneous injury with grave consequences can occur.

Uppers

Cocaine and amphetamines are considered uppers or stimulant drugs. Their stimulant effect will synergize with the stimulant effect of epinephrine in local anesthetics.

Downers

Alcohol and marijuana are downers/depressant drugs. They alter the potency of anti-seizure drugs and antidepressants. Alcohol hastens the utilization of local anesthetics.

Ideally, the patient must be drug-free for 24 hr before you decide to use a local anesthetic containing epinephrine.

HERBAL MEDICATIONS

Herbals can have harmful side effects that can interfere with surgery and anesthesia (Table 37.1). The herbal medication acts as a powerful blood thinner that inhibits clotting.

All herbal medications cause platelet dysfunction. Thus, it is important to stop all herbal medications at least 7 days prior to major surgery.

Specific herbals that promote bleeding or drowsiness or cause cardiovascular side effects are of concern in any surgical setting.

IX
Endocrinology

Diabetes: Type 1 and Type 2 Diabetes: Assessment, Analysis, and Associated Dental Management Guidelines

DIABETES OVERVIEW, FACTS, AND TESTS

Diabetes Overview

The β cells of the pancreas produce the anabolic storage hormone insulin. Insulin plays a very important role in the metabolism of carbohydrates, proteins, and fats. Insulin enhances the conversion of glucose to glycogen, amino acids to proteins, and fatty acids to triglycerides. Absence of insulin causes elevated glucagons levels, muscle wasting, and high levels of acetoacetic acid and β hydroxybuteric acid in the blood.

Excessive glucose (hyperglycemia) in the blood causes it to spill into the urine resulting in glycosuria and frequent urination.

Insulin is produced and released in response to eating, to utilize the sugars and store excess amounts for use during starvation.

Type 1 Diabetes

The exact etiology of type 1 diabetes is not known. Autoimmune attack on the β cells of the pancreas is thought to cause destruction of the cells and consequent lack of insulin production. An environmental stimulus, however, is not discounted. The patients are usually younger, thin, and prone to ketosis, weight loss, and blackouts.

Type 2 Diabetes

These patients have a combination of insulin resistance and insulin deficiency. 90% of diabetics encountered suffer from type 2 diabetes. Type 2 diabetes has a higher genetic predisposition compared to type 1 diabetes.

The patients are usually obese and older at the time of disease onset. This fact, however, has changed, with the obesity epidemic affecting populations globally. It is not uncommon now to encounter obese patients in their teens or twenties suffering from type 2 diabetes.

Diabetes Symptoms and Signs

The following are symptoms and signs of diabetes:

- Polyuria (excessive urination), polydipsia (excessive thirst), and polyphagia (excessive appetite) are the hallmark symptoms associated with diabetes. Patients with type 1 diabetes experience these symptoms a lot more frequently compared to the type 2 diabetic patient.

- It is not uncommon for these patients to experience weight loss, fatigue, and blurred vision due to the elevated blood sugar levels.
- A weight loss history is a lot more common in the type 1 patient compared to the type 2 diabetic. The blurred vision is caused by adherence of sugar to the optic lens. The blurring of vision does improve when the sugar levels improve with treatment.
- Poor wound healing and opportunistic infections occur with chronic elevation of the blood sugar values.

Diabetes Diagnostic Tests

Diagnosis of diabetes is made utilizing the tests outlined in the following sections.

Fasting Blood Sugar (FBS)

A diagnosis of diabetes is made when the fasting blood sugar (FBS) is ≥126 mg/dL. With treatment, the FBS should be maintained between 70–100 mg/dL. The FBS should be maintained above 60–70 mg/dL to avoid precipitation hypoglycemia.

Impaired FBS

A patient is said to have **prediabetes** or impaired fasting glucose when the FBS is 100–125 mg/dL. The patient can normalize the impaired FBS sugar levels with stringent implementation of proper diet control and exercise.

Postprandial Blood Sugar (PPBS)

For optimal control the PPBS or the 2-hr postmeal blood sugar should be maintained between 100–140 mg/dL.

Random Blood Sugar

A diagnosis of diabetes is made when a random blood sugar is >200 mg/dL.

Oral Glucose Tolerance Test (OGTT)

The OGTT measures the patient's ability to utilize glucose in a laboratory setting. The patient's FBS is checked and the patient is made to drink 75–100 g of glucose. The blood sugar levels are then monitored at half-hour intervals for 2 hr. The patient is said to be prediabetic if the blood sugar at 2 hr ranges between 140–200 mg/dL. Values >200 mg/dL indicate diabetes definitely.

HemoglobinA$_1$C (HbA$_1$C)

The normal reference range of HbA$_1$C is: **4–5.9%**. Hemoglobin A in the RBCs combines with glucose, forming a glycated hemoglobin molecule, HbA$_1$C. The percentage of HbA that turns into HbA$_1$C increases as the blood glucose concentration increases. The HbA$_1$C percentage indicates the blood glucose level averaged over the half-life of red blood cells, which is typically 50–55 days. Poor diabetes control is associated with an elevated HbA$_1$C level, and effective treatment is associated with a declining HbA$_1$C level towards normal.

Table 38.1. HbA₁C and average blood sugar level comparison

HbA$_1$C	Comparison to Average Blood Sugar Level
6% HbA$_1$C	Reflects an average sugar level of 120 mg/dL
7% HbA$_1$C	Reflects an average sugar level of 150 mg/dL
8% HbA$_1$C	Reflects an average sugar level of 180 mg/dL
9% HbA$_1$C	Reflects an average sugar level of 210 mg/dL

The American Diabetes Association states that for optimal control it is best to maintain the HbA$_1$C below 7%. The International Diabetes Federation and American College of Endocrinology, however, support that the HbA$_1$C should be maintained below 6.5% for optimal control.

Table 38.1 shows the American Diabetes Association recommended comparison list of the HbA$_1$C and the corresponding average blood sugar value.

ACUTE MEDICAL EMERGENCIES ASSOCIATED WITH DIABETES

Hypoglycemia and hyperglycemic coma are the two acute complications associated with diabetes.

Hypoglycemia

Acute hypoglycemia reaction can occur in both the diabetic and the nondiabetic patient. The brain is totally dependent on the glucose supply for its energy requirements. The brain can sustain itself only for less than 3 min when the patient collapses because of hypoglycemia. Thus, the treatment has to be immediate to avoid brain damage or other negative consequences.

Please refer to Chapter 9, "Management of Medical Emergencies in the Dental Setting: Assessment, Analysis, and Associated Dental Management Guidelines," for a complete discussion on predisposing factors, clinical features, and management of hypoglycemia.

Hyperglycemia

Diabetic ketoacidosis (DKA) and coma can occur because of infection, poor intake of medications, etc. The patient must be sent to the emergency room where treatment is provided with fluids and Insulin.

Please refer to Chapter 9, "Management of Medical Emergencies in the Dental Setting: Assessment, Analysis, and Associated Dental Management Guidelines," for a complete discussion on predisposing factors, clinical features, and management of hyperglycemia.

CHRONIC MEDICAL COMPLICATIONS OF DIABETES

Microvascular Disease: Retinopathy and Nephropathy

Retinopathy- and nephropathy-associated microvascular disease is specific for diabetes. Retinopathy is the leading cause of blindness and should be differentiated from the blurring of vision caused by excessive sugar getting attached to the lens in the eyes. Diabetes accounts for 25% of all kidney failure and diabetes is the leading cause for dialysis.

Macrovascular Disease

Macrovascular disease is associated with an increased incidence of CVA/stroke and myocardial infarction (MI) that is often silent because of underlying autonomic neuropathy.

Macrovascular disease also affects the peripheral circulation causing peripheral vascular disease and narrowing of the blood vessels, and this can lead to amputation of the limbs.

Neuropathy

Poor diabetes control is associated with sensory and autonomic neuropathy, and the neuropathy has a classic glove-and-stocking type of presentation.

Autonomic neuropathy causes gastroparesis, which is associated with a slowing down of the stomach. The patient feels full after a few bites and experiences gastric reflux, halitosis, and vomiting. Because of the small food intake there is a greater likelihood of hypoglycemia if the patient skips eating often. This patient therefore will do better when given **shorter dental appointments** and treatment is provided in a semi-sitting position.

Skin or Mucus Membrane Infections

Yeast infections affect the oral cavity and it is not uncommon for the uncontrolled diabetic to have oral candidiasis and/or esophageal candidiasis. Always ask the patient about dysphagia (difficulty swallowing) or odynophagia (painful swallowing) whenever you see oral candidiasis and/or elevated blood sugar values. Esophageal candidiasis is associated with dysphagia and odynophagia.

Urinary tract infection is another complication of hyperglycemia and it affects the female diabetic patient more commonly.

Staphylococcal infections of the hair follicles cause chronic skin problems in the uncontrolled diabetic. It is not uncommon, therefore, to find frequent small pustules on the skin in general or between the shoulder blades.

DIABETES MANAGEMENT

Type 1 Diabetes

The type 1 diabetic is treated with daily insulin by subcutaneous (SC) injections or via an insulin pump.

Type 2 Diabetes

The type 2 diabetic patient is treated with diet, exercise, oral antidiabetic medications, insulin, or a combination of oral agents and insulin.

Diabetes Medical Management

Insulin is used in the management of type 1 diabetes and some cases of the uncontrolled type 2 diabetes. The patient is always on specific insulin preparations and doses, as dictated by the patient's physician. Tables 38.2 and 38.3 list the specifics for the most commonly used insulin preparations and oral agents.

Table 38.2. Time course of action of insulin preparation

Insulin Type	Onset	Peak	Duration
Regular Insulin	30–60 min	2–4 h	6–10 h
NPH (Novolin)	0.5 h	2–12 h	24 h
Lente Insulin	1–2.5 h	8–12 h	18–24 h
Ultralente	4–8 h	16–18 h	>36 h
Insulin Anologs:			
1. **Lispro (Humalog)**	5–15 min	1–2 h	4–6 h
2. **Insulin Aspart (Novolog)**	5–15 min	1–2 h	4–6 h
3. **Glargine (Lantus)**	1.5 h	None	20–24 h
4. **Insulin Glulisine (Apidra)**	15–30 min		4–6 h
5. **Insulin Determir (Levemir)**	1–2 h	Flat	24 h

Table 38.3. Oral agents for the management of type 2 diabetes

Category and Mech. of Action	Generic (Trade) Name	Side Effects, Special Facts
Sulphonylureas: Stimulate the pancreas to secrete more insulin.	**First generation:** Chlorpropamide (Diabinese) **Second generation:** 1. Glyburide (Glynase) 2. Glimepiride (Amaryl) 3. Glyburide (DiaBeta) 4. Glyburide (Glynase) 5. Glyburide (Micronase) 6. Glipizide (Glucotrol) 7. Glipizide (Glucotrol XL)	All sulfonylureas may cause hypoglycemia and sun sensitivity. Contraindicated during pregnancy and lactation. Diabinese can cause a flushing reaction with alcohol use and may also cause low blood sodium problems. Glucotrol XL cannot be chewed, crushed, or divided.
Meglitinides: Act by causing the pancreas to secrete more insulin.	1. Repaglinide (Prandin) 2. Nateglinide (Starlix)	Prandin may be used with kidney disease. Prandin is shorter- and faster-acting than sulfonylureas. Prandin can cause hypoglycemia, but less than sulfonylureas. Contraindicated with pregnancy/lactation.
Biguanides: Act by decreasing the liver glucose production.	1. Glucophage (Metformin) 2. Metformin generic 3. Glucophage XR (Metformin long acting) 4. Metformin oral solution (Riomet)	Rarely cause hypoglycemia. Contraindicated with pregnancy/lactation. Contraindicated with kidney disease, active liver disease, elderly, heart failure.

Table 38.3. *Continued*

Category and Mech. of Action	Generic (Trade) Name	Side Effects, Special Facts
Alpha-Glucosidase Inhibitors: Act by working in the intestines to slow the digestion of some carbohydrates and thus the after-meal blood glucose peaks are not so high.	1. Acarbose (Precose) 2. Miglitol (Glyset)	These drugs block the action of enzymes in the digestive tract that break down carbohydrates. The sugars are absorbed more slowly into the blood, which helps prevent the rapid rise in blood sugar that usually occurs right after a meal. They cause abdominal bloating, flatulence, and diarrhea. They are contraindicated with pregnancy/lactation. Hypoglycemia may occur when used with Prandin, insulin, or sulfonylureas. Treat the hypoglycemic reaction with **pure glucose tablets/gel or milk because** Precose or Glyset **delay** absorption of other carbohydrates.
Thiazolidine-diones (TZDs or Glitazones): These drugs help the muscle cells respond to insulin and use glucose.	1. Rosiglitazone maleate (Avandia) 2. Pioglitazone HCL (Actos)	TZDs require normal liver function. LFTs are done frequently. Contraindicated during pregnancy, lactation, and CHF. Rarely cause hypoglycemia.
Combination Drugs	1. Glyburide + Metformin (Glucovance) 2. Glipizide + Metformin (Metaglip) 3. Rosiglitazone + Metformin (Avandamet) 4. Pioglitazone + Metformin (Actoplus Met) 5. Rosiglitazone + Glimepiride (Avandaryl)	
Newer Drugs: **Incretin Mimetics**	1. Exenatide (Byetta)	Injectable Incretin hormone analog, injected SC bid 1 h prior to meals. Used in combination with Sulfonylurea and/or Metformin. **Category C agent.** Affects absorption of oral medications, so take antibiotics or OCs **1 h prior** to taking Byetta.

Table 38.3.   *Continued*

Category and Mech. of Action	Generic (Trade) Name	Side Effects, Special Facts
2. **Cannabinoid Receptor Antagonist**	Rimonabant (Acomplia or Zimulti)	
3. **Pramlintide (Symlin)**		Injectable.
4. **Inhaled Insulin (Exubera)**	Recently withdrawn due to poor demand	
5. **DPP-4 Inhibitors:** DPP-4 inhibitors release insulin in the presence of elevated blood sugar level. They decrease glucagon when needed thus minimizing hypoglycemia.	Sitaglyptin Phosphate (Januvia)	Stuffy nose, headaches.

DIABETES DENTAL ALERTS AND SUGGESTED MANAGEMENT GUIDELINES FOR DENTISTRY

The following are dental alerts and guidelines for diabetes:

1. Elevated sugar levels can predispose to the development of caries, periodontal disease, xerostomia, and parotid gland inflammation. Periodontal inflammation occurs because of poor blood sugar control. The patients have elevated C-reactive protein (CRP) levels and this indicates inflammation. The inflamed periodontal tissues have very high counts of anaerobic bacteria.

    There is a definite improvement in the patient's blood sugar and HbA$_1$C levels with periodontal treatment. Excessive periodontal inflammation is associated with an increased risk of death from cardiovascular and renal disease.

    Xerostomia predisposes to dental caries and oral candidiasis.

2. Know the type of diabetes and the duration of the diabetes and determine the patient's diabetes treatment.

3. Assess the laboratory tests—FBS, PPBS, HbA$_1$C—to determine the degree of disease control.

4. Avoid treating an uncontrolled diabetic. Elevated blood sugars can increase the risk of infection.

5. Determine the meal and snack times of the patient and always treat the patient on a full stomach.

6. Ideally, morning appointments are best following a regular breakfast. It does not make sense, however, to schedule a morning appointment if the patient eats minimally or not at all in the morning! Always check the patient's meal and snack times. Determine what the patient consumes and how much before you schedule the patient. The idea is always to treat the patient on a full stomach.

7. Always plan breaks for snack times so the patient can eat. Snack times are usually around 10:00am/3:00pm.

8. For outpatient routine dentistry, the type 1 patient **does not** need to cut back on the insulin dose. You need to check the blood sugars particularly during longer major surgical procedures.

9. A well-controlled patient will have an FBS <126 mg/dL, a PPBS <140 mg/dL, and an HbA$_1$C <7%.

10. An HbA$_1$C level >8% indicates that the patient has been uncontrolled for the past 1–2 months or 50–55 days.

11. Treat even a small infection aggressively with antibiotics for 5–7 days. Failure to treat an infection can promote the occurrence of acute or chronic osteomyelitis, and this in turn can worsen the diabetes control.

12. Always provide aggressive pain management immediately.

13. Pain, infection, and inflammation cause epinephrine release. Epinephrine causes glycogen breakdown to glucose and this results in the precipitation of hyperglycemia.

14. An insulin-dependent diabetic therefore must follow "sick-day rules of insulin" during these temporary states of hyperglycemia to bring the diabetes under control and to have a better outcome with the pain, infection, or inflammation.

15. **"Sick-day rules of insulin"**: The patient needs to monitor the blood sugar levels in the presence of infection, inflammation, bleeding, trauma, or fever. If the levels are elevated, the patient contacts the physician and the physician orders short-term changes in insulin therapy to correct the temporary rise in the blood sugar values.

16. Delayed healing and increased incidence of opportunistic infections are common with uncontrolled diabetes.

17. Neutrophil action is decreased and WBC migration to the site of the lesion is sluggish in patients with uncontrolled diabetes. These patients need antibiotics to promote the healing process.

18. Use stress management whenever needed to reduce anxiety.

19. Maintain hygiene recall at 3–4 month intervals.

20. Use nonabsorbable suture materials.

21. Patients on oral agents should take their normal dosage for all routine procedures done in a dental office.

22. Do not use NSAIDS or corticosteroids long-term in diabetics because they promote hyperglycemia. Chronic NSAIDS and corticosteroids use raises the blood sugar levels by promoting the breakdown of glycogen to glucose.

Suggested Modifications in Insulin Therapy for Major Surgery in the Dental Office (Outpatient Setting)

The following are insulin therapy modifications:

1. Remember that the patient will be slow in resuming food intake postoperatively.

2. The usual recommended protocol is for the patient to take **half** the dose of the intermediate or long-acting insulin and the **full dose** of the rapid or very rapid-acting insulin, prior to a full breakfast.

3. Following the procedure, when the patient is ready to resume meal consumption, the patient checks the sugar level prior to injecting insulin. The amount of

insulin injected postoperatively is dictated by the blood sugar level obtained at this time.
4. Once fully recovered, the patient gets back onto the routine insulin regimen.

Suggested Diabetes Management Protocol for a Type I Diabetic Undergoing Inpatient Major Surgery Under General Anesthesia

Use the following protocol for a type 1 diabetic:

1. The patient is kept NPO (nil by mouth) overnight.
2. **Half** of the intermediate or long-acting insulin is given on the morning of the surgery and **all** rapid or very rapid insulin is **withheld**.
3. The basal insulin is continued with IV 5% dextrose in water.
4. The blood glucose is checked frequently intraoperatively and is maintained between 100–150 mg/dL. Blood glucose, when kept in this range intraoperatively, ensures better postoperative recovery and healing.
5. If the intraoperative blood glucose levels increase beyond 200 mg/dL, the patient is given a bolus dose of Humalog/Novolog at a dose of 0.1 unit/kg body weight (BW). This is followed by a continuous drip of 1–2 units of Humalog or Novolog/hr. The dosage per hour is calculated as follows:

    Total Daily Dose (TDD) ÷ 24 hr = units given per hour.

6. The blood glucose is monitored every 1–2 hr during the postoperative period. Once meal consumption is resumed, the patient goes back on the routine insulin regimen as discussed previously.

Diabetes Management and Insulin Pumps

Patients on insulin pumps use Humalog or Novolog insulin only **and** continuous basal insulin is infused subcutaneously. The patient tests his/her blood sugar prior to every meal and adds more insulin if needed.

NPO Surgical Procedures and the Insulin Pump

The patient is put on an insulin drip as described under inpatient insulin protocol and the pump is temporarily stopped.

Suggested Major Surgery Management Guidelines and Type 2 Diabetes

Use the following guidelines for a Type 2 diabetic:

1. If a Type 2 patient is to undergo major surgery the patient is kept NPO (nil by mouth) overnight.
2. The patient **does not take** the oral agent on the morning of the surgery.
3. During surgery, the patient's blood glucose levels are monitored and maintained with infusion of IV insulin as done with the type 1 diabetic, discussed earlier.
4. Following surgery, when full meal intake is ready to be resumed, the patient monitors the blood sugar level **before** taking the oral agent. If the postop sugars are low, the patient can skip taking the oral agent. The patient resumes the routine oral agent intake on full recovery.

Blood Sugar Values and Suggested Dental Management Guidelines

The following are dental management guidelines for blood sugar values:

1. **The Well-Controlled Patient Will Have FBS <126 mg/dL, PPBS <140 mg/dL, and HbA₁C <7%:**
   - **Local Anesthetics:** Use 2% lidocaine (Xylocaine), 2% mepivacaine (Carbocaine) with 1:20,000 levonordefrin (NeoCobefrin), 0.5% bupivacaine (Marcaine) or 4% prilocaine HCL (Citanest Forte), maximum 2 carpules.
2. **The Moderately Uncontrolled Patient Can Have an FBS range of 125–140 mg/dL, a PPBS range of 140–200 mg/dL, and a HbA₁C range of 7–8%:**
   - **Local Anesthetics:** Decrease the amount of epinephrine in the local anesthetic. Use 4% prilocaine HCL (Citanest Forte) or 0.5% bupivacaine (Marcaine) local anesthetics with 1:200,000 epinephrine only, maximum 2 carpules.
   - **Antibiotics:** If antibiotics are needed following major surgery, **full** dose can be used.
3. **The Severely Uncontrolled Patient Will Have an FBS >140 mg/dL, a PPBS >200 mg/dL, and an HbA₁C >8%:**
   - The patient is treated dentally **only** if oral assessment indicates the presence of an **acute** dental infection. Infection worsens the diabetes control and treatment of the acute dental infection will improve the blood sugar levels during the postrecovery period.
   - Defer routine dental treatment in this stage for *all* patients with poor sugar controls until the diabetes is brought under better control.
   - Any dental emergency is treated using only 3% mepivacaine HCL (Carbocaine) or 4% prilocaine HCL (Citanest Plain). Give **low dose** antibiotic coverage to promote healing, for 3, 5, or 7 days.

39

Thyroid Gland Dysfunctions, Hyperthyroidism and Hypothyroidism: Assessment, Analysis, and Associated Dental Management Guidelines

HYPERTHYROIDISM

Hyperthyroidism Etiology

The patient can present with hyperthyroidism that can be due to a toxic nodular goiter, toxic adenoma, or excess thyroid hormone intake. Graves' disease (an autoimmune disorder) can also be associated with hyperthyroidism.

Hyperthyroidism Clinical Features

Hyperthyroidism can be associated with agitation, restlessness, anxiety, heat intolerance, fine tremors, polyphagia (excess appetite) with weight loss, excess perspiration of the hands and feet, warm skin, and frequent runs or diarrhea.

Graves' disease is associated with proptosis or protruding eyes because the Mueller's muscles are affected. This inflammation process can lead to double vision.

Graves' disease patients also have dermopathy that presents as pretibial myxedema or hypopigmentation of the skin. The gland is firm and smooth in Graves' disease.

Hyperthyroidism Vital Signs and Cardiac Findings

The following are vital signs and cardiac findings for patients with hyperthyroidism:

- **Pulse:** The patient can have a rapid heart rate/tachycardia with irregular heartbeats and resting tachycardia, which is an increased pulse rate during sleep.
- **Blood pressure:** The systolic blood pressure (SBP) is elevated because the BMR is increased. The diastolic blood pressure (DBP) is decreased in the uncontrolled hyperthyroid patient. Thus, the pulse pressure (PP), which is the difference between the SBP and the DBP is widened in hyperthyroidism and the PP is >40 mmHg (normal: 40 mmHg).
- **Cardiac findings:** Auscultation of the heart may often reveal a functional systolic murmur, which is a consequence of the hyperdynamic circulation secondary to the increased BMR and associated anemia. Arrhythmias can occur and this is the reason why hyperthyroid patients often take lanoxin (Digoxin) and/or warfarin (Coumadin) long-term.

Hyperthyroidism Diagnosis

Blood tests will show high T_3 and T_4 and low TSH. The high levels of T_3 and T_4 inhibit the release of the thyroid-releasing hormone (TRH) from the hypothalamus and this in turn inhibits the release of thyroid-stimulating hormone (TSH) from the pituitary.

Hyperthyroidism Treatment Options

Hyperthyroidism treatment options consist of the following:

1. **Antithyroid drugs:** Propylthiouracil (PTU), Tapazole, or Methimazole. These drugs interfere with thyroid hormone production.
2. **Radioactive iodine (I^{131}):** I^{131} causes gradual destruction of thyroid gland cells.
3. **Surgery:** Thyroidectomy can be an option for any age patient, and removal of part of the gland restores the euthyroid (normal thyroid) status.

Hyperthyroidism Treatment Option Selection Protocol

The treatment option selected depends on the patient's age:

1. **Childbearing age:**
   a. **First option—Antithyroid drugs:** Treatment with Propylthiouracil (PTU), Methimazole, or Tapazole constitutes the first option.
   b. **Second option—Surgery:** A part of the gland is removed and normal gland function is subsequently restored. Overtreatment with surgery can lead to hypothyrodism. Once the patient becomes hypothyroid, synthroid (L-thyroxine) is given as replacement therapy for life.
2. **Non-childbearing age:**
   Radioactive I^{131}: This treatment is reserved for the non- childbearing age patient or patients who have had failures of antithyroid drug therapy. Radioactive I^{131} is given as a drink. In the first 2 weeks following I^{131} treatment, the patient is isolated from pregnant patients and children to prevent radiation. 25% of these patients can go on to develop hypothyroidism 1 year later. An important fact to remember is that I^{131} concentrates in the **salivary glands** and can cause xerostomia, caries, and salivary gland swelling.

HYPERTHYROIDISM DENTAL FACTS AND SUGGESTED DENTAL GUIDELINES

The following are dental facts and guidelines for hyperthyroidism:

1. Accelerated tooth development occurs in children with hyperthyroidism.
2. Malocclusion can occur if eruptions of secondary teeth are precocious.
3. **Local Anesthetics:** Epinephrine in the local anesthetic and epinephrine cords must absolutely be avoided during the time the patient is on PTU/Methimazole/Tapazole. Once the patient is off these drugs, the use of local anesthetics with epinephrine can resume; however, limit it to two carpules only.
4. PTU has anti–Vit K activity and causes agranulocytosis and thrombocytopenia. Always check the CBC with platelet count and PT/INR when doing major dental work on such patients.

5. Calculate the absolute neutrophil count (ANC) in the patient with a decreased WBC count and follow the ANC guidelines for antibiotic coverage. Antibiotics are needed to prevent infection and promote healing in the presence of agranulocytosis.
6. Sympathetic overactivity in the hyperthyroid patient is suppressed medically with the use of β-blockers. β-blockers decrease the associated tachycardia, agitation, and elevation of the BP.
7. β-blockers mask hypoglycemic symptoms, and sweating is the only symptom that occurs. Therefore, always consider a hypoglycemic reaction occurring if the patient starts to sweat in the chair and you are aware that the surroundings are not hot.

HYPOTHYROIDISM

Hypothyroidism Etiology

Autoimmune-associated Hashimoto's thyroiditis is the most common form of hypothyroidism. Hypothyroidism can also occur as a consequence to postradioactive iodine treatment or posthyperthyroid surgery.

Hypothyroidism Symptoms

These patients are lethargic, slow to react, have coarse dry skin, feel cold, suffer from constipation, have puffiness around the face and complain of fatigue, weight gain, and cold intolerance. Cretinism occurs with congenital hypothyroidism.

Hypothyroidism Signs

The pulse is slow and the SBP is decreased because the BMR is decreased. The DBP is elevated because of severe vasoconstriction. The pulse pressure in an uncontrolled hypothyroid patient is <40 mmHg.

Hypothyroidism Diagnosis

Blood tests show low T_4 and high TSH.

Hypothyroidism Treatment

Levo-Thyroxine (Synthroid) is the treatment of choice. The half-life of Synthroid is 12 days.

Drug-Drug Interactions (DDIs) with Synthroid

The following are drug-drug interactions with Synthroid:

- L-Thyroxin (Synthroid) decreases the effectiveness of digoxin (Lanoxin), so dose adjustments are needed in patients taking both these drugs.
- Synthroid enhances the catabolism of warfarin (Coumadin) in patients taking both these drugs.

HYPOTHYROIDISM ADDITIONAL FACTS AND SUGGESTED DENTAL GUIDELINES

The patient with cretinism presents with maxillary prognathism and retardation of tooth development. Excessive caries, macroglossia, and swollen lips can occur due to myxedema.

Hypothyroidism and Local Anesthetics

Use the following guidelines for local anesthetics:

1. **Uncontrolled hypothyroid patient:** Do not use epinephrine in the uncontrolled hypothyroid patient. The epinephrine will stay in the system longer because the BMR is decreased, plus the epinephrine can tax a sluggish heart.
2. **Controlled hypothyroid patient:** Use xylocaine with epinephrine, but limit it to 2 carpules.

Hypothyroidism and Sedatives, Hypnotics, and Narcotics

Use the following guidelines for sedatives, hypnotics, and narcotics:

1. The uncontrolled patient will have exaggerated response to narcotics and barbiturates.
2. Do not use diazepam (Valium), codeine, or other sedatives, hypnotics, or narcotics in the uncontrolled hypothyroid patient, because myxedema coma can occur.
3. The controlled hypothyroid patient can get diazepam (Valium), Tylenol #1–3, or other sedatives, hypnotics, or narcotics.

40

Adrenal Gland Cortex and Medulla Disease States: Assessment, Analysis, and Associated Dental Management Guidelines

ADRENAL GLAND PHYSIOLOGY AND ADRENAL GLAND HORMONES

Adrenal Cortex Hormones

The adrenal cortex produces the following main hormones:

- Glucocorticoids
- Mineralocorticoids
- Androgens

Glucocorticoids

Cortisol is released daily from the adrenal cortex and it helps the body regulate the protein, carbohydrate, and fat metabolism. Additionally, cortisol release also helps fight stress and suppress inflammation.

The Normal Mechanism of Cortisol Production (Figure 40.1)

The hypothalamus releases the corticotropin hormone (CRH). CRH stimulates the pituitary to release the adrenocorticotropic hormone (ACTH). ACTH stimulates the adrenal cortex to release cortisol, which is also called *hydrocortisone*. Cortisol, in turn, provides the negative feedback to the pituitary and the hypothalamus when adequate cortisol level is reached.

Cushing's syndrome is associated with **excess** cortisol production, and Addison's disease is associated with a **deficiency** of cortisol and aldosterone.

Normal Cortisol Amounts Released and Corresponding Prednisone Equivalents

In a normal healthy patient **20 mg Cortisol** is released in the early morning every day between **2–8am** and this is equivalent to **5 mg prednisone**. The maximum output of endogenous cortisol released in response to severe stress by a **normal** gland is around **100–150 mg**; this is equivalent to about **25–40 mg prednisone**.

The antiinflammatory potency of prednisone is *four times* that of hydrocortisone (Solu-Cortef). Thus, the *maximum* amount of steroid replacement given *during stressful* times should be about **25–40 mg prednisone PO or 100–150 mg hydrocortisone PO/IV**.

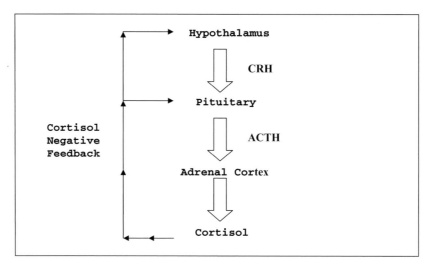

Figure 40.1. The hypothalamus-pituitary–adrenal cortex cortisol release cycle.

Mineralocorticoids

Aldosterone is the main hormone that helps maintain the plasma sodium and potassium balance. Aldosterone secretion is regulated by the renin-angiotensin system, the ACTH, and the plasma sodium and potassium levels. With a drop in the blood pressure, renin is released from the kidneys and renin triggers the release of aldosterone. Aldosterone, in turn, causes retention of sodium and a washout of potassium, which then causes the blood pressure to rise.

Androgens

The androgens released by the adrenal cortex help with protein anabolism and growth.

The Adrenal Medulla

The adrenal medulla produces the following:

- **Catecholamines:** The catecholamines regulate the myocardial contraction, myocardial excitability, blood pressure, sympathetic tone, and metabolisms.
- **Two Main Hormones:** epinephrine and norepinephrine.

CUSHING'S SYNDROME

Cushing's Syndrome Etiology

Endogenous Causes

Pituitary, adrenal, or ectopic tumors in the lungs produce excess cortisol.

Exogenous Causes

Excessive steroid intake given for the management of asthma, rheumatoid arthritis, etc., can increase cortisol levels in the blood.

Cushing's Syndrome Symptoms and Signs

Fatigue, weakness, ankle edema, central obesity, moon faces, "buffalo hump" around the neck, acne, hirsutism, menstrual dysfunction or amenorrhea, hypertension, easy bruising, osteoporosis, and peripheral muscle wasting are common presenting features.

Cushing's Syndrome Treatment

Treatment options are surgery, radiation, or medication.

CUSHING'S SYNDROME–ASSOCIATED DENTAL ALERTS

The following are dental alerts associated with Cushing's syndrome:

1. Patients with Cushing's syndrome have an increased risk for osteoporosis (because cortisol lowers bone formation), hypertension, heart failure, peptic ulcer, and diabetes (cortisol is antagonistic to insulin). The status of any of these conditions when present must be assessed and dental management accordingly modified following the disease/condition-specific suggested dental guidelines in appropriate sections where discussed.
2. The blood pressure (BP) should be routinely monitored during dentistry.
3. Aspirin and NSAIDS should be avoided because of the high incidence of peptic ulcer.
4. Patients with Cushing's syndrome also have an increased risk for periodontitis, oral candidiasis, and easily bleeding gums.
5. Excess steroids in the system lower the immune system activity and this increases the risk of infections and poor wound healing.
6. The practitioner should also provide adequate antibiotic coverage for 5–7 days following a major surgical procedure to promote the healing process.
7. The practitioner should assess and treat the oral cavity for oral and esophageal candidiasis when present.
8. Generalized osteoporosis can also affect the mandible and patients with dentures may need frequent readjustments.

ADDISON'S DISEASE

Addison's disease is associated with a lack of adrenal hormones cortisol and aldosterone.

Addison's Disease Etiology

The etiological factors associated with Addison's disease are autoimmune insult, TB affecting the adrenal gland, metastatic tumor, and bilateral adrenal cortical hemorrhage.

Addison's Disease Symptoms and Signs

Addison's disease patients experience tiredness, weakness, anorexia, weight loss, nausea, vomiting, lethargy, postural hypotension and oral pigmentation. Blotchy melanin patches occur on the oral mucosa and skin. The melanocyte stimulating hormone (**MSH**) is co-secreted **along with ACTH** causing the pigmentation. The pigmentation occurs on the buccal mucosa and spreads backward from the commissures.

Addison's Disease Diagnosis

Blood tests show low levels of cortisol and aldosterone and high levels of ACTH.

ADDISON'S DISEASE–ASSOCIATED DENTAL ALERTS AND SUGGESTED DENTAL GUIDELINES

The following are dental alerts and guidelines for Addison's disease:

1. Patients with Addison's disease have to be compensated with steroids to fight the stress associated with infection; inflammation; excessive bleeding; postprocedure starvation; pre- and postop pain (**very high risk factor**); and trauma associated with surgery, due to the lack of cortisol and aldosterone.
2. The dentist must consult with the patient's physician during the above-mentioned circumstances and provide adequate steroid coverage to compensate for the stress. Failure to provide coverage will precipitate acute adrenal insufficiency and collapse.
3. Patients taking steroids for more than 2 weeks may have adrenal insufficiency and consequently require additional steroid coverage for up to 2 years after treatment.
4. Oral infections must be aggressively treated in the Addison's disease patient to prevent hypoadrenal crisis or acute adrenal insufficiency from happening.
5. Addison's patients benefit when given stress management with benzodiazepines or $O_2 + N_2O$ because stress reduction decreases cortisol demand.
6. It is best to treat the patient as the **first** appointment of the day because the cortisol secretion is at its highest in the morning between **2–8am**. Cortisol secretion is **lowest** toward the **end** of the day.
7. Individuals working the night shift have a circadian rhythm reversal, and maximum cortisol release occurs during early evening, when they are awake.
8. If the patient is **currently** on steroids it is best for the patient to take the steroid for that day, **2 hr prior** to dentistry.
9. Avoid barbiturates because they decrease cortisol levels.
10. Typically for minor procedures, no extra steroids are needed.
11. For major procedures, give **25–40 mg prednisone** PO, 1 hr prior to treatment on the day of surgery and taper over 2 days. Alternatively, you can give **100–150 mg IV/IM hydrocortisone**, 1 hr prior to the procedure, if the patient has to be nil-by-mouth (NPO) on the day of the surgery. This is followed by a taper back to baseline within 48 hr once surgery is completed.

CORTICOSTEROIDS ADDITIONAL DETAILS AND SUGGESTED DENTAL GUIDELINES

The following are additional details and dental guidelines for corticosteroids:

1. During history-taking always evaluate for a history of corticosteroid therapy and determine:

"**The rule of twos**": Ask whether the patient is currently on steroids or has been on corticosteroids for 2 weeks or longer within the past 2 years. You must go back 2 years in the history because it can take **2 weeks to 2 years** for the adrenal glands to bounce back to **normal** function.

2. When exogenous steroids are taken by mouth or by injections, an inhibition of the endogenous cortisol release occurs because of a negative feedback and associated decreased ATCH release.

3. Normal cortisol release occurs around 2–8am daily. Individuals working the night shift (discussed earlier) have a circadian rhythm reversal and maximum cortisol release occurs in the late afternoon and early evening, when they are awake.

4. Exogenous corticosteroids will cause *minimal* endogenous corticosteroid suppression when the exogenous dose is given **prior to 9am**.

5. Patients needing steroids prior to dentistry will benefit when treated as the **first** appointment in the morning.

6. Patients needing steroids will also benefit when given stress management with benzodiazepines or $O_2 + N_2O$ because stress reduction decreases cortisol demand.

7. In the dental setting a patient with a history of steroid intake may need **extra** steroids in the presence of infection, fever, inflammation, bleeding, pain, or trauma due to surgery. Always consult with the patient's physician under such circumstances to determine the need for supplementation.

8. Corticosteroids decrease inflammation by inhibiting the migration of polymorphonuclear (PMN) leukocytes and causing a reversal of increased capillary permeability.

9. The antiinflammatory potency of prednisone is *four times* that of hydrocortisone (Solu-Cortef). This becomes important during a dental emergency when hydrocortisone (Solu-Cortef) is used instead of prednisone: 5 **mg prednisone = 20 mg Hydrocortisone**.

10. Prednisone, hydrocortisone, and dexamethasone are the most commonly used steroid preparations.

11. Dexamethasone is **40 times** stronger than hydrocortisone.

12. When extra steroids are needed for planned procedures, the intake or boost must begin **48 hr prior** to the surgery and, as discussed earlier, the *maximum* amount of steroid replacement given *during stressful* times is about 25–40 mg **prednisone** PO or 100–150 mg **hydrocortisone** PO/IV.

13. For planned surgical procedures, the prednisone dose is increased gradually in a step-up pattern preoperatively and decreased gradually in a step-down pattern postoperatively, as shown in Figure 40.2.

Alternate-Day Steroid Intake and Dentistry

Patients are often on alternate-day steroid intake because this method of care is associated with a lesser degree of endogenous steroid secretion inhibition. It is best to schedule surgery on the day of steroid intake. In most cases depending on the intensity of the procedure and the amount of steroid boost required, one can double the steroid dose on the day of treatment and taper the dose post operatively.

The step-up and step-down corticosteroid protocols using **10 mg/20 mg/40 mg** prednisone **on the day** of the surgical procedure in a patient on **0-5-0 mg** alternate-day steroid intake therapy are illustrated in Figure 40.3.

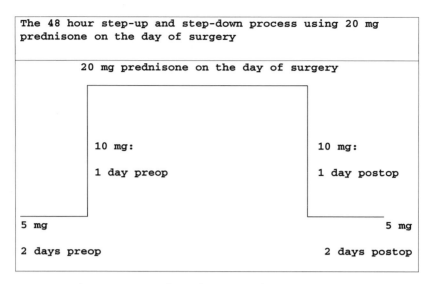

Figure 40.2. Prednisone step-up and step-down protocol.

Surgery Day Dose	10 mg/20 mg/40 mg prednisone boost protocol with 0-5-0 alternate day prednisone therapy
10 mg	Doubling of dose on the day of intake: 0 5 0 **10** 5 0 5 0 5 0 5 0 5 0 5 0 5 0 5 0 5 0 5
20 mg	0 5 0 **10 20 10** 5 0 5 0 5 0 5 0 5 0 5 0 5 0
40 mg	0 5 **10 20 40 20 10** 5 0 5 0 5 0 5 0 5 0 5 0

Figure 40.3. Suggested step-up and step-down corticosteroid protocols.

Discussion: Suggested Steroid Dose Guidelines for Mild/Moderate/Severe Stress-Associated Dentistry

Mild Stress

This could be about four or less extractions or one quadrant flap surgery. Double the steroid dose if the patient is currently on steroids or give 25 mg hydrocortisone PO/IV or 6.25 mg (round off to 6.0 mg) of prednisone PO, 1 hr prior to surgery if the patient is not currently on steroids but needs steroids. Giving 5 mg prednisone will also suffice.

Moderate Stress

This could be about 5–16 extractions or two quadrants flap surgery. Prescribe 50–75 mg hydrocortisone PO/IV or 12.5–18.75 mg (round off to 15–20 mg) of prednisone PO, 1 hr prior to surgery.

Severe Stress

This could be about 17 or more extractions or three or more quadrants flap surgery: Prescribe 100–150 mg hydrocortisone PO/IV or 25–37.5 mg (round off to 25–40 mg)

Table 40.1. Suggested steroid dose guidelines for mild/moderate/severe stress-associated dentistry

Stress Level	Suggestions
Mild stress: Stress equivalent to 1–4 extractions or 1 quadrant flap surgery	If patient is currently on steroids: Depending on the procedure, double the steroid dose. If patient is **not** currently on steroids: **Use 1 of 3 choices 1 h before surgery:** **1.** 6 mg prednisone PO **2.** 25 mg Hydrocortisone PO/IV **3.** 5 mg prednisone PO
Moderate stress: Stress equivalent to 5–16 extractions or 2 quadrants flap surgery	**Use 1 of 2 choices 1 h before surgery:** **1.** 15–20 mg prednisone PO **2.** 50–75 mg Hydrocortisone PO/IV
Severe stress: Stress equivalent to 17 or more extractions or 3 or more quadrants flap surgery	**Use 1 of 2 choices 1 h before surgery:** **1.** 25–40 mg prednisone PO **2.** 100–150 mg Hydrocortisone PO/IV

prednisone PO, 1 hr prior to surgery. It is always best to err on the side of giving more steroids than giving lesser amounts of steroids when needed (Table 40.1).

Prednisone or Hydrocortisone Boost Protocol During Dental Emergency

Follow these steps:

1. During a dental emergency, the treatment cannot be delayed to incorporate the step-up protocol of steroid intake. Thus, the step-up protocol is completely skipped.
2. Dependent on the patient's needs and the major surgical procedure performed, approximately 25–40 mg prednisone is given PO/IV/IM. The PO and IV dose are given **1 hr** prior to surgery.
3. Alternately the patient can be given PO/IV hydrocortisone (Cortef/Solu-Cortef) and, as discussed earlier, the dose given is *four times* the prednisone dose required for the major dental procedure.
4. The postoperative steroid step-down is never skipped and is done with prednisone or hydrocortisone PO in the outpatient dental setting. Hydrocortisone IV is used for step-down in the inpatient dental setting.
5. Failure to give extra steroids when needed will result in greatly lowered cortisol levels, triggering a circulatory collapse due to acute adrenal insufficiency.

Acute Adrenal Insufficiency Attack

In the presence of acute infection, inflammation, pain, trauma, or massive bleeding, acute adrenal insufficiency can occur if the patient is not given a steroid supplementation when needed. Please refer to Chapter 9, "Management of Medical Emergencies in the Dental Setting: Assessment, Analysis, and Associated Dental Management Guidelines," for discussion on clinical features and management of acute adrenal insufficiency.

Parathyroid Dysfunction Disease States: Assessment, Analysis, and Associated Dental Management Guidelines

PARATHYROID GLAND PHYSIOLOGY, FACTS, AND DYSFUNCTION OVERVIEW

Parathyroid dysfunction is frequently associated with disturbances in the bone. Presence of some form of bone pathology may prompt a dentist to evaluate tests to measure serum calcium, phosphorus, and alkaline phosphatase levels. These tests are primarily used to diagnose hyperparathyroidism, Paget's disease, metastatic bone disease, and disturbances in calcium absorption (Figure 41.1).

Calcium Metabolism and Homeostasis

All normal adult patients should consume 800–1,500 mg/day of calcium. About 800–1,200 mg is absorbed and most of the absorbed calcium is retained in the bones.

The parathyroid hormone (PTH) activates vitamin D that affects bones and the kidneys. Most of the vitamin D is produced by the skin via absorption of the ultraviolet rays, but some vitamin D is also obtained from the diet. The inactive form of vitamin D is 25(OH)-D and it is stored in the liver. The active form of vitamin D is 1, 25 dihydroxy D and the activation occurs in the kidneys.

Increases in serum calcium levels usually result from mobilization of calcium from the bones into the blood. This is a common finding with hyperparathyroidism, dietary and absorption disturbances, and vitamin D toxicity.

Parathyroid hormone regulates the excretion of phosphate by the kidneys and hyperparathyroidism is associated with low phosphorous levels. Phosphorous levels are increased in patients with hypoparathyroidism and renal disease.

Alkaline phosphatase is an enzyme mainly found in the liver and the bones. Biliary stasis, pregnancy, growing bones, Paget's disease, metastatic bone disease, and renal and intestinal tumors all cause increases in the alkaline phosphatase levels.

Hyperparathyroidism

Hyperparathyroidism is associated with high calcium levels and high PTH. It usually manifests as a single adenoma but all four parathyroid glands may be affected.

Disease State(s):	Parathyroid Hormone (PTH); Calcium and Phosphorus patterns
Hyperparathyroidism:	↑ PTH, ↑ Calcium, ↓ Phosphorus
Hypoparathyroid or Renal Disease:	↓ PTH, ↓ Calcium, ↑ Phosphorus
Secondary Hyperparathyroidism:	↑ PTH, ↓ Calcium, ↑ Phosphorus

Figure 41.1. PTH, calcium, and phosphorus changes and associated disease states.

Hypoparathyroidism

Hypoparathyroidism is associated with low calcium and low PTH levels. The condition is usually autoimmune. Hypoparathyroidism may be associated with oral candidiasis, hypoplasia of enamel, dentin, short roots, and delayed eruption of the teeth.

Osteomalacia

Osteomalacia is associated with vitamin D deficiency and it can be familial or acquired.

Renal Osteodystrophy

The active form of vitamin D, 1,25 dihydroxycholecalciferol is not formed because of kidney failure, and this failure to form the active metabolite of vitamin D results in inhibition of calcium absorption from the gut. Low calcium absorption triggers secondary hyperparathyroidism and for the body to maintain adequate calcium hemostasis, calcium is drawn out from the bones. Patients with renal osteodystrophy are therefore prone to accelerated alveolar bone loss and it is not uncommon to discover Brown tumors in the jaws of such patients.

During dentistry, follow the AAA guidelines suggested for kidney disease in patients presenting with renal osteodystrophy.

Vitamin D Excess

Excess vitamin D is associated with an excess of calcium.

Endogenous Causes of Vitamin D Excess

Endogenous causes include sarcoidosis, lymphoma, or TB. The immune cells make vitamin D in excess and this causes the calcium levels to be high.

Exogenous Causes of Vitamin D Excess

The exogenous cause is the presence of too much vitamin D in the milk.

Hypercalcemia from Tumors

Hypercalcemia can be caused by calcium-producing tumors from the lungs or breast.

OSTEOPOROSIS

Risk Factors Associated with Osteoporosis

Thin body, Caucasian or Asian patient, low calcium intake, and hyperthyroidism, which accelerates bone metabolism. Osteoporosis is most common in postmenopausal women. Osteoporosis is diagnosed by measurement of the bone density, mass, and volume of the lumbar spine and hip.

Osteoporosis Treatment

Calcium and vitamin D supplementation, antiresorptive agents (bisphosphonates) and recombinant parathyroid hormone (rPTH) are used in the treatment of osteoporosis.

BISPHOSPHONATES

Bisphosphonates Facts and Overview

Bisphosphonates decrease bone resorption, thus slowing down bone loss. They have long been used to prevent bone fractures in patients with osteoporosis and to control bone pain. Bisphosphonates, however, **interfere** with the natural **bone-rep**air process.

Bisphosphonates, when started, **accumulate slowly** in the bone due to minimal absorption in the gut. They also **come out slowly**, later, when stopped. The bones retain bisphosphonates for a long time. Bisphosphonates coat the bone and depress overall bone turnover, thus causing too much bone formation and overall bone destruction. Short- or long-term use may therefore result in bone necrosis.

Recent studies done in the medical field have shown that patients on bisphosphonates for 5–7 years were found to be at risk for fractures in the long bones of the leg. Thus, many medical bone centers the world over, suggest a "drug holiday" for 1–2 years, after about 5 years of bisphosphonate therapy. The endpoint of this drug holiday is reached when the blood test, like the serum C-terminal cross-linking telopeptide (CTX) reference value, (CTX test), shows an increase in bone-turnover markers.

The serum CTX test assesses the rate of bone renewal, clinical healing, and risk level for bisphosphonate-induced osteonecrosis. The patient has to fast for 12 hr prior to the test and results are obtained in 4–7 days.

Intravenous bisphosphonates are most used in patients with myeloma, breast cancer, and prostate cancers because these tumors are most susceptible to the effects of systemic bisphosphonates. They can also be used to prevent some cancers of the breast or lymphoma from spreading to the bone.

Bisphosphonate-Related Osteonecrosis of the Jaw (BRONJ) or Bisphosphonate-Induced Osteonecrosis of the Jaw (BIONJ)

Of late, bisphosphonates have been implicated in the nonhealing of bone at extraction sites, leading to osteonecrosis. Intravenous zoledronic acid (Zometa) and pamidronate (Aredia/Pamisol) have been most implicated. The exact risk of BRONJ/BIONJ with oral bisphosphonates—alendronate (Fosamax), risedronate (Actonel), and Ibandronate (Boniva)—is not known, but it is thought to be less than that for systemic bisphosphonates. Literature shows that oral intake of bisphosphonates, has been implicated in some sporadic cases.

BRONJ/BIONJ affects the mandible most often, followed by the maxilla. The maxilla, however, is found to have more multifocal or bilateral involvement when compared with the mandible. Most lesions occur on the posterior lingual mandible near the mylo-hyoid ridge.

BRONJ/BIONJ Clinical Presentation

When it occurs, BRONJ/BIONJ presents as an intraoral lesion containing exposed bone that appears yellow-white, with ragged margins. Sinus tracts may or may not be associated with the lesion. Painful ulcers frequently surround the lesion and are present in the adjacent soft tissues.

Suggested Treatment of BRONJ/BIONJ

Treatment of BRONJ/BIONJ consists of the following:

1. Temporarily stop the bisphosphonate therapy.
2. Avoid any further dentoalveolar trauma.
3. Use oral antibiotic plus rinses and allow time for healing. Systemic and topical antibiotic therapy with oral penicillin VK or amoxicillin is suggested along with the use of 0.12% chlorhexidine gluconate oral rinses. This regimen is quite effective in controlling the pain associated with BRONJ/BIONJ. It is important to remember that there is no resolution of the lesion with this regimen.
4. Dental gingival flap placement may help stimulate healing.
5. Hyperbaric oxygen may need to be used in some cases to counteract osteonecrosis.

BRONJ/BIONJ Prevention

Patients on bisphosphonates must maintain good oral hygiene and the dentist must implement preventative dentistry and prevent the need for extractions in the future.

Dental extractions, dentoalveolar surgery, and ill-fitting dentures have been most implicated as causative procedures or factors for BRONJ/BIONJ.

BRONJ/BIONJ can be prevented by completing all these procedures when needed, **prior** to the start of bisphosphonate therapy or **within** the first 3 years of therapy. The serum CTX test should be done **prior** to major dentistry, especially if bisphosphonate therapy has gone **beyond** 3 years. The CTX test will indicate the risk level for BRONJ/BIONJ.

Serum CTX values <100 pg/mL are associated with a **high risk** of developing BIONJ; values between 100–150 pg/mL have a **moderate risk** of BIONJ and values >150 pg/mL have **no risk** of developing BIONJ.

Patients at high risk are usually advised to stop the intake of the bisphosphonate temporarily for 4–6 months and a repeat CTX level is done to identify the endpoint of the temporary cessation and the go-ahead for major dentistry.

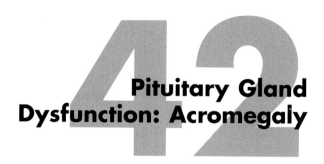

Pituitary Gland Dysfunction: Acromegaly

ACROMEGALY FACTS

The following summarizes acromegaly seen in dentistry:

- Acromegaly is associated with excess growth hormone (GH) from a pituitary tumor. The hands and feet are big, the patient often complains of excessive sweating, and there is an increased incidence of colonic polyps and colon cancer.
- Accelerated tooth eruption occurs in children.
- Enlarged jaw with prognathism is common, the teeth are spaced and tipped outward, and the facial features are coarse. The patient has larger maxillary sinuses, and this is the cause of a booming voice in these patients.

ACROMEGALY TREATMENT

Acromegaly treatment options are, surgery, radiation or somatostatin therapy (an inhibitor of GH), and GH receptor blockade.

X

Seizure Disorders

Classic Seizures, Petit Mal and Grand Mal Epilepsy: Assessment, Analysis, and Associated Dental Management Guidelines

SEIZURE CLASSIFICATION, OVERVIEW, AND TREATMENT OPTIONS

Seizure Classification

Conditions associated with seizures are:

1. Vasovagal syncopal reaction
2. Orthostatic hypotension
3. Hyperventilation syndrome
4. Hypoglycemic reaction
5. Grand mal epilepsy
6. Petit mal epilepsy

The first four causes are discussed in Chapter 9, "Management of Medical Emergencies in the Dental Setting: Assessment, Analysis, and Associated Dental Management Guidelines." Causes 5 and 6 are major seizure disorders discussed in this chapter.

General Introduction

Seizures are caused because of abnormal electrical discharges in the brain, and they can occur as grand mal seizures, petit mal seizures, or temporal lobe seizures. Occurrence of repeat seizures leads to a diagnosis of epilepsy.

The seizure is said to be **generalized** if the abnormal electrical discharges cross over the midline in the brain. When the seizures involve only a few muscles on the face, arms, or legs it is called a **focal** seizure. A grand mal seizure or a tonic-clonic seizure is characterized by loss of consciousness associated with the patient falling down, loss of bowel or bladder control, and rhythmic-to-arrhythmic convulsions.

Seizure Etiology

The following are etiological factors associated with seizures:

- **Familial:** Seizures can be familial affecting several members in the family.
- **Unknown Etiology:** Often the etiology is unknown and there is no associated family history.

- **Metabolic Disturbances:** Seizures can occur from chemical imbalance due to liver or kidney disease or due to very low levels of sodium, calcium, or magnesium.
- **Trauma:** Head injuries can cause seizures.
- **Space-Occupying Lesions:** Tumors or arterial-venous malformations in the brain can trigger seizures.
- **Cerebrovascular Accidents (CVA) or Strokes:** CVA can cause seizures in older patients.
- **Drug Addiction:** Recreational drug withdrawal can be associated with seizures.
- **Cerebral Infection:** Meningitis or encephalitis can trigger a seizure.
- **Other Causes:** Seizures can also be triggered by stress, lack of sleep, flickering lights, alcohol, or touch.

Seizure Diagnosis

Seizure diagnosis is established with the following:

1. **History and Physical (H&P) Examination:** A good H&P can reveal the etiology and presenting symptoms and signs of the seizure.
2. **Electroencephalography (EEG):** EEG measures the electrical activity in the brain and can show areas of increased activity.
3. **Magnetic Resonance Imaging (MRI):** MRI can detect brain pathology.

Seizure Treatment

Management of seizures consists of the following:

1. Treatment of the underlying cause, if known.
2. **Surgery:** Surgery is an option when a tumor or vascular malformation is the cause of the seizure. Surgery is also an option when the patient does not respond to medications and has such frequent seizures that it compromises the patient's life style on a major scale.
3. Antiseizure medications.

SEIZURE MEDICATIONS

Grand Mal Seizure Medications

The most common medications used for grand mal epilepsy are phenytoin sodium (Dilantin); carbamazepine (Tegretol); phenobarbital (Barbita/Luminal); primidone (Mysoline); gabapentin (Neurontin); clonazepam (Klonopin); oxcarbazepine (Trileptal); and benzodiazepines, lorazepam (Ativan) or diazepam (Valium).

Petit Mal Seizure Medications

The following are petit mal medications:

1. **Older medications:** Valproic acid (Depakene), divalproex (Depakote), and ethosuximide (Zarontin)
2. **Newer medications:** Lamotrigine (Lamictal), topiramate (Topamax), and zonisamide (Zonegran).

SEIZURE MEDICATIONS DETAILED DISCUSSION

To better manage a patient with a history of seizures, it is important to understand the medications used to treat the disorder, as presented in the next sections. Significant facts relevant to dentistry have been highlighted with each drug.

Phenytoin Sodium (Dilantin)

Dilantin Facts

Phenytoin (Dilantin) is used in the management of grand mal epilepsy, and chronic use is associated with **gingival hyperplasia.** Dilantin **inhibits** the absorption of **folic acid** from the gut and predisposes the patient to develop folic acid deficiency/megaloblastic anemia. Evaluate the CBC and follow the suggested AAA guidelines for anemia, if detected on the CBC. Chronic **alcohol** use or abuse decreases the serum levels of Dilantin and predisposes the patient to have more **frequent seizures.**

Dilantin and Drug-Drug Interactions (DDIs)

The following are Dilantin drug-drug interactions:

- Avoid the use of salicylates or diazepam (Valium) because these drugs can increase the serum levels of Dilantin.
- Avoid using doxycycline (Vibramycin) because the efficacy of doxycycline is impaired in the presence of Dilantin.

Carbamazepine (Tegretol)

Carbamazepine (Tegretol) is used for the management of grand mal seizures **and** trigeminal neuralgia.

Tegretol and DDIs

The following are Tegretol drug-drug interactions:

- Avoid using doxycycline (Vibramycin) because carbamazepine (Tegretol) decreases the half-life of doxycycline.
- Macrolides and propoxyphene (Darvon) use should be restricted because these drugs raise Tegretol level.

Phenobarbital (Barbita/Luminal)

Phenobarbital Facts

Phenobarbital is the oldest and most widely used medication in the world and it is used for the management of generalized and partial seizures. Due to its sedative and hypnotic effects, phenobarbital is less preferred compared to the benzodiazepines.

Phenobarbital (Barbita/Luminal) and DDIs

The following are phenobarbital drug-drug interactions:

- Do not prescribe doxycycline with phenobarbital because phenobarbital induces the CYP450 enzymes in the liver, enhancing the utilization of doxycycline.

- Phenobarbital increases the effectiveness of sedatives, hypnotics, narcotics, and acetaminophen. It is suggested you avoid using sedatives, hypnotics, and narcotics with phenobarbital and also use only regular-strength Tylenol, not extra-strength Tylenol.

Primidone (Mysolin)

Primidone Facts

Primidone is used for the management of grand mal, complex, and focal seizures. Primidone is the first-line drug (along with Propranolol) for the management of benign tremors. It is a GABA receptor agonist that also causes sedation because of its active metabolites, phenobarbital and phenylethylmalonamide. Primidone is associated with folic acid deficiency and poor calcium absorption. Evaluate the CBC and the radiographs for bone density in patients on primidone. Follow the AAA suggested guidelines for anemia if the CBC shows anemia. Primidone induces the enzymes in the liver and accelerates the metabolism of several medications.

Primidone (Mysolin) and DDIs

The following are primidone drug-drug interactions:

- Primidone hastens the metabolism of doxycycline, dexamethasone, and other steroids due to liver enzyme induction and consequently decreases their effect.
- Avoid fentanyl use as Primidone causes increase in fentanyl levels.

Gabapentin (Neurontin)

Neurontin is used for seizure disorders, trigeminal neuralgia, leg cramps, and postherpetic neuralgia. Alcohol increases the risk of side effects with Neurontin.

Gabapentin (Neurontin) and DDIs

The following are gabapentin drug-drug interactions:

- Antacids decrease Neurontin absorption and an interval of **at least 2 hr** must be maintained to avoid this DDI.
- Neurontin increases the effects of antihistamines, sedatives, centrally acting pain medications, benzodiazepines, and muscle relaxants, causing profound drowsiness. Avoid dispensing these medications during dentistry.

Clonazepam (Klonopin)

Clonazepam is a benzodiazepine and is used for the treatment of petit mal seizures, restless leg syndrome, panic disorders, and neuralgia. Klonopin causes increased salivation.

Clonazepam (Klonopin) and DDIs

Avoid clarithromycin and metronidazole because they increase Klonopin levels via inhibition of the CYP3A4 enzyme.

Oxcarbazepine (Trileptal)

Trileptal is used in the management of partial seizures in adults and children. Trileptal works by decreasing impulses in the nerves that cause seizures and it is associated with significant xerostomia.

Valproic Acid (Depakene)

Valproic acid is used in the treatment of petit mal epilepsy. Valproic acid increases the effect of pain medications and anesthetics. Depakene causes hypofibrinogenemia; thrombocytopenia; inhibition of platelet aggregation; leukopenia; eosinophilia; and macrocytic, folic acid–associated anemia.

Always monitor the CBC, platelet count, and coagulation tests **prior** to major dental surgery in patients on Depakene. Always check the **LFTs** and avoid using other hepatotoxic drugs with valproic acid.

Valproic Acid (Depakene) and DDIs

Avoid aspirin, NSAIDS, barbiturates and diazepam.

Ethosuximide (Zarontin)

Ethosuximide is an antiseizure medication used in the management of petit mal epilepsy.

Zarontin can cause pancytopenia, so always assess CBC prior to major dental surgery.

Divalproex (Depakote)

The liver- and pancreas-associated side effects are similar to valproic acid. Depakote causes excessive sunburns.

Lamotrigene (Lamictal)

Lamictal is used for the treatment of partial seizures, generalized seizures in adults and children over 16, and bipolar disorder. Lamictal has relatively few side effects.

Topiramate (Topamax)

Topamax is used for the treatment of partial seizures plus tonic-clonic seizures in children and adults. Topamax causes taste change, feeling of pins and needles in the head and limbs, osteoporosis, gingivitis, xerostomia, and hyperthermia in children.

Zonisamide (Zonegran)

Zonegran is used for the treatment of partial seizures.

SEIZURE MEDICATIONS AND SUGGESTED DENTAL ALERTS

The following are medications and dental alerts:

1. Always check for a history of alcohol use during history-taking because alcohol decreases the potency of seizure medications.
2. All antiseizure drugs can increase the effectiveness of pain medications and muscle relaxants, causing drowsiness.

3. Avoid centrally acting pain medications, sedatives, hypnotics, narcotics, and sedating antihistamines with antiseizure medications because they enhance sedation.
4. Use regular-strength acetaminophen (Tylenol) only.
5. Phenytoin (Dilantin), carbamazepine (Tegretol), primidone (Mysolin), and phenobarbital are the most potent hepatic enzyme inducers at therapeutic doses and as discussed above, use doxycycline, clarithromycin, steroids, and metronidazole with extreme caution if you plan on using any one of them. It is best to avoid these medications.
6. Most of the seizure medications cause xerostomia.
7. Dilantin and primidone cause folic acid deficiency and macrocytic anemia. Obtain the **CBC** prior to dental treatment. Follow the AAA suggested guidelines for anemia if CBC indicates changes associated with folic acid deficiency.
8. Phenytoin (Dilantin) additionally causes gingival hyperplasia. It is best to schedule hygiene recall every 3–4 months to control the hyperplasia.
9. Primidone (Mysoline) and topiramate (Topamax) cause osteoporosis. Always check the bone density on the dental radiographs. Presence of bone loss may cause frequent denture adjustments if the patient has removable appliances.
10. Topiramate (Topamax) additionally causes taste changes and parasthesias in the head and limbs. Always confirm the presence of any such symptoms prior to injecting the local anesthetic.
11. Valproic acid enhances the effects of pain medications and anesthetics, so use decreased doses or decreased amounts of the drugs.
12. Check the CBC, calculate the ANC, and determine the PT/INR if the patient is on valproic acid for reasons discussed earlier. The patient may need antibiotics to prevent and/or treat an infection.
13. Check the CBC for pancytopenia if the patient is on Ethosuximide. The patient may need antibiotics to prevent and/or treat an infection.
14. Antiseizure medications, particularly phenobarbital and primidone (Mysolin), depress the CNS and the patient could be sleepy in the chair.

GRAND MAL SEIZURE ATTACK

Refer to Chapter 9, "Management of Medical Emergencies in the Dental Setting: Assessment, Analysis, and Associated Dental Management Guidelines," for discussion on clinical features and management of a grand mal seizure.

PETIT MAL SEIZURE

Petit Mal Seizure Facts

Petit mal seizure is also called *absence seizure*, and it is a type of seizure that occurs most often in children. An abnormal electrical discharge in the brain causes the seizure.

A petit mal seizure is brief and there is a sudden lapse of conscious activity, but the patient never falls to the ground. Each seizure lasts a few seconds or minutes and hundreds of seizure attacks may occur each day.

There may be occasional jerking of the facial muscles or hands or lip smacking during the seizure phase. The patient usually resumes normal activities following the seizure and experiences no confusion but has no recall of the seizure or the lost activity.

Petit mal seizures often occur when the child is inactive or alone, and thus the diagnosis can often be delayed or missed if no adult supervision exists during the attacks. An observant mother will often state that the child has a "blank look" or is "staring at the TV without blinking."

Some children can outgrow the seizures and go on to discontinue the medications in adulthood. Others, however, may progress to develop grand mal seizures in adult life.

Petit Mal Epilepsy Etiology

The etiology is the same as with grand mal epilepsy.

Petit Mal Epilepsy Diagnosis

The diagnosis is the same as with grand mal epilepsy.

Petit Mal Epilepsy Treatment
Older Medications

Though older, Valproic acid (Depakene) and Ethosuximide (Zarontin) have been excellent standard drugs for the management of petit mal epilepsy.

Newer Medications

Lamotrigine (Lamictal), Topiramate (Topamax) and zonisamide (Zonegran) are the newer medications available for petit mal epilepsy treatment.

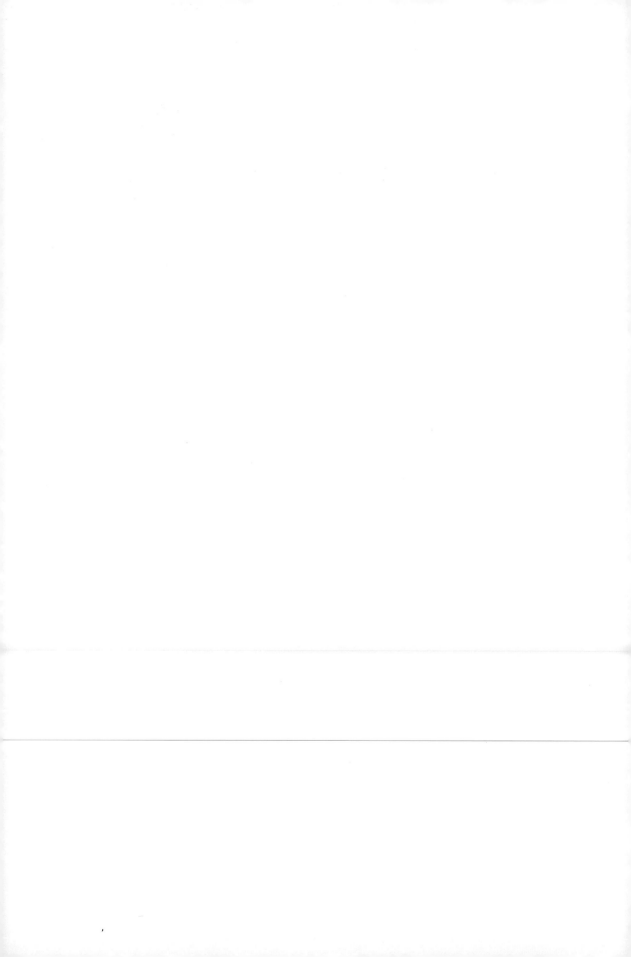

XI
Gastrointestinal Conditions/Diseases

Gastrointestinal Disease States and Associated Oral Cavity Lesions: Assessment, Analysis, and Associated Dental Management Guidelines

ANGULAR CHEILITIS

Angular cheilitis is associated with cracking at the corners of the mouth, pain, and bleeding in severe cases.

Angular Cheilitis Predisposing Factors

Nutritional anemias, and very particularly iron deficiency anemia; ill-fitting dentures; improper bite; HIV/AIDS; cold weather; and constant lip-smacking are common etiological factors.

Superinfection with candidiasis is very common at the corners of the mouth. Some patients may have associated esophageal candidiasis and may complain of dysphagia, and/or odynophagia.

Angular Cheilitis Treatment

Prescribe topical antifungal therapy, pain medications in severe cases, and lip balm for those suffering because of the cold weather. Additionally, always treat the underlying cause of angular cheilitis.

APHTHOUS ULCERS

Aphthous Ulceration Etiology

Aphthous ulceration is often brought on by stress, local trauma, prolonged fever, or Crohn's disease (Table 44.1). 4–15% of Crohn's disease patients have aphthous ulcers. Aphthous ulceration is a rare finding with celiac disease.

Aphthous ulcers can also occur in patients suffering from immunological conditions such as Sjögren's syndrome, systemic lupus erythematosus (SLE), and scleroderma.

Aphthous Ulceration Treatment

The severity of the ulceration determines the type of treatment provided. Some of the treatment options available are listed in Table 44.1. For a complete list, refer to Chapter 48, "Therapeutic Management of Oral Lesions in the Immune-Competent and the Immune-Compromised Patient in the Dental Setting."

Table 44.1. Treatment options for aphthous ulcerations

Disease	Generic (Trade) Name	Treatment Instructions
Mild Disease	1. **Topical 0.15 Benzydamine** (Difflam or Tantum) oral rinse	Apply to the ulcers 4 times/day for 2 weeks or until the ulcers heal.
Mild Disease	2. **Protective Bioadhesives: Topical Carellose** (Orabase: Pectin plus Gelatin)	Apply to the ulcers 4 times/day for 2 weeks or until the ulcers heal.
Mild Disease	3. **Topical Corticosteroids, in adhesive base or as a spray/cream/pellet:** a. **1% Triamcinalone dental paste** (Adrortyl or Kenolog in Orabase) b. **Hydrocortisone, 2.5 mg pellets** (Corlan) c. **0.12% or 0.2% Chlorhexidine gluconate aqueous mouthwash** (Peridex) or 1% Chlorhexidine gluconate gel	With any of the preparations for mild disease: Apply to the ulcers 4 times/day for 2 weeks or until the ulcers heal.
Severe Disease	1. **Systemic Corticosteroids:** Tablets/capsules	30–60 mg prednisone daily for 1 week, followed by a 1-week dose taper.
Severe Disease	2. **Thalidomide** (Thalomid)	50–200 mg daily for 4–8 weeks.

PEUTZ-JEGHER'S SYNDROME

Peutz-Jegher's Syndrome Etiology

Peutz-Jegher's syndrome is associated with mucocutaneous hyperpigmentation and gastrointestinal hamatomatous polyps. The polyps can appear throughout the GI tract.

Peutz-Jegher's Syndrome Clinical Manifestations

The macules appear in infancy and childhood and fade over time. The macules over buccal mucosa, however, do not fade over time. 95% of the lesions occur on the lips; 83% on the buccal mucosa; and occasional macules are seen on the palms, soles, digits, eyes and mouth.

Peutz-Jegher's Syndrome Complications

Complications associated with Peutz-Jegher's Syndrome are intestinal obstruction, abdominal pain. and gastrointestinal (GI) bleeding.

ESOPHAGEAL CANCER

Esophageal cancer can be a squamous cell cancer or an adenocarcinoma. Both, however, have poor prognosis.

Squamous cell cancer is not associated with Barrett's esophagus. The cancer is usually located in the middle to proximal esophagus, and it may coexist with oropharyngeal cancer.

Esophageal Cancer Risk Factors

Risk factors for esophageal cancer are smoking and alcohol use. The additional risk factors for adenocarcinoma of the esophagus are GERD, Barrett's esophagus, and a white 40-year-old male patient.

GASTROESOPHAGEAL REFLUX DISEASE (GERD)

GERD Etiology

Gastroesophageal reflux disease occurs when the lower esophageal sphincter (LES) does not close properly and stomach contents leak back into the esophagus, causing heartburn, or the contents go into the back of the mouth, causing a water brash.

A hiatal hernia may contribute to GERD. A hiatal hernia can happen at any age and is not uncommon in people over 40–50. Obesity and pregnancy are often aggravating factors for GERD. Heartburn that occurs more than twice per week may be considered GERD.

GERD Clinical Features

Patients with GERD experience substernal heartburn associated with burning, belching, water brush (acid and water), and regurgitation. Heartburn may indicate severe disease. The symptoms occur after a meal and are aggravated by any change in position. The symptoms are also aggravated by certain foods: fatty foods, spicy foods, and tomato-based foods.

Extraesophageal Manifestation of GERD

GERD-associated extraesophageal manifestations can be oral dental erosions, chronic cough and constant clearing of the throat, atypical chest pain, epigastric pain, and nausea.

GERD Complications

Complications associated with GERD are esophagitis associated with linear ulcers seen on endoscopy, strictures caused by partially healed ulcers, and Barrett's esophagus that is diagnosed by barium swallow.

GERD TREATMENT

GERD Medical Management

GERD treatment includes the following medical management:

1. **Proton pump inhibitors (PPIs):** PPIs are acid suppressants and they are the most effective drugs prescribed to treat GERD. Esomeprazole (Nexium), lansoprazole (Prevacid), omeprazole (Prilosec), and pantoprazole (Protonix) are the most commonly prescribed PPIs.
   - **Proton pump inhibitors (PPIs) side effects:** PPIs can interfere with the absorption of calcium because of the hypochlorhydria and they also reduce bone

resorption through inhibition of osteoclastic vacuolar-proton pumps. There is an increased risk of fractures associated with long-term PPI therapy or with high doses of PPIs.

2. **H_2 blockers:** H_2 Blockers provide short-term relief and should not be used for more than a few weeks. Cimetidine (Tagamet), famotidine (Pepcid), and ranitidine (Zantac) are the commonly used H_2 blockers.

GERD Surgical Management

GERD treatment includes the following surgical management:

1. **Surgery:** The goal with surgery is to tighten the stomach by fundoplication where the top part of the stomach is wrapped around the esophagus. Surgical management is not always efficient.
2. **Implant:** The FDA recently approved an implant for patients who want to avoid surgery. Enteryx is a solution that becomes spongy and reinforces the lower esophageal splinter (LES), thus preventing the stomach acid from flowing into the esophagus. Enteryx is injected during endoscopy. The implant has been approved for people who have GERD that has responded to proton pump inhibitors. The long-term effect of the implant therapy is unknown.

GERD Adjunct Treatment

Adjunct treatment guidelines for GERD are:

1. The patient should sleep with the head end elevated.
2. There should be no food consumption for **3 hr** prior to sleeping.
3. The patient should stop smoking and avoid alcohol, caffeine, and mint-containing foods.
4. The patient should also avoid aspirin and NSAIDS to avoid further aggravation of symptoms.

PEPTIC ULCER DISEASE

Peptic Ulcer Etiology

Heliobacter pylorus (H. pylori) is most often implicated as the leading cause of peptic ulcer. H. pylori can reside in the mucosal lining and cause no problem in some patients. When implicated however, it is found to erode the mucosa and cause ulceration.

The next leading cause is chronic NSAIDS use. Peptic ulcers can also be due to ischemia consequent to smoking. Stress and diet are no longer thought to be causative factors.

Peptic Ulcer Classification

Peptic ulcers named according to their location in the GI tract are:

*   **Gastric Ulcer:** A peptic ulcer found in the stomach
*   **Duodenal Ulcer:** A peptic ulcer found in the duodenum

Peptic Ulcer Symptoms

The following are peptic ulcer symptoms:

- Pain: The most common type is a burning pain caused by the stomach acid coming in contact with the ulcer. The pain varies in location and can also be gnawing or hungerlike. The pain can last for a few minutes or a few hours. It is often relieved with food.
- Nausea and vomiting with/without blood.
- Black tarry stools or dark blood in the stools.
- Indigestion, anorexia, early satiety, and bloating.

Peptic Ulcer Diagnosis

Peptic ulcer diagnosis is made with the following:

1. **Barium studies:** Barium studies detect the location of the ulcer(s) and identify the ulcer status.
2. **Endoscopy:** Endoscopy visually detects the location of the ulcer(s) and identifies the ulcer status.
3. **Blood test:** The blood test is done to detect the presence of H. pylori antibodies. This test has a disadvantage because it cannot differentiate between past exposure and current infection with the bacteria. The test may be positive for several months after the bacteria have been eradicated.
4. **Breath test:** During the breath test a radioactive carbon atom as a part of urea is consumed as a clear liquid and 30 min later the patient is asked to exhale in a small plastic bag. H. pylori when present breaks down the urea consumed and the radioactive carbon atom is detected in the form of CO_2 in the exhaled air.

    The advantage of the breath test is its ability to detect bacteria eradication with treatment.
5. **Stool antigen test:** This test helps identify the presence of H. pylori in the stool. It also helps detect eradication, with treatment.

Peptic Ulcer Treatment

The treatment goal is to promote healing by eradicating H. pylori and decreasing the acid production that aggravates the ulcer. Successful treatment takes just a few weeks; the treatment options are the following:

1. **Antibiotics:** H. pylorus is eradicated with antibiotic treatment and antibiotic treatment reduces the recurrence rate down to 10–20%. Antibiotic treatment options are the following:
    a. **Combination Antibiotics:** Combination antibiotics work best; the ones commonly prescribed for **2 weeks are** amoxicillin (Amoxil), clarithromycin (Biaxin), and metronidazole (Flagyl).
    b. **Commercial Preparations:** Commercial preparations containing two of the antibiotics along with a cytoprotective or acid suppressant are available under the names Helidac and Prevpac.
2. **Proton Pump Inhibitors (PPIs):** The PPIs shut down the tiny pumps in the acid-secreting cells in the stomach and promote healing. The PPIs are also found to inhibit H. pylori activity.
3. **Acid Blockers:** H_2 blockers reduce the amount of acid released in the GI tract and promote healing.

4. **Cytoprotective Medications:** Sucralfate (Carafate), misoprostol (Cytotec), or bismuth subsalicylate (Pepto-Bismol) are often prescribed. These medications protect the tissue lining of the stomach and duodenum, plus they appear to inhibit H. pylori activity.

Peptic Ulcer Complications

Complications associated with peptic ulcer are: bleeding, perforation, or obstruction. Note that bleeding ulcers don't perforate and perforated ulcers don't bleed.

ESOPHAGITIS, GERD, AND PEPTIC ULCER SUGGESTED DENTAL ALERTS

The following are dental alerts for esophagitis, GERD, and peptic ulcer:

1. Always check for a history of chronic intake of aspirin, NSAIDS, and corticosteroids because any one of these drugs can trigger peptic ulcer disease.
2. Aspirin, NSAIDS, or steroids therefore should not be prescribed in patients with history of peptic ulcers because these agents cause GI mucosal irritation.
3. Check whether the patient is on antacids such as Mylanta, Maalox, or Gelusil. Always be aware that these agents contain aluminum hydroxide, which inhibits the absorption of all tetracyclines.
4. H_2 blockers such as cimetidine (Tagamet), famotidine (Pepcid), or ranitidine (Zantac) prolong the absorption of diazepam (Valium) or lorazepam (Ativan), and these stress-management drugs should be avoided in patients taking the mentioned H_2 blockers.
5. Omeprazole (Prilosec) decreases the acid production in the stomach. Avoid the use of ampicillin in these patients because ampicillin needs the presence of acid in the stomach for absorption.
6. Sucralfate (Carafate) coats the stomach and promotes healing, and it often causes constipation, so avoid the use of codeine with sucralfate (Carafate).
7. Carafate can also decrease the bioavailability of certain drugs by binding with them. Dental use drugs affected are H_2 blockers and tetracyclines.
8. Always check the dental radiographs for bone density in patients on PPIs because PPIs affect calcium absorption.

PANCREATIC DISEASE: ACUTE PANCREATITIS

Gallstones and ETOH are responsible for a majority of the cases of acute pancreatitis. Other factors responsible could be bile stones, bile duct obstructing tumors, drugs such as diuretics, protease inhibitors, trauma, infections, hypercalcemia, or genetic predisposition.

Acute Pancreatitis Clinical Features

Acute pancreatitis is associated with epigastric pain radiating to the back, nausea, and vomiting.

Acute Pancreatitis Laboratory Tests

The following are acute pancreatitis tests:

1. **Amylase test:** Amylase level assessment has a low specificity and cannot be used alone.
2. **Lipase test:** Lipase level determination has a high specificity and is more sensitive compared to the amylase test.

Acute Pancreatitis Diagnosis

Diagnosis of acute pancreatitis is made by evaluation of the clinical picture and laboratory tests.

Acute Pancreatitis Treatment

Treatment options are the following:

1. Bowel rest and parenteral nutrition is paramount and the patient is not allowed to consume any food orally.
2. Aggressive IV hydration is implemented to compensate for the loss of fluids from the pancreas.
3. Aggressive pain control is implemented immediately.
4. Treatment of the underlying condition precipitating the acute pancreatitis is simultaneously addressed.

CELIAC SPRUE

Celiac sprue is also called *gluten-sensitive enteropathy* or *nontropical sprue*. It is a genetic disease that causes the patient to be sensitive to wheat, rye, and barley. Caucasians are mostly affected with celiac sprue.

Celiac Sprue Clinical Features

The clinical features for celiac sprue can vary. Symptoms may occur in the digestive system or in other parts of the body. Typically, the patient presents with crampy, abdominal pain; chronic diarrhea; bloating; weight loss; and steatorrhea.

Celiac disease prevents the body from absorbing nutrients appropriately. The patient can experience glossitis, burning mouth, large bruises, and deep tissue bleeding.

To compensate for nutritional loss, the patient needs to receive supplementation for iron, folic acid, B vitamins, fluids, and electrolytes along with calcium, potassium, and magnesium.

Celiac Disease Diagnosis

Diagnosis is established with the following:

1. **Biopsy:** Biopsy of the small intestine is the gold standard test that shows blunting of the villi in the small intestinal mucosa.
2. **Blood tests:** Diagnosis can be established with the detection of antigliadin antibody, antiendomysial antibodies, and tissue transglutaminase.

Celiac Disease Treatment

Treatment options are a gluten-free diet along with nutritional supplements iron, vitamin D, calcium, folic acid, and vitamin B_{12}.

Celiac Disease and Suggested Dental Alerts

The following are dental alerts for celiac disease:

1. The status of the iron deficiency anemia, osteoporosis due to poor calcium absorption, easy bruising due to malabsorption of vitamin K, and peripheral neuropathy due to poor absorption of folic acid and vitamin B_{12} should be assessed prior to dentistry by evaluating the CBC, PT/INR, and dental radiographs for bone density.
2. Both men and women with low bone density may require vitamin D replacement.
3. Associated conditions, such as lactose intolerance or diabetes, may need to be treated. Evaluate the FBS, PPBS, and Hb_1AC if the patient has associated diabetes.
4. These patients have underfunctioning immune systems and may not handle infections well. Use antibiotics to **promote** the healing process following major surgical procedures.
5. The patient may need less or sometimes even more of a particular vitamin, mineral, or medication because of inadequate absorption.
6. The dentist must work with the patient's physician; the M.D. will help determine the appropriate doses for specific antibiotics that can work optimally for the patient's infection.

IRRITABLE BOWEL SYNDROME (IBS)

IBS is the most commonly diagnosed condition that is chronic, recurrent, and involves the small intestines. The diagnosis is made by exclusion.

Women are more commonly affected compared to men.

Symptoms experienced are abdominal pain, disturbed bowel movements with constipation or diarrhea, abdominal bloating, and abnormal peristalsis.

The symptoms are not explained by any structural or biochemical abnormalities.

IBS Diagnosis

Diagnosis is established using the following:

1. **The Manning Criteria:** The Manning criteria of diagnosis contains the following: pain that is relieved with defecation; more frequent bowel movements, occurring at the onset of pain and associated with lesser amount of stools; visible abdominal distention; passage of mucus; and a sensation of incomplete evacuation.
2. **The Rome III Criteria:** The Rome III diagnosis criteria are more widely used, consisting of recurrent abdominal pain or discomfort at least 3 days/month in last 3 months. This pain or discomfort is associated with at least two or more of the following: improvement of pain with defecation, onset associated with change in the frequency of stools, or onset associated with a change in the form or appearance of the stools.

IBS Medical Management

Treatment options for IBS are the following:

1. **Dietary modifications:** IBS is treated with lactose-free, gas-reducing food items that are high in fiber.

2. **Antispasmodic drugs:** Hyoscyamine (Levsin), an anticholinergic drug may be prescribed.
3. **Antidiarrheal agents:** Diphenoxylate (Lomotil) or loperamide (Immodium) could be prescribed to control the diarrhea.
4. **Promotility: Tegaserod (Zelnorm)** is used for the short-term treatment of constipation only in women.
5. **Psychosocial therapy:** Behavior modification therapy could alleviate or lessen symptoms.
6. **Antidepressants:** Antidepressants are often prescribed as adjunct therapy.

CLOSTRIDIUM DIFFICILE INFECTION (CDI)

CDI Facts

Pseudomembranous colitis is antibiotic-associated colitis that occurs after antibiotic use. Any antibiotic when used in high doses or for a prolonged period can cause c. difficile colitis. Clindamycin has often been implicated as the antibiotic most responsible for c. difficile colitis, but recent literature has shown otherwise. Colonic bacterial flora is altered during c. difficile colitis.

C. Difficile Symptoms and Signs

C. difficile colitis is associated with fever and an elevated WBC count detected on the CBC. The patient is symptomatic for three or more unformed stools over 24 hr for 2 successive days and shows positive stool test results or the presence of pseudomembranes in the stools.

C. Difficile Diagnosis

The initial test done to detect CDI is the enzyme immunoassay (EIA) test. The EIA accesses for toxins A and B and it is 79–97% sensitive.

The cell culture toxin assay, considered the gold standard test, is done when the EIA is positive. The assay is observed for 24–48 hr.

C. Difficile Treatment

Treatment measures are the following:

1. **Prevention:** Prevention is the best course of action and special attention should be placed on the dose, duration, and frequency of antibiotic prescriptions. The patient should be encouraged to use probiotics or acidophilus-containing yogurt with antibiotic intake to maintain the intestinal flora. Bleach-based disinfectants are very effective in destroying c. difficile spores.
2. **Medical management:** Treatment provided is based on the extent of the disease, which can be mild, moderate, or severe CDI. Mild or moderate CDI is associated with WBC < 15,000 cells/mm^3 and serum creatinine < 1.5 times the level, **prior** to the CDI.

Severe CDI is associated with WBC ≥ 15,000 cells/mm^3 or serum creatinine > 1.5 times the level, **prior** to the CDI.

Metronidazole, 500 mg TID for 10–14 days, is the first-line therapy for an **initial or first recurrence** of mild or moderate CDI. A second recurrence is treated with oral vancomycin. Oral vancomycin therapy is extremely effective in treating mild, moderate, or severe disease, but oral vancomycin is quite expensive compared to metronidazole.

There is **no difference** in the effectiveness of metronidazole and oral vancomycin for a new or first recurrence mild/moderate CDI, but oral vancomycin is clearly **superior** for a second recurrence or severe CDI.

Patients respond within 3 days with oral vancomycin compared to 4–6 days with metronidazole, plus intestinal levels are higher with oral vancomycin because it is not absorbed by the colon.

Oral vancomycin, 125 mg QID for 10–14 days, is the first-line therapy for **initial** or recurrence of **severe** disease. **Second recurrence** is treated with oral vancomycin taper over 4 weeks, with or without pulse dosing when 125 mg oral vancomycin is given q2–3 days, for 2–8 weeks.

INFLAMMATORY BOWEL DISEASE (IBD)

IBD Epidemiology

Crohn's disease and ulcerative colitis are the two most commonly occurring IBD states that affect the large bowel, causing significant disease. There is an increased incidence of IBD in industrialized nations.

Peak onset of IBD occurs between the ages of 15–25 and a second peak occurs between the ages of 50–65. Males and females are equally affected.

CROHN'S DISEASE

Crohn's disease is an inflammatory bowel disease that can affect any area of the GI tract, from the mouth to the anus. It most commonly, however, affects the lower part of the small intestine, the ileum.

All layers of the intestine may be involved and normal healthy bowel can be found between sections of diseased bowel. White blood cells accumulate in the lining of the intestines, producing chronic inflammation, which leads to ulcerations and bowel injury.

Crohn's disease affects men and women equally and seems to run in some families. Crohn's disease is more often diagnosed in people between the ages of 20 and 30. People of Jewish heritage have an increased risk of developing Crohn's disease; African-Americans are at decreased risk for developing Crohn's disease.

Some people with Crohn's disease also report that they experience a flare in disease when they are dealing with a stressful event or situation.

Always provide **stress management** if dentistry is stressful for the patient.

Crohn's Disease Clinical Features

The most common symptoms experienced are abdominal pain, often in the lower right area, and diarrhea. Rectal bleeding, weight loss, arthritis, skin problems, and fever may also occur. Bleeding may be serious and persistent, leading to anemia. Always evaluate the CBC **prior** to dental treatment.

The swelling can cause pain and can make the patient have frequent bowel movements resulting in diarrhea.

Crohn's can sometimes present with intestinal obstruction and appendicitis-like right-sided acute inflammation. 50% of the cases present with ileocolitis, 30% of the cases present with ileitis, and 20% of the cases present with colitis.

Extracolonic manifestations of Crohn's include uveitis, iritis, arthritis, rash, and hepatitis.

Crohn's is characterized by rectal sparing, perianal disease, fistulization, and cobblestone appearance on endoscopy.

Crohn's Disease Diagnosis

Diagnosis is established with the following:

1. A thorough physical exam and a series of tests may be required to diagnose Crohn's disease.
2. Blood tests may be done to check for anemia, which could indicate bleeding in the intestines.
3. Blood tests may also show a high white blood cell count, which is a sign of inflammation.
4. An upper GI series will show the status of the small intestine.
5. Sigmoidoscopy can be done to examine the lining of the lower part of the large intestine, or a colonoscopy can be done to examine the lining of the entire large intestine.

Crohn's Disease Complications

The following are complications of Crohn's disease:

- Deficiencies of proteins, calories, and vitamins caused by inadequate dietary intake
- Low protein levels, which can be associated with intestinal loss of protein due to malabsorption
- Arthritis, skin problems, inflammation in the eyes or mouth, kidney stones, gallstones, or other diseases of the liver and biliary system

Crohn's Disease Drug Therapy

The following are drugs used for Crohn's disease:

1. **Antiinflammatory Drugs:** Most patients are first treated with drugs containing mesalamine that helps control inflammation. Patients who have no relief from mesalamine or who cannot tolerate it are put on other mesalamine-containing drugs, such as mesalamine (Asacol), olsalazine (Dipentum), or mesalamine (Pentasa).
2. **Corticosteroids:** Prednisone is usually prescribed in a large dose during the worst stage of the disease. Once symptoms resolve, the dose is decreased. Follow "the rule of twos" for major dentistry when the history is positive for steroid intake.
3. **Immune Suppressants:** 6-Mercaptopurine or Azathioprine are usually prescribed. Always evaluate the CBC and determine the ANC counts prior to dental treatment.
4. **Infliximab (Remicade):** Infliximab (Remicade) is a tissue necrosis factor (TNF) drug that blocks the body's inflammation response. The U. S. Food and Drug Administration approved the drug for the treatment of moderate to severe Crohn's disease that does not respond to standard therapies (listed above) and for the treatment of open, draining fistulas.

5. **Antibiotics:** Ampicillin, sulfonamide, cephalosporin, tetracycline, or metronidazole may be prescribed to treat intestinal infections. Before you prescribe an antibiotic for an oral infection, always determine whether the antibiotic the patient is receiving is bactericidal or bacteriostatic in action.

6. **Antidiarrheal Drugs:** Diarrhea and abdominal cramps often resolve when the inflammation subsides, but additional medication may also be necessary. Diphenoxylate (Lomotil) or loperamide (Immodium) could be used to control the diarrhea. Do not prescribe codeine because it will be additive in action promoting constipation.

7. **Fluid Replacements:** Patients dehydrated because of diarrhea need treatment with fluids and electrolytes.

ULCERATIVE COLITIS

Ulcerative colitis is also called *colitis, distal colitis, pancolitis,* or *ulcerative proctitis.* Ulcerative colitis causes inflammation and ulcers in the mucosal lining of the rectum and colon. Ulcers form where inflammation has killed the cells that usually line the colon.

Ulcerative colitis can happen at any age, but it usually starts between the ages of 15 and 30. It tends to run in families.

Ulcerative Colitis Symptoms

The most common symptoms experienced are pain in the abdomen (very particularly on the left side), bloody diarrhea, urgency, fever, nocturnal diarrhea, and frequent small-volume bowel movements.

Other symptoms may include anemia, severe tiredness, weight loss, loss of appetite, bleeding from the rectum, sores on the skin, and joint pain.

Some patients have long periods of remission during which they are free of symptoms. In severe cases the colon may be removed and there is a higher incidence of colon cancer in these patients.

Ulcerative Colitis Diagnosis and Medical Management

The diagnosis and medical management of ulcerative colitis and Crohn's Disease is essentially the same with specific focus on the large intestines. All alerts suggested for Crohn's disease apply to ulcerative colitis.

CROHN'S DISEASE AND ULCERATIVE COLITIS SUGGESTED DENTAL GUIDELINES

The following are dental guidelines for Crohn's disease and ulcerative colitis:

1. Provide stress management, when needed, for an anxious patient.
2. Always assess the CBC, serum creatinine, and LFTs in patients with Crohn's disease, prior to dentistry.
3. Avoid codeine in patients already taking antidiarrheal medications because severe constipation may occur.
4. Determine what medications the patient is on for Crohn's disease or ulcerative colitis. With specific antibiotic intake, you need to determine whether the antibiotic is cidal/static. Match the cidal/static status with an antibiotic you may need to give

the patient for treatment of an oral infection. If the two antibiotics don't match with their status, keep a 6-hr interval between the two.

5. Check whether the patient has been on steroids within the past 2 years or whether the patient is currently on steroids. You need to follow "the rule of twos" for major dentistry if the history is positive.

6. As with all chronic GI conditions, delay routine dentistry during the acute flare-up phase of the disease.

DIVERTICULITIS

Diverticulitis mainly affects the descending and pelvic colon and symptoms include abdominal pain, constipation, and flatulence.

Diverticulitis and Suggested Dental Alerts

The following are dental alerts for diverticulitis:

1. Avoid codeine in these patients to prevent further worsening of the constipation.

2. Determine what medications the patient is on for the management of diverticulosis or diverticulitis. With any specific antibiotic intake, you need to determine whether the antibiotic is cidal/static. Match the cidal/static status with an antibiotic you may need to give the patient for treatment of an oral infection. If the two antibiotics don't match with their status, keep a 6-hr interval between the two.

3. Check whether the patient has been on steroids within the past 2 years or if the patient is currently on steroids. You need to follow "the rule of twos" for major dentistry if the history is positive.

4. As with all chronic GI conditions, delay routine dentistry during the acute flare-up phase of the disease.

COLON CANCER

Colon Cancer Facts

Colon cancer presents as colon polyps; there are two types of polyps:

- **Hyperplastic:** A hyperplastic polyp has no cancer risk.
- **Adenomatous:** An adenomatous polyp is premalignant.

Colon cancer is the second most common fatal cancer in the U.S. A high-fiber and low-fat diet are protective against colon cancer. The right colon is most affected and the transverse colon is least affected with colon cancer.

All individuals above age 50 should have a colonoscopy and flexible sigmoidoscopy to check the colon status for polyps, abnormal areas, or cancer.

Colon Cancer Diagnosis

Biopsy specimens obtained from suspect areas are viewed under a microscope to check for signs of cancer.

Colon Cancer Treatment

Treatment options depend on the following: The stage of the cancer, whether the cancer has recurred, and the patient's general health.

GI DISEASES ADDITIONAL ALERTS AND SUGGESTIVE DENTAL GUIDELINES

The following are additional alerts for GI diseases:

1. Bleeds in the upper GI tract cause black tarry stools and the **Guiac test** will be positive showing the presence of blood in the stools in such patients.
2. Lower GI bleeds cause the presence of fresh blood in the stools.
3. No dental treatment should be done during an acute intestinal flare-up. Delay routine dental treatment by 4–6 weeks in the presence of an acute flare-up.
4. Do not prescribe codeine for **any** patient that has a history of **chronic constipation** or in the presence of diverticulitis, as discussed earlier.
5. Always obtain the CBC with platelet count and WBC differential if the patient is on immune-suppressant drugs, and always calculate the absolute neutrophil count (ANC) before proceeding with dentistry.

XII

Hepatology

Liver Function Tests (LFTs), Hepatitis, and Cirrhosis: Assessment, Analysis, and Associated Dental Management Guidelines

LIVER FUNCTION TESTS (LFTS)

Liver Function Tests Overview

LFTs indicate how well the liver is functioning. LFTs should always be evaluated along with the patient's history and physical examination. LFTs are not very sensitive, nor are they very specific.

Albumin, bilirubin, and PT/INR are true indicators of the biosynthetic capacity of the liver. ALT (SGPT), AST (SGOT), and alkaline phosphatase all indicate the status of hepatocellular damage.

LIVER STATUS ASSESSMENT COMPONENTS

The components that typically assess the liver status are the total protein, serum albumin, serum globulin, prothrombin time/international normalized ratio (PT/INR), alanine aminotransferase (ALT/SGPT), aspartate aminotransferase (AST/SGOT), total bilirubin, conjugated plus unconjugated bilirubin, alkaline phosphatase, and gamma-glutamyltransferase (GGT).

When LFTs are requested, most laboratories provide information on all componants listed above with the **exception** of the PT/INR. The PT/INR always has to be requested separately, when needed.

The PT/INR and the partial thromboplastin time (PTT) are provided together when coagulation studies are requested for surgical preoperative assessment.

For discussion purposes, PT/INR will be included in the next section because it assesses liver function.

LIVER FUNCTION TESTS (LFTS) DETAILED DISCUSSION

Total Protein

The total protein constitutes the amount of albumin and globulin in the blood. The total protein value helps with the diagnosis of kidney disease, liver disease, liquid (blood) cancer, or malnutrition. The normal albumin to globulin ratio is 2:1; with cirrhosis the ratio is reversed to 1:2. Normal total protein reference range is 6.5–8.2 g/dL.

Albumin

Albumin is a true indicator of liver function and it is exclusively synthesized by the liver. The half-life of albumin is 20 days. Low albumin results in fluid leakage from the blood vessels into the tissues causing edema of the extremities. Albumin levels are always normal in acute liver disease and decreased in cirrhosis. Decreased levels, however, are not specific to liver disease, because protein-losing intestinal disease, colitis, acute or chronic infection, malnutrition, or chronic kidney disease can also cause a lowering of the albumin level. The normal albumin range is 3.9–5.0 g/dL.

Globulin

Globulins are made by the immune system and the liver cells. Globulins help fight infections. Globulin levels are increased in cirrhosis.

Low Albumin and Normal LFT Profile

Low albumin and normal LFTs are associated with proteinuria; acute inflammatory states caused by trauma, sepsis, burns; and a chronic inflammatory state caused by active rheumatic disorders.

   Note: Albumin values are lower in pregnancy.

Prothrombin Time/International Normalized Ratio: PT/INR

PT/INR, like albumin, is a true indicator of liver function:

- The liver produces Clotting Factors II, V, VII, IX, and X. An elevated PT/INR can result from a vitamin K deficiency in patients with chronic cholestasis (bile flow obstruction) or fat malabsorption from disease of the pancreas or small bowel and blood-thinning medications. Thus, a prolonged PT/INR is not specific to liver disease. The PT/INR does not become abnormal until more than 75–80% of liver synthetic capacity is lost. An abnormal PT/INR prolongation may be a sign of serious liver dysfunction. Bleeding will occur with INR >1.5.
- Factor VII has a short half-life of about 6 hr and it is sensitive to rapid changes in liver synthetic function. In fact, compared to other Clotting Factors, Factor VII has the shortest half-life. Thus, PT/INR is very useful for following liver function in patients with acute liver failure. Normal PT/INR range is 0.9–1.2, average 1.

The ALT and AST

The ALT and AST help the liver metabolize amino acids and thus make proteins. The ALT and AST show liver damage and are sensitive indicators of liver injury, especially acute liver injury. The ALT and AST are present in low levels in the normal patients. ALT (SGPT) is predominately found in liver and is present in the cytosol of the hepatocytes. The normal ALT range is 5–60 IU/L.

   AST (SGOT) is found in the liver, cardiac and skeletal muscle, kidney, brain, pancreas, lungs, RBCs, and WBCs, and in the cytosol and mitochondria of the hepatocytes. The normal AST range is 5–43 IU/L.

   Mild elevations of ALT or AST in asymptomatic patients can be evaluated by initially considering alcohol abuse, hepatitis B, or hepatitis C.

ALT, AST Levels of Elevation and Hepatocellular Necrosis Etiology

The following are ALT and AST elevation levels:

- **Mild ALT and AST elevation (<250 IU/L):** Mild elevations can be due to drugs, bile stones, viral infection, alcohol, or exercise.
- **Moderate ALT and AST elevation (250–1,000 IU/L):** Moderate elevations can be due to EBV or HSV infection or NSAIDS.
- **Severe ALT and AST elevation (>2,000 IU/L):** Severe elevations can be drug- or toxin-induced or due to an acute viral infection, choledocolithiasis, or primary graft failure.

Bilirubin

Total bilirubin indicates the status of bile transportation, and bilirubin is the product of hemoglobin breakdown. Conjugated and unconjugated bilirubin are measured when LFTs are ordered.

Unconjugated Hyperbilirubinemia Etiology

Gilbert's syndrome is the most common cause of benign hyperbilirubinemia and it is associated with impaired uptake or impaired conjugation of bilirubin.

Conjugated Hyperbilirubinemia Etiology

Hepatocellular disease, intra- or extrahepatic bile duct obstruction or sepsis are common causes of conjugated hyperbilirubinemia.

Alkaline Phosphatase (AP)

Alkaline phosphatase is found in the liver, bone, placenta, kidney, intestine, and WBCs. AP metabolizes phosphorus and thus is an energy source for the body. AP levels are higher in men than in women. The normal range of AP is 30–115 IU/L.

AP is a marker of chronic cholestasis disease due to bile duct obstruction caused by stricture/stones *or* infiltrative disease caused by sarcoidosis/TB/cancer. Nonpathologic elevations of AP may occur during the 3rd trimester of pregnancy, during adolescence, or as a normal part of aging. With cholestasis, alkaline phosphatase is markedly elevated when compared to the aminotransferases or bilirubin levels. The total bilirubin will be increased with cholestasis disease.

AP and GGT are often labeled "the cholestatic enzymes" because they spill from the liver into the bloodstream, with obstruction. The AP and gamma-glutamyltransferase (GGT) levels typically rise to several times the normal level after several days of bile duct obstruction or intrahepatic cholestasis. GGT helps differentiate if AP is coming from the liver or bone. With biliary obstruction, the GGT will be increased. With bone disease the GGT is unaltered.

The highest AP levels, often greater than 1,000 U/L or more than six times the normal value, are found in diffuse infiltrative diseases of the liver, such as infiltrating tumors and fungal infections.

Both AP and GGT levels are elevated in about 90% of patients with cholestasis. An elevated AP value originating from the liver is usually accompanied by an elevated GGT value, an elevated 5'-nucleotidase value, and other LFT abnormalities. Please note that nucleotidase is a subset of alkaline phosphate.

Cholestasis Etiology

Etiological Factors associated with cholestasis are

1. **Obstructive causes:** partial bile duct obstruction, primary biliary cirrhosis, primary sclerosing cholangitis, and drug-induced cholestasis
2. **Infiltrative causes:** sarcoidosis, TB, and primary or metastatic liver cancer

Isolated Elevation of AP Level Assessment in an Asymptomatic Patient with Normal GGT Level

Consider bone growth or injury, or primary biliary cirrhosis. AP levels rise in late pregnancy.

Gamma-Glutamyltransferase (GGT)

GGT is found in the hepatocytes and the biliary epithelial cells and brings oxygen to tissues. GGT is a sensitive indicator of hepatobiliary disease. It is **not** elevated in bone disease. GGT is most useful for confirming the hepatic origin of elevated alkaline phosphatase.

Isolated Elevation of GGT Level Assessment

Isolated elevation of GGT level is induced by alcohol and there is usually no actual liver disease. The elevation of GGT alone, with no other LFT abnormalities, often results from enzyme induction by alcohol or seizure medications in the absence of liver disease. The GGT level is often elevated in persons who take three or more alcoholic drinks per day. A mildly elevated GGT level is a typical finding in patients taking anticonvulsants and by itself does not necessarily indicate liver disease. The normal GGT level is 5–80 IU/L.

LFTs and Coagulation Studies Medical Case Note/Medical Record Lattice Recording

LFTs, PT/INR, and PTT are often recorded in a standardized lattice pattern in medical records or medical case notes, and every practitioner should be able to read the tests when written as such. Figures 45.1 and 45.2 show the LFTs and coagulation studies lattice recordings.

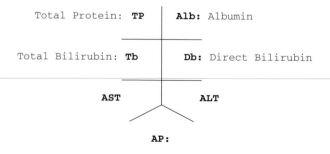

Figure 45.1. Liver function tests lattice recording.

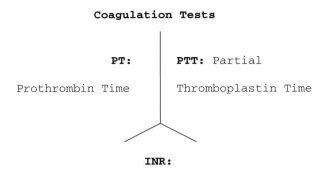

Figure 45.2. Coagulation tests lattice recording.

ACUTE VIRAL HEPATITIS: HEPATITIS A AND E

Acute and Chronic Viral Hepatitis Introduction

Viral hepatitis can present as an acute or chronic disease state and viral infections of importance in the dental setting are hepatitis A, B, C, D, and E. Hepatitis A and E are grouped as the acute types of hepatitis. Hepatitis B, C, and D are grouped as the chronic types of hepatitis.

Hepatitis A and E General Overview

Hepatitis A and E are caused by the hepatitis A virus (HAV) and the hepatitis E virus (HEV), respectively. Hepatitis A is universal in occurrence and is associated with endemic outbreaks. Hepatitis A affects all age groups and jaundice is common.

Hepatitis E occurrence in the U.S. is very rare; it is, however, prevalent in South Asia and North Africa. Hepatitis E is more prevalent among pregnant women and is especially a big concern during the third trimester.

The incubation period is 2–6 weeks for hepatitis A and 2–9 weeks for hepatitis E. There is no chronic state, nor is there any sexual transmission with either type of hepatitis.

Hepatitis A and E Transmission

Transmission of both types is by contaminated food and water. Person-to-person transmission is more common with hepatitis A than with hepatitis E.

Symptoms and Signs of Hepatitis A and E

Nausea, vomiting, abdominal pain, loss of appetite, fatigue, dark urine, and jaundice occur with both types of hepatitis.

Hepatitis A and E Infection Markers

The occurrence of jaundice heralds the start of recovery, especially with hepatitis A. Jaundice usually occurs in 70% of the cases infected with the hepatitis A virus.

Infection with hepatitis A or E is indicated by the presence of anti-HAV IgM or anti-HEV IgM in the blood, respectively. The patient is infected and infectious to others during this phase. Presence of anti-HAV IgG or anti-HEV IgG indicates immunity to hepatitis A and E, respectively. The antibodies provide **lifelong** immunity to hepatitis A; lifelong protection with the hepatitis E antibody is questionable.

Acute Viral Hepatitis LFT Profiles

ALT levels often rise to several thousand units per liter in patients with acute viral hepatitis. The highest ALT levels, often more than 10,000 IU/L, are usually found in patients with acute toxic injury subsequent to acetaminophen overdose. AST and ALT levels usually fall rapidly after an acute insult. In typical viral or toxic liver injury, the serum ALT levels rise more than the AST value, reflecting the relative amounts of these enzymes in hepatocytes.

Hepatitis A and E Vaccinations

Hepatitis A infection can be prevented with the hepatitis A vaccine, which is given in two doses, 6–18 months apart. The vaccine is recommended for children in day-care settings, cafeteria workers, and those traveling to areas with a high risk of transmission.

Of adults vaccinated, 94–100% develop antibodies 1 month after the first injection, and 100% of the vaccinated adults develop protective antibodies after the second dose. Hepatitis A vaccine gives **lifelong** immunity. Immune globulin (IG) is given after the first dose to travelers who plan to travel in less than 1 month after the first dose of the vaccine. There is **no** vaccine for Hepatitis E.

CHRONIC HEPATITIS: HEPATITIS B, C, AND D

General Overview

Hepatitis B is caused by the hepatitis B virus (HBV).
Hepatitis C is caused by the hepatitis C virus (HCV).
Hepatitis D is caused by the defective, hepatitis D virus (HDV) that needs the presence of the hepatitis B virus to exist. Hepatitis D virus (HDV) is thus found associated with a first infection with HBV or with an HBV carrier state.

Hepatitis B, C, and D Transmission

Hepatitis B, C, and D are chronic or gradual in onset; the transmission is via contaminated blood.

Hepatitis B, C, and D Symptoms and Signs

Nausea, vomiting, diarrhea, constipation, fever, skin rash, anorexia, weight loss, joint pains, dark-colored urine, yellowing of the skin or eyes, and aversion to smoking are the common complaints.

Hepatitis B Detailed Discussion

The incubation period for hepatitis B is 2–6 months. Hepatitis B virus is transmitted by exposure to contaminated blood and with IV drug use. Mother-to-child transmission can occur and there is a high rate of sexual transmission with the virus.

Jaundice occurs in 30% of the patients. For most adults it is a form of infection that ultimately resolves; for most children it is a form of infection that persists as a chronic state of infection. HBV attacks the liver and it can cause lifelong infection, cirrhosis, liver cancer, and even death. Of adult patients, 1–3% are affected with chronic hepatitis. Hepatitis B can predispose to liver cancer, in the absence of cirrhosis.

Hepatitis B Serological Markers

Hepatitis B virus is associated with three distinct antigen markers: HBsAg, HBeAg, and HBcAg. Each antigen has a definite time line of appearance during the infection cycle and each triggers the appearance of a corresponding antibody in the blood indicating recovery or otherwise. Anti-HBs, anti-HBe, and anti-HBc are the antibodies triggered by the antigens HBsAg, HBeAg, and HBcAg, respectively.

The Hepatitis B Antigen-Antibody Cycle Graph

Figure 45.3 depicts the sequential pattern of the rise and fall of the hepatitis B–associated antigen-antibody markers. Each of the markers is discussed next, using Figure 45.3 as a reference.

Serological Markers Facts

HBsAg (Surface Antigen)

The presence of HbsAg on hepatic serology indicates the presence of current infection. HBsAg is the first marker to appear in the blood, roughly around the 7th week from the start of an acute infection.

In patients with a resolving infection, the HBsAg disappears completely from the blood by about the 20th week from the start of infection.

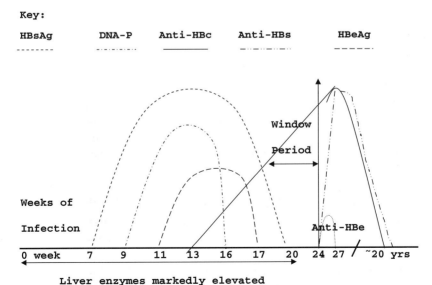

Figure 45.3. Classic hepatitis B antigen-antibody cycle.

A patient is said to be a simple "carrier" patient when the HBsAg does not disappear as expected and continues to be detected on serology beyond the 24th week of infection. The carrier state occurs more commonly in children than adults.

Anti-HBs (Surface Antibody)

The presence of anti-HBs on hepatic serology indicates immunity. Anti-HBs presence can be a consequence of hepatitis B immunization or it can appear in the blood **after** HBsAg from a natural infection that has completely cleared the system.

With natural infection anti-HBs appears around the 24th week from the start of the infection and persists for 15–20 years, providing the patient with immunity during that time. It might be present with anti-HBc IgG following recovery from a natural infection.

Anti-HBs is the only antibody formed with hepatitis B immunization. Anti-HBc IgM or anti-HBc IgG are not formed with vaccination.

HBcAg (Hepatitis B Core Antigen)

HBcAg resides inside the infected hepatocytes only and does **not** make its appearance in the blood. Hepatic serology does not record HBcAg, a marker of infection, and it is detected only on liver biopsy.

Anti-HBc IgM (IgM Core Antibody)

The presence of anti-HBc IgM indicates current infection **and** infectious status. Anti-HBc IgM develops **during the acute state** of hepatitis B and is generated consequent to a natural infection. Anti-HBc IgM is **not** associated with hepatitis B immunization.

Anti-HBc IgM is the only marker present during the "window period" of the typical hepatitis B cycle.

The window period is the time interval during the cycle when the patient has shed the HBsAg but has not yet developed the Anti-HBs. During the window period the patient is negative for HBsAg, DNA-P, HBeAg, and anti-HBs.

Anti-HBc IgM typically appears in the blood around the 13th week from the start of infection and stays till about the 24th week when anti-HBc IgG is formed.

Anti-HBc IgG (IgG Core Antibody)

Anti-HBc IgG is formed beyond the 24th week or 6 months after the start of the hepatitis B infection. Once anti-HBc IgG appears in the blood, it can persist for 15–20 years. Isolated presence of anti-HBc IgG on hepatic serology does not indicate recovery. It indicates only that the patient was infected with the hepatitis B virus **more than** 6 months ago. When anti-HBc IgG is found along with anti-HBs on hepatic serology, it indicates definite recovery and immunity from a natural infection.

HBeAg (Hepatitis B e-antigen)

The presence of HBeAg on hepatic serology indicates active replication of the virus, and the patient is highly infectious at this time. During a typical cycle, HBeAg appears in the blood around the 11th week from the start of infection and completely disappears from the blood around the 17th week from the start of infection.

A carrier patient positive for HBsAg, who also continues to shed the HBeAg beyond the 24th week is called a *super infective carrier* patient.

During the acute state of Hepatitis B, the patient will be positive for HBsAg, HBeAg, DNA-polymerase (DNA-P/viral DNA), anti-HBc IgM, and very high levels of ALT plus AST. Additionally, the patient will have symptoms associated with an acute infection.

Anti-HBe (Hepatitis B e-antibody)

The presence of anti-HBe on hepatic serology indicates that the virus has ceased to replicate and there is an improvement in the patient's infectivity status compared to before. Anti-HBe usually appears around the 24th week and disappears by the 27th week from the start of the infection.

The Hepatitis B Carrier Patient

As stated above, the simple carrier patient continues to shed HBsAg and the super infective carrier continues to shed HBsAg and HBeAg beyond the 24th week/6 months from the start of infection. Both these types of carrier patients do **not** develop anti-HBs, the marker of immunity, till the time HBsAg is detected on serology.

When the virus stops replicating and HBeAg is no longer detected on hepatic serology, the super infective status is lost but the patient will continue to be infective and infected till the time HBsAg is detected on hepatic serology.

The carrier patient's liver enzymes or LFTs will be normal or near normal. Past history assessment will in most cases indicate infection with the hepatitis B virus.

The carrier rate is inversely proportional to the age of the patient. The carrier rate is 80–85% among children, and pediatric patients are usually asymptomatic when infected. Adult patients are usually symptomatic and have a 10–20% carrier rate. Carrier patients can develop very severe hepatitis and about 25% of adult carriers go on to develop cirrhosis of the liver.

The Carrier Patient and Dentistry

Dental treatment is not contraindicated in the simple or super infective carrier patient. Always evaluate the LFTs prior to dentistry to determine whether the carrier patient has underlying hepatitis or cirrhosis. Then follow the AAA suggested dental guidelines for either one of the two disease states.

Hepatitis B Vaccine

Two single antigen hepatitis B vaccines are licensed in the United States for persons of any age. The vaccine is given in three doses at 0, 1, and 6 months. The second dose is given 1 month after the first dose and the third is given 5 months after the second dose. If the series is interrupted after the first dose, the second dose should be given immediately. The third dose should be given at least 2 months after the second. A delayed third dose should be given immediately.

When the vaccine is given according to the protocol of 0, 1, and 6 months, 30–50% protection occurs after the first dose. 50–75% protection occurs after the second dose and 90% protection occurs after the third dose.

HIV patients may need several more shots, beyond the routine three, to gain immunity. Individuals who do not respond to the primary vaccine series may have to complete a second three-dose series and be tested subsequent to that.

Hepatitis B Postvaccination Testing

Testing for antibody response is **not** indicated after completion of the injections at 0, 1, and 6 months. Postvaccination testing after completion of the routine series or interrupted series **may** be indicated in the following:

1. **Health care workers (HCW):** HCW coming in close contact with blood or body fluids **may** be tested 1–2 months after the last dose.
2. **Chronic hemodialysis patients**: Chronic hemodialysis patients may be tested 1–2 months after the last dose.
3. **Sex partners of hepatitis B–infected persons**: Sex partners of hepatitis B–infected persons may be tested 1–2 months after the last dose.
4. **Infants born to hepatitis B–infected mothers**: Infants born to hepatitis B–infected mothers may be tested at 9–15 months of age.

Combined Hepatitis A and B Vaccine

Twintrix is the combined vaccine approved by the FDA for adults. Three doses of the combined vaccine are given over 6 months.

Hepatitis B Needle-Stick Exposure Rate

The transmission rate of hepatitis B by a single needle-stick is 6–30%, and this is the reason why immunization against hepatitis B is required for dentists and others working in the dental setting.

HEPATITIS C (HCV)

Hepatitis C Detailed Discussion

HCV infection is universal in occurrence. The incubation period for hepatitis C is 15–150 days. HCV is spread through the sharing of needles (accounting for 40% of infections), needle-sticks or sharps exposures on the job, from an infected mother to her baby during birth, and through sexual transmission. The sexual transmission rate is quite low when compared with that for hepatitis B.

Hepatitis C can be acute or chronic and the chronic rate of hepatitis C is higher. Hepatitis C usually has a silent acute onset (80%). Only 5–10% of patients are symptomatic and experience nausea and jaundice. Thus, the occurrence of jaundice is rare. The patient has a better chance of clearing the infection in the presence of symptoms.

Hepatitis C has a high rate (55–85%) of progression to silent chronic hepatitis. Aggressive progression (70%) to chronic hepatitis occurs in the presence of coinfection with hepatitis B or HIV, at an older age, in male patients, and in the presence of alcohol use. Of chronic hepatitis patients, 20% develop cirrhosis and 2–3% of patients with cirrhosis develop liver cancer.

Hepatitis C is thus associated with a slow evolution (~20–40 years) to end-stage liver disease and is the leading cause for liver transplant.

Within 8 weeks from the start of the infection, anti-HCV antibody is formed. Anti-HCV antibody, unlike other antibodies, is *not* a protective antibody.

Hepatitis C Needle-Stick Exposure Rate

Incidence of Hepatitis C with a single needle-stick in health care workers is <5.0%.

Hepatitis C Blood Tests

The five most common tests for Hepatitis C are:

1. **Anti-HCV Test**
2. **HCV RIBA Test**
3. **HCV-RNA Test**
4. **Viral Load or Quantitative HCV Test**
5. **Viral Genotyping**

HCV Antibody Tests

The Anti-HCV Test and The HCV RIBA Test are the two tests that detect the antibody associated with hepatitis C. The anti-HCV testing is done by enzyme immunoassay (EIA). The RIBA Test is the recombinant immunoblot assay. Both the anti-HCV Tests (anti-HCV and RIBA) are reported as positive when they detect the presence of antibodies to the hepatitis C virus. The tests indicate only exposure to the virus in the past. They are unable to indicate whether the patient still has an active viral infection.

Anti-HCV Test

HCV antibodies usually appear about 8 weeks into an infection and are always present in the later stages of the disease. A patient with a weakly positive anti-HCV antibody test should get the HCV RIBA test before final results are reported. The HCV RNA must be done if the hepatitis C antibody is positive. False negative results can occur in HIV or other immune-compromised patients. These patients also must be confirmed with the hepatitis C RNA test.

HCV RIBA Test

This test also confirms the presence of antibodies to the virus and, like the anti-HCV test, the RIBA test cannot determine whether the patient is currently infected. It indicates only that the patient has been exposed to the virus. A positive anti-HCV is reconfirmed with the RIBA test.

- **RIBA Positive:** Confirms exposure to HCV. Check the hepatitis C RNA by PCR in RIBA-positive patients.
- **RIBA Negative:** Indicates the positive anti-HCV was a false positive test.

HCV-RNA Test

The HCV RNA Test is a more reliable test and is positive 1 week after infection. The test is also used posttreatment to see whether the virus has been eliminated with therapy. This test detects the presence of the virus in the blood and indicates an active HCV infection. It is reported as HCV-RNA positive when the virus is detected.

- Conclusion: Positive HCV RNA: Patient is chronically infected.
- Negative HCV RNA: **Patient has cleared the infection.**

Viral Load or Quantitative HCV Test

This test measures the number of viral RNA particles in the blood. The Viral Load Test is often used before and during treatment to help determine response to therapy by comparing the amount of virus present before and after treatment, and it is usually done after a period of 3 months. Successful treatment is associated with a decrease of 99% or more (2 logs) in the viral load within 1–3 months of starting treatment. Successful treatment usually leads to the viral load becoming undetected.

Viral Genotyping

This test is used to determine the virus genotype. Genotyping is often ordered before treatment is started to get a heads-up on the likelihood of treatment success and the length of time for which the treatment would be needed. There are six major types of HCV detected by genotyping. The most common genotype is genotype 1, and it is less likely to respond to treatment than genotypes 2 or 3. Genotype 1 usually requires **48 weeks** of therapy compared to **24 weeks** for genotype 2 or 3.

HCV Tests Summary

- If the antibody test result is positive, the patient probably has been infected with hepatitis C.
- A positive RIBA confirms that the patient has been exposed to the virus.
- A negative RIBA indicates that the first test was probably a false positive and the patient has never been infected by HCV.
- A positive HCV RNA means that the patient is **currently** infected by HCV.

Hepatitis C and Associated LFTs

The serum ALT level correlates only moderately well with liver inflammation in hepatitis C. Liver cell death in hepatitis C occurs by a programmed cell death process or apoptosis and by necrosis. Liver cell death by apoptosis is associated with lesser amounts of AST and ALT because the liver cells wither away with time.

This accounts for why one-third of patients infected with the hepatitis C virus have persistently normal serum ALT levels despite the presence of inflammation on liver biopsy.

Hepatitis C Treatment

Mild Hepatitis C Treatment

Mild hepatitis C is treated with diet, exercise, no alcohol, and regular visits with the specialist to monitor the disease.

Chronic Hepatitis C Treatment

Two regimens have FDA approval and the goal of therapy is to have a negligible viral load on completion of treatment. The two types of therapy are

1. **Monotherapy:** Monotherapy care is provided using IV interferon. Intron A, Roferon-A, Infergen, or PEG-Intron are the four interferon preparations approved by the FDA. Intron A, Roferon-A, and Infergen are injected three times/day. PEG-Intron is injected once/week. Ribavirin can be combined only with Intron-A or PEG-Intron.
2. **Combination Therapy:** Combination therapy is done with IV interferon and PO ribavirin (Rebetol). The combination therapy works better than interferon alone.

Rebetol with PEG-Intron has shown better results compared with Rebetol and Intron A. The relapse rate with monotherapy is higher compared with the combination therapy.

See Tables 45.1 and 45.2 for summaries of hepatitis vaccine protocols and LFT changes. See also Table 45.4.

ALCOHOLIC LIVER DISEASE

Alcoholic Liver Disease Facts

Alcoholic hepatitis leads to alcoholic cirrhosis, and 20% of chronic alcoholics develop advanced hepatitis or cirrhosis. Alcoholic fatty liver develops with transient alcohol use over days, with binge drinking or chronic use. The patient is asymptomatic and the process is reversible with abstinence. With continued alcohol use, however, 20–30% develop alcoholic hepatitis or cirrhosis.

Alcoholic Hepatitis

Alcoholic hepatitis develops after years of alcohol abuse. The patient develops fever; a tender, enlarged liver; and leukocytosis.

Alcoholic Liver Disease Laboratory Tests

Testing for alcoholic liver disease involves the following:

- Minimal elevations of AST and ALT often occur. AST is always greater than ALT and the AST/ALT ratio is >2–3.
- The serum AST level is almost never greater than 500 U/L and the serum ALT value is almost never greater than 300 U/L. The reasons for these limits on AST and ALT elevations are not well understood.
- The higher the AST-ALT ratio, the greater the likelihood that alcohol is contributing to the abnormal LFTs.
- The elevated AST-ALT ratio in alcoholic liver disease results in part from the depletion of vitamin B_6 (pyridoxine) in chronic alcoholics. ALT and AST both use pyridoxines as a coenzyme, and the synthesis of ALT is more strongly inhibited by pyridoxine deficiency compared to AST. Alcohol also causes mitochondrial injury, which releases the mitochondrial isoenzyme of AST.

Note: **ALT > AST** in nonalcoholic fatty liver disease.

Alcoholic Liver Disease LFT Conclusion

AST:ALT > 2:1 plus AST is <500 U/L and ALT is <300 U/L.

CIRRHOSIS OF THE LIVER

Cirrhosis Symptoms and Signs

The symptoms and signs associated with cirrhosis are jaundice; flailing hands when the arms are raised out in front; muscle wasting, particularly in the temple area and the extremities; spider angiomas on the body and face; palmer erythema; caput medusa

Table 45.1. Hepatitis A, B, and C summary with vaccine protocols and post-needle-stick exposure testing and prophylaxis

Indicators	Hepatitis A	Hepatitis B	Hepatitis C
Incubation	2–6 weeks	2–6 months	2–24 weeks
Jaundice	Affects all ages and jaundice is common.	Jaundice occurs in 30% of cases.	Jaundice occurrence is rare.
Course	It is an acute type of hepatitis.	Acute for most adults, chronic for most kids.	Can be acute or chronic, chronic rate is higher.
Mode of Transmission	Contaminated food and water.	Exposure by contact with contaminated blood and IV drug use.	Exposure by contact with contaminated blood and IV drug use.
Mother to Child Transmission	No mother to child transmission.	Mother to child transmission is possible.	Mother to child transmission is possible.
Sexual Transmission	No sexual transmission.	High rate of sexual transmission.	Sexual transmission rate is quite low.
Prevalence	Universal with endemic outbreaks.	Universal	Universal
Clinical Features and Prognosis	**Pediatric patients:** Have a silent infection. **Adult patients:** Are more symptomatic with flulike symptoms.	**Pediatric patients:** Are asymptomatic and have 90% carrier rate **Adult patients:** Are symptomatic, can get very severe hepatitis and have a 10–20% carrier rate.	Hepatitis C usually has a silent acute onset (80%). Only 5–10% patients are symptomatic, having nausea and jaundice. The patient has a better chance of clearing the infection in the presence of symptoms. Hepatitis C has a high rate of progression to silent chronic hepatitis (55–85%). Aggressive progression to chronic hepatitis occurs in the presence of coinfection with hepatitis B or HIV, older age, male patient, and alcohol use (70%). Hepatitis C is associated with a slow evolution (~20–40 years) to end-stage liver disease (1–5%).

Laboratory Tests and/or Hepatic Serology

Anti-HAV IgM: Indicates acute infection.

Anti-HAV IgG: Indicates recovery and lifelong immunity.

1. **Acute Infection:**
   HBsAg: Positive
   Anti-HBs: Negative
   Anti-HBc IgM: Positive
   HBeAg: Positive
   Anti-HBe: Negative

2. **Recovery:**
   HBsAg: Negative
   Anti-HBs: Positive
   Anti-HBc IgM: Negative
   Anti-HBc IgG: Positive
   HBeAg: Negative
   Anti-HBe: Positive

3. **Chronic Carrier with viral replication:**
   HBsAg: Positive
   Anti-HBs: Negative
   Anti-HBc IgM: Negative
   Anti-HBc IgG: Positive
   HBeAg: Positive
   Anti-HBe: Negative

4. **Chronic Carrier without replication:**
   HBsAg: Positive
   Anti-HBs: Negative
   Anti-HBc IgM: Negative
   Anti-HBc IgG: Positive
   HBeAg: Negative
   Anti-HBe: Positive

5. **Vaccine:**
   HBsAg: Negative
   Anti-HBs: Positive
   Anti-HBc IgM: Negative
   Anti-HBc IgG: Negative
   HBeAg: Negative
   Anti-HBe: Negative

1. **Anti-HCV Antibody Test:** Positive antibody test indicates the patient probably has been infected with hepatitis C.

2. **RIBA Test:** RIBA positive confirms exposure to the virus. Next, check hepatitis C RNA by PCR RIBA.
   Negative: Indicates the positive anti-HCV was a false positive test.

3. **HCV RNA Test:**
   Positive HCV RNA indicates current chronic infection.
   Negative HCV RNA: Patient has cleared the infection.

4. **Viral Load or Quantitative HCV test:** This test determines the number of viral RNA particles in the blood.

5. **Viral Genotyping Test:** This test determines the virus genotype.

6. **LFTs:** In chronic hepatitis C the serum ALT level correlates only moderately well with liver inflammation.
   One-third of patients infected with hepatitis C virus have persistently normal serum ALT levels.

(Continued)

Table 45.1. *Continued*

Indicators	Hepatitis A	Hepatitis B	Hepatitis C
Complications	Some severe infections need hospitalization. Full recovery following infection occurs in most cases and no chronic state exists.	**Chronic Hepatitis:** 1–3% patients are affected with chronic hepatitis. Hepatitis B predisposes to liver cancer, in the absence of cirrhosis.	Chronic hepatitis C is the number one reason for liver transplant. 20% of the patients go on to develop cirrhosis. 2–3% patients with cirrhosis develop liver cancer.
Needle-Stick Exposure Rate	No exposure via needle-stick.	6–30% chance of exposure with single needle-stick.	<5% exposure rate with single needle-stick.
Post-needle-stick Blood Tests and Follow-up	None	**For Provider:** Check anti-HBs titer for immunity status. Hepatitis B vaccine and/or HBIG is given dependent on provider's vaccination & antibody status. **Source:** Source is tested for HBsAg and HBeAg.	**For Provider:** Check baseline anti-HCV status. **Source:** Source tested for Anti-HCV and Hepatitis C RNA. **If Source Is Positive:** Provider has follow-up serology tests at 6 and 12 weeks. With conversion, provider is referred to MD for evaluation and treatment.
Vaccine	2 doses of Hepatitis A vaccine given 6 months apart. Vaccine gives lifelong immunity. 1st shot given 1 month prior to travel to endemic area. Immune Globulin (IG) also given with vaccine if travel will be in less than 1 month.	**Primary Vaccine:** 3 shots. First 2 shots given at least 1 month apart. 3rd shot given 6 months from start or at least 2–4 months after 2nd shot. No booster shots needed anymore.	No vaccine is available.

Table 45.2. LFT changes with acute and chronic viral hepatitis

LFT Markers	Acute Hepatitis	Chronic Hepatitis
Total Protein	Normal	Normal
Albumin (A)	Normal	Normal
Globulin (G)	Normal	Normal
A:G ratio	Normal	Normal
ALT/SGPT	>2,000 IU/L	Mild increase or normal
AST/SGOT	>2,000 IU/L	Mild increase or normal
ALT:AST ratio	ALT > AST	ALT > AST
GGT	Normal	Normal
Alk Phos (AP)	Increased	Increased
PT/INR	Normal	Normal
Total Bilirubin	Increased	Increased or normal
Direct-B	Increased	Increased or normal
Indirect-B	Increased	Increased or normal

around the umbilicus and umbilical hernia; enlarged liver; testicular atrophy; chronic scarring; fibrosis of the liver; and portal hypertension and ascites. With ascites there is fluid buildup in the peritoneal cavity. The patient is treated with diuretics and a diet low in sodium. With **ascites, premedication** prior to dentistry is a must.

Cirrhosis Complications

The following are complications associated with cirrhosis:

- **Pressure changes:** Pressure changes include increased portal hypertension, decreased systemic BP, and esophageal varices that can be life threatening if they bleed.
- **Hepatic encephalopathy:** The liver is unable to clear the toxins that develop. Infection, GI bleeds, narcotics, and sedatives can trigger encephalopathy.
- **Hepatorenal syndrome:** The liver is unable to clear toxins that affect the kidneys, causing renal failure.
- **Hepatopulmonary syndrome**
- **Hepatocellular carcinoma:** α-fetoprotein is measured for carcinoma of the liver.

Cirrhosis and Associated LFTs

The following are cirrhosis associated LFTs:

- Patients with cirrhosis often have normal or only slightly elevated serum AST and ALT levels. The levels do not rise beyond 300 U/L with both, and AST level is greater than ALT.
- AST and ALT levels tend to be higher in cirrhotic patients with continuing inflammation or necrosis than in those without continuing liver injury.
- An increased AST-ALT ratio is often found in patients with cirrhosis.

Cirrhosis Treatment

Treatment is as follows:

1. Cirrhosis patients are treated with a low-protein diet.
2. Lactulose and antibiotics are given to kill the ammonia-producing bacteria in the gut. When lactulose is broken down by bacteria in the gut, H^+ is produced and the hydrogen binds to ammonia, producing ammonium that cannot be absorbed by the gut. It thus gets excreted, decreasing the toxins in the blood.

SUGGESTED DENTAL GUIDELINES WITH HEPATITIS OR CIRRHOSIS

The following are dental guidelines for hepatitis or cirrhosis:

1. Always obtain the complete blood count (CBC) with platelets, hepatic serology, viral load, LFTs, and PT/INR, as discussed below.
2. Evaluate the laboratory results and determine the type of hepatitis or cirrhosis the patient has. The patient may have a history of one or more types of viral hepatitis.
3. Recovery is 100% with hepatitis A, and you do not need to obtain hepatic serology to confirm recovery if the patient is certain that it was hepatitis A.
4. Obtain the hepatic serology and viral load for each type of blood-transmitted hepatitis (B, C, or D) to determine current viral activity status for the virus infecting the patient.
5. Obtain the liver function tests (LFTs) in all patients with a history of any type of hepatitis or cirrhosis.
6. Look at the serum albumin level. The level will be normal with hepatitis and decreased with cirrhosis.
7. Elevated liver enzymes with a normal albumin indicates active hepatitis.
8. Normal or mild elevation of liver enzymes with a normal albumin indicates chronic hepatitis.
9. Decreased albumin and AST > ALT is seen with cirrhosis.
10. In the presence of cirrhosis, always obtain the PT/INR prior to probing.
11. Prolongation of PT/INR depends on the **frequency and amount** of blood loss experienced by the cirrhotic patient and **not by the duration** of the disease.
12. Consult with the patient's M.D. if the PT/INR is prolonged or increased. The M.D. may give you the go-ahead to proceed with minor dentistry without transfusion therapy if the PT/INR is <2.
13. The patient will need blood plasma transfusion (Fresh Frozen Plasma/FFP or whole blood) for major and minor dentistry if the PT/INR is >2.
14. Cirrhosis can be associated with thrombocytopenia (decreased platelets) due to sequestration of the platelets by the spleen and/or decreased production by the liver.
15. Follow the platelet guidelines for dentistry (discussed in the hemopoietic section) and consult with the patient's M.D. for platelet replacement therapy, when required.
16. Calculate the absolute neutrophil count/ANC (discussed in the hemopoietic section) for all patients with hepatitis or cirrhosis. Follow the ANC guideline recommendations if the ANC is <1,500 cells/mm^3
17. Follow the suggested anesthetic, analgesic, antibiotic (AAAs) guidelines listed in Table 45.3.

Table 45.3. Anesthetics, analgesics, and antibiotics (AAAs) guidelines for hepatitis and cirrhosis

Medications	Prescriptions: Normal and Altered	Drug Alerts/Advice
LOCAL ANESTHETICS		
1. **2% Lidocaine (Xylocaine)** with 1:100,000 epinephrine	Any local anesthetic can be used. Use only 2 carpules per visit for hepatitis or cirrhosis.	Amide LAs toxicity can occur with significant liver disease. Liver disease does not increase the duration of the amides. Dental treatment with cirrhosis must be completed **over multiple visits** to minimize the total amount of local anesthetic used per visit.
2. **4% Prilocaine HCL (Citanest Forte)** with 1:200,000 epi		
3. **4% Septocaine (Articaine)** with 1:100,000 & 1:200,000 epi		
4. **0.5% Bupivacaine (Marcaine)** with 1:200,000 epi		
5. **2% Mepivacaine (Carbocaine)** with 1:20,000 levonordefrin		
6. **3% Mepivacaine HCL** (Carbocaine)		
7. **4% Prilocaine HCL** (Citanest Plain)		
ANALGESICS		
1. **Acetaminophen** (Tylenol)	1. **Chronic Inactive Hepatitis Dose:** 325–650 mg q6h 2. **Chronic Active Hepatitis/Cirrhosis Dose:** 325–650 mg q8h	Avoid chronic use. Use low-dose therapy with liver disease. Maximum daily dose should be <2 g/day with cirrhosis or chronic active hepatitis. Absolutely avoid with alcoholic liver disease.
2. **Aspirin**	Avoid use because aspirin promotes bleeding.	Truly only contraindicated with severe liver disease.
3. **NSAIDS**	All NSAIDS are contraindicated with hepatitis and cirrhosis.	Avoid aspirin and Ibuprofen with any liver disease. Patients with cirrhosis are at increased risk of kidney damage with NSAIDS.
4. **COX-2 inhibitors**	Avoid COX-2 inhibitors with any hepatic impairment.	
5. **Hydromorphone (Dilaudid)**	**Normal Dilaudid Dose: Oral:** 2–4 mg q4h **IV:** 1.5 mg q4h	Recommended for use in liver failure.
6. **Fentanyl**	**Normal Oral Fentanyl Dose:** Start with one 200 µg lozenge and use it over 15 min. Wait 15 min and use a second 200 µg lozenge if the pain does not immediately subside. Do not use more than 2 lozenges at a given time.	Recommended for use in liver failure.

Table 45.3. *Continued*

Medications	Prescriptions: Normal and Altered	Drug Alerts/Advice
7. **Codeine**	**Dose for Mild or Chronic Inactive Hepatitis:** Use the normal Codeine dose: 30–60 mg: Dispense 1–2 Tylenol #3 q4h PRN. **Dose for Moderate-Severe or Active Hepatitis:** Use 50% of the full dose of Codeine (15–30 mg): Dispense 1–2 Tylenol #2 q6h PRN. **Dose for Cirrhosis:** Use 25% of the full dose of Codeine (7.5–15 mg): Dispense 1–2 Tylenol #1 q8h PRN.	Use caution with hepatitis and cirrhosis. Lower the dose and prolong the interval if an opioid has to be used in a patient with liver disease.
8. **Oxycodone + Acetaminophen (Percocet)**	**Hepatitis Dose:** One 2.5/325 tablet q6h PRN. **Cirrhosis Dose:** One 2.5/325 tablet q8h PRN.	Limited, low-dose therapy for 2–3 days is usually well tolerated in hepatitis or cirrhosis.
9. **Hydrocodone + Acetaminophen (Vicodin)**	**Dose Schedule for Hepatitis:** Dispense 1 tab q6h PRN. **Cirrhosis Dose:** Dispense 1 tab q8h PRN.	Limited, low-dose therapy for 2–3 days is usually well tolerated in hepatitis or cirrhosis. **Avoid chronic use.**
10. **Morphine** 11. **Meperidine** (Demerol) 12. **Propoxyphene** (Darvon) 13. **Pentazocine** (Talwin) 14. **Tramadol** (Ultram)	No doses specified because the drugs listed from 10–14 are contraindicated with any type of liver disease.	Avoid with any form of liver disease.
ANTIBIOTICS		
1. **Penicillin VK**	**Rx:** 250 mg/500 mg/tab. **Normal Dose:** 250 mg or 500 mg q6h/qid × 5–7 days	Safe to use and no dose alteration needed with hepatitis or cirrhosis.
2. **Amoxicillin**	**Rx:** 250, 500 or 875 mg/capsules. **Normal Dose:** 250/500 mg q8h or 500–875 mg PO q12h × 5–7 days.	Safe to use and no dose alteration needed with hepatitis or cirrhosis Can be used with 50% dose adjustment in a patient with **both** kidney and liver disease.
3. **Ampicillin**	**Rx:** 250 mg or 500 mg/capsules. **Normal Dose:** 250–500 mg q6h for 5–7 days.	Use caution in the presence of any liver disease; **best to avoid.**
4. **Dicloxacillin**	**Normal Dose:** 250–500 mg qid × 5–7 days	Safe; use normal dose with hepatitis or cirrhosis.

Table 45.3. *Continued*

Medications	Prescriptions: Normal and Altered	Drug Alerts/Advice
Cephalosporins: 5. **Cephalexin** (Keflex) 6. **Cefadroxil** (Duricef)	**Cephalexin (Keflex):** **Rx:** 250 or 500 mg/capsule. **Normal Dose:** 250–1,000 mg q6h/qid × 5–7 days, maximum 4.0 g/day. **Cefadroxil (Duricef): Rx:** 250 or 500 mg/capsules. **Normal Dose:** 1–2 g/day in two divided doses × 5–7 days.	Safe; use normal dose with hepatitis or cirrhosis. Decrease the dose by 50% in patients with ***both*** kidney and liver disease.
7. **Clarithromycin** (Biaxin)	**Rx:** 250 or 500 mg/capsules. **Normal Dose:** 250 or 500 mg bid for 5–7 days.	No dose adjustment is needed with ***any*** liver disease ***as long as*** the renal function is ***normal.***
8. **Azithromycin** (Zithromax)	No prescriptions given because it is contraindicated with hepatitis/cirrhosis.	Avoid in patients with all forms of liver disease.
9. **Clindamycin** (Cleocin)	**Rx:** 150 or 300 mg/tablet. **Normal Dose:** 150–450 mg q6–8h/qid PO × 5–7 days. Prescribe the lower dose of Clindamycin (150 mg tid or q8h) routinely to minimize adverse side effects.	No dose adjustment required with hepatitis. Decrease the dose by 50% in patients with cirrhosis. Decrease the dose by 50% in a patient with ***both*** kidney and liver disease.
10. **Tetracycline HCl**	No Prescriptions given because Tetracycline is contraindicated.	Contraindicated with liver disease, kidney disease, or both liver and kidney disease.
11. **Doxycycline** (Vibramycin)	**Doxycycline, 100 mg/ capsule Normal Dose:** 200 mg PO 2 h prior to bed on day 1; 100 mg 2 h prior to bed/day: days 2–10. **Doxycycline, 50 mg/ capsule Normal dose:** 100 mg PO 2 h prior to bed on day 1; 50 mg 2 h prior to bed/day: days 2–10.	No Doxycycline dose change is needed with any form of liver disease. Use Doxycycline without dose change in a patient with ***both*** kidney and liver disease.
12. **Metronidazole** (Flagyl)	**Rx:** 250 or 500 mg/tab. **Normal Dose:** 250 mg q6h or 500 mg q8h × 5–7 days **OR** **Rx:** 7.5 mg/kg BW, maximum 1 g **Normal Dose:** Take q6h × 7 days.	No dose alteration is needed with ***mild*** liver disease. The dose should be decreased in ***moderate*** and ***severe*** liver disease. Use 250 mg q12h. Can be used in the presence of ***both*** liver and kidney disease but with a ***reduced*** dose, 250 mg q12h.

Table 45.4. LFT changes with alcoholic hepatitis, cirrhosis, and cholestatic disease

LFT Markers	Alcoholic Hepatitis	Cirrhosis	Cholestatic Disease
Total Protein	Normal	Decreased	Normal or decreased with chronic disease
Albumin (A)	Normal	Decreased	Normal or decreased with chronic disease
Globulin (G)	Normal	Increased	Normal or increased with chronic disease
A:G ratio	Normal	Reversed	Normal or reversed with chronic disease
ALT/SGPT	Mild increase: <300 IU/L	Normal/mild increase: <300 IU/L	>2000 IU/L
AST/SGOT	Mild increase: <500 IU/L	Normal/mild increase: <300 IU/L	>2000 IU/L
ALT:AST ratio	AST > ALT (>2:1)	AST > ALT	ALT > AST
GGT	Increased	Normal or increased with alcoholic cirrhosis	Severely increased
Alk. Phos (AP)	Normal	Increased	Severely increased
PT/INR	Normal	Normal/prolonged	Normal/prolonged with chronic disease
Total Bilirubin	Normal	Increased	Increased
Direct-B	Normal	Decreased or normal	Severely increased
Indirect-B	Normal	Increased or normal	Increased

18. Premedicate a cirrhotic patient presenting with ascites to prevent bacterial growth in the ascetic fluid.
19. Minimize bleeding with dentistry and use the suction aggressively to prevent the swallowing of blood in the presence of cirrhosis. Swallowed blood is protein, which the cirrhotic patient's liver is unable to handle and this can lead to hepatic encephalopathy.

BILIARY DISEASE

Primary Biliary Cirrhosis (PBC)

Primary biliary cirrhosis is an autoimmune disease associated with destruction of intra-hepatic bile ducts. Many patients are asymptomatic and subsequently go on to develop jaundice and cirrhosis. Middle-aged women are most affected with biliary cirrhosis.

Classic symptoms experienced are intense itching, jaundice, and cirrhosis in the long term.

Primary Biliary Cirrhosis (PBC) Blood Test

Antimitochondrial antibody (AMA) is a sensitive and specific test for PBC. It is 95% positive with this disease. Additionally, the AP is markedly increased.

Primary Sclerosing Cholangitis

Primary sclerosing cholangitis is also an autoimmune disease, but it is more common in men around age 40. It is often associated with ulcerative colitis.

Primary Sclerosing Cholangitis Pathology

Primary sclerosing cholangitis is associated with stricture of the intra- or extrahepatic bile ducts and cirrhosis is a long-term complication.

Primary Sclerosing Cholangitis Diagnosis

Primary sclerosing cholangitis is diagnosed with endoscopic retrograde cholangiopancreotography (ERCP). There is no cure, and transplant is the only option for this disease state.

XIII

Postexposure Prevention and Prophylaxis

Needle-Stick Exposure Protocol and Associated Management Prophylaxis in the Dental Setting

NEEDLE-STICK EXPOSURE OVERVIEW

Needle-stick exposure in the dental setting can predispose to hepatitis B, hepatitis C, or HIV infection. Every effort should be made to minimize the risk and prevent such accidents from happening.

Exposure Risks with Percutaneous and Mucocutaneous Exposures

The risk of exposure with percutaneous injury is 0.3% and with mucocutaneous exposure is 0.09%. The risk increases with deep exposures and/or large volume exposure.

Risk Reduction Steps

The two steps that can decrease the risk of infection are accident prevention protocol and having a percutaneous and mucocutaneous exposure protocol.

ACCIDENT PREVENTION PROTOCOL

An ideal accident prevention protocol should have the following steps implemented at all times during patient care:

1. Plan ahead and collect all instruments needed prior to the start of treatment. This is of particular importance in a dental school setting where the student has to collect the instruments needed and this increases the chances of injury when the provider is rushed.
2. Do not have two hands in the mouth at any time. Use the hand mirror to assist with the local anesthetic injection.
3. Do not recap the needles with two hands. Unfasten the needle using the disengaging guard. Cover the burr after use with an inverted clean plastic cup to prevent injury.
4. Lay instruments in appropriate slots in the instruments box after use or in a single layer on the dental tray. Do not pile the instruments one over the other after use.
5. Never reach for instruments without looking.
6. Do not be distracted by others. Focus on the procedure being done.

All steps listed above should periodically be reviewed and reenforced, particularly in a student setting.

PERCUTANEOUS AND MUCOCUTANEOUS EXPOSURE PROTOCOL

In the event of an injury, every health care setting must have a written percutaneous/needle-stick and mucocutaneous exposure protocol that must be implemented immediately. It is necessary to test and treat the exposed person within *1 hr* of the exposure.

The dental office must designate in advance a neighboring physician's office or hospital emergency room as the site responsible for providing immediate and follow-up care for both the provider/health care worker (HCW) and the source patient.

Every member of the office should be familiar with the protocol and it should be visibly posted in the clinical care areas with all the appropriate telephone numbers listed.

The needle-stick exposure protocol should be periodically discussed among the office staff to ensure awareness. In the event of an accident, noninjured members can actively help and this, in turn, decreases the anxiety experienced by the injured HCW.

EXPOSURE PROTOCOL

Postexposure Steps

Following an exposure, implement these steps immediately:

1. Stop dental treatment immediately, deglove, and wash the injured area with soap and tepid water. If the oral mucosa or eyes have gotten contaminated, rinse the mouth or splash tepid water into the eyes, accordingly. Do **not** be overly aggressive with the washing.
2. Inform your patient about the accident once you have completed the washing. Also inform the patient about your percutaneous and mucocutaneous protocol. The patient **needs to consent** for the blood tests that will be completed at the location implementing your protocol.

Postexposure Tests Protocol for the Source and the Provider/Health Care Worker (HCW)

Postexposure Tests for the Source

The source patient's status for HIV, hepatitis B, and hepatitis C are determined by conducting the following tests: Rapid HIV Test, HBsAg and HBeAg, Anti-HCV, and Hepatitis C RNA.

The Rapid HIV test results are obtained within 20 min. If the source is positive for hepatitis C, the provider has to be tested at baseline and have follow-up serology tests at 6 and 12 weeks. If conversion occurs the provider/HCW is referred to an infectious disease specialist for hepatitis C infection evaluation and treatment.

Known HIV/AIDS-Positive Source

If the source patient is a **known** HIV-infected patient, the **HIV PCR or viral load** is determined stat for that source patient. The viral load is also determined if the source tests positive with the Rapid HIV Test. In this case, it is clear that the source was unaware of the HIV status prior to the Rapid HIV Test. The designated physician will, in this case, inform the CDC (1.800.893.0485) about a new HIV case, because it is mandatory for the M.D. to report all HIV seroconversions.

Tests for the Provider/Health Care Worker (HCW)

The provider must be tested for **baseline** HCV and HIV infections using the Anti-HCV and the Rapid HIV Tests, respectively. Additionally, the anti-HBs titer test is done to determine the provider's immunity status with the hepatitis B vaccine. The hepatitis B vaccine and/or HBIG (hepatitis B immune globulin) are given dependent on the provider's vaccination and antibody status.

The provider must be reevaluated at 6 weeks, 12 weeks, and 6 months. If the provider seroconverts for HIV or HCV, the testing is continued for an additional 6 months, for a total of 12 months from the time of exposure.

Postexposure Medications

When the source patient is a **known** HIV/AIDS patient or the HIV/AIDS status of the source is unknown, the HCW must be protected immediately with postexposure medications.

With a known positive Source, the medications are given for 28 days or 4 weeks. With the **unknown** source, once the HIV/AIDS status of the source is confirmed to be negative, the medications can be stopped immediately.

The recommended drugs that should be started immediately within **1 hr** of the exposure are:

1. **2-Drug Regimen:** The 2-drug regimen consists of Lamivudin/Epivir (3TC) or Emtriva (FTC) plus Zidovudin (AZT) or Zerit/Stavudin (d4T) or Tenofovir (TDF).
2. **3-Drug Regimen:** The 3-drug regimen consists of Lopinavir + Ritonavir/Kaletra (LPV/r) [Preferred drug] or Atazanavir/reyataz (ATV), Fosamprenavir (FPV), Indinavir (IDV/r), Saquinavir (SQV/r), or Nelfinavir (NFV). EFV is considered if the source demonstrates resistance and the provider is not pregnant.

An infectious disease expert should be consulted if treatment has been delayed by more than 24–36 hr or the provider is pregnant or breast-feeding.

THE CDC OCCUPATIONAL POSTEXPOSURE PROPHYLAXIS (PEP) GUIDELINES

The CDC PEP guidelines to help the M.D. select the 2- or 3-drug regimen for the **exposed provider** are:

1. **If the source is HIV-positive, asymptomatic, and with a viral load <1.500 c/mL:** Two drugs are given for solid needle puncture or a superficial injury or if only a few drops splashed on the mucocutaneous areas.

   Three or more drugs are given for puncture with a large bore hollow needle or when deep injury occurs or there was visible presence of blood on the needle or instrument.

   Two or three drugs are given if there has been a major splash affecting the mucocutaneous areas.

2. **If the HIV-positive source is symptomatic or has AIDS or has acute retroviral syndrome or has a known high viral load:** Three or more drugs are used immediately for all major or minor percutaneous or mucocutaneous exposures. Immediate consultation with an infectious disease expert is required if the source has demonstrated resistance to HIV medications. In some cases of known multidrug resistance to medications in the source, the physician will have to contact the CDC for further guidance or help in obtaining experimental/newer drugs that may prove to be beneficial.

3. **If the source is unknown:** The option is to use no medication for a low- or no-risk source or use 2–3 drugs, dependent on the extent of exposure.

PEP Therapy Side Effects

The main symptoms experienced are nausea, malaise, and fatigue.

PEP Guidelines for Toxicity Monitoring and Transmission Protection

The provider's CBC and LFTs are done at baseline and at 2 weeks.

If protease inhibitors (PIs) are used, the provider's fasting blood sugar (FBS) is also done at baseline, on the day of exposure and start of treatment.

The provider's urinanalysis is done at baseline if IDV is used.

The provider is asked to report any fever, rash, vomiting, body pain, hematuria (blood in the urine), dysuria (painful urination), or symptoms of hyperglycemia.

The provider is also reminded to use protection during sex to prevent pregnancy, in the first 6–12 weeks after exposure. The provider is also asked not to donate blood or body tissues during the prophylaxis period.

The physician-generated protocol has been outlined to empower any provider accidentally injured during patient care. Realizing that the drug intake should be started immediately, it alleviates anxiety knowing you have the CDC PEP protocol on hand to share with the M.D.

It is beneficial for the physician, too, because it is not very often an M.D. treats percutaneous or mucocutaneous exposures.

XIV

Infectious Diseases

47

Human Immunodeficiency Virus (HIV) and Sexually Transmitted Diseases (STDs): Assessment, Analysis, and Associated Dental Management Guidelines

HUMAN IMMUNODEFICIENCY VIRUS (HIV)

Human Immunodeficiency Virus (HIV) Specifics

HIV is an infection caused by the human immunodeficiency virus that was formerly called the *human T-lymphotropic virus-III (HTLV-III)*. HIV-1 and HIV-2 are the two species of HIV that infect humans. HIV-1 is the more aggressive of the two and it accounts for the majority of the infections worldwide. HIV-2 is less aggressive and is limited to western Africa.

The reverse transcriptase enzyme in the virus helps with the transfer of viral RNA into the DNA of the host cell. The virus attacks the CD_4 T cells causing them to become infected. The infected cells are destroyed in one of three ways: direct viral killing, death by poptosis, and death through the cytotoxic effects mediated by the CD_8 lymphocytes.

The T_4 lymphocytes are like the "pilots" of immunity that also govern the quality and quantity of the B lymphocytes.

Defective cell-mediated and lymphokine-mediated humoral immunity consequently occurs. Impaired immunity accounts for the increased incidence of opportunistic infections when the patient becomes symptomatic.

In addition to the CD_4 cells the virus affects the monocytes, macrophages, neural cells, or glial cells and crosses the blood brain barrier. The virus has been isolated from almost all bodily fluids as free viral particles or embedded in cells specified above. Isolation is most pronounced from the blood and the seminal fluid.

Gradual decline in immunity over time ultimately leads to the patient developing the acquired immunodeficiency syndrome (AIDS). The patient is said to have AIDS when the CD_4 count is <200 cells/μL.

With the implementation of HIV/AIDS treatment, the CD_4 count can improve and rise >200 cells/μL. The patient will, however, retain the diagnosis of AIDS. It is important to remember that throughout the asymptomatic phase the CD_4 count is on a steady decline.

Modes of HIV Transmission

HIV transmission can occur with the following:

1. Blood or Clotting Factors transfusion.
2. Intravenous drug use (IVDU)
3. Exchange of body fluids: unprotected homosexual or heterosexual sex can transmit the virus. Worldwide, the transmission rate by heterosexual sex is now greater than the transmission occurring by homosexual sex.
4. Vertical transmission from mother to child: Transmission mostly occurs during birth, but there is data showing that some transmission may be intrauterine. Vertical transmission is now prevented with implementing elective cesarian section prior to the rupture of membranes in the HIV-positive mother.
5. The virus can also be transmitted through breast-feeding.

Epidemiology of HIV

Epidemiology of HIV in the Developed Nations

Initially in the developed world men having sex with men (MSM) was the leading cause of HIV transmission. With increased awareness of risk practices and prevention strategies, those numbers have declined.

Recently, there has been an increased rate of transmission of the virus in the heterosexual population because of unprotected sex and among people of color because of IV drug use (IVDU).

Vertical transmission from mother to child is now rare in the developed world because of initiation of treatment during pregnancy and the implementation of elective cesarian section around the 38th week of pregnancy.

Epidemiology of HIV in the Developing Nations

In the developing nations the highest rate of transmission has been encountered among the heterosexual population because of unprotected sex and IVDU.

Mother-to-child vertical transmission is another leading cause for the increased numbers of infected cases.

There is a dire need to provide antiretroviral therapy (ART) in the developing nations along with improved prevention strategies to decrease the numbers.

Prevention can be achieved by educating the population about HIV infection and the modes by which the virus is transmitted.

HIV Natural History

Listed in the following sections are the ways in which the viral infection can progress, following exposure.

Acute Retroviral Infection

An acute retroviral infection progresses as follows:

1. Some patients on seroconversion experience infectious mononucleosis type symptoms, about 2–4 weeks postexposure. The mononucleosis-type illness simulates an actual mononucleosis attack and it lasts for 10–14 days. The patient usually recovers

from the acute attack and progresses through an asymptomatic phase for years before becoming symptomatic again.

2. The majority of patients, however, are asymptomatic.

The Asymptomatic Patient

This patient has CD_4 >250 cells/uL and viral load up to 50–100 K/mL. The patient can stay asymptomatic up to 10 years while the CD_4 count gradually declines over time. No treatment is recommended in the presence of established disease if the patient is asymptomatic.

The Symptomatic Patient

The patient presents with AIDS defining conditions (ADC). Weight loss, oral candidiasis, opportunistic infections, tumors, etc., occur. The opportunistic infections that occur must be diagnosed and treated appropriately.

The Early Symptomatic Stage

The CD_4 count is >200/uL and the usual range at this stage is 250–300 cells/uL. MTB, candida infections, cryptococcus infection, histoplasmosis, and recurrent bacterial infections occur.

The Late Symptomatic Stage

Pneumocystis carinii pneumonia (PCP), now called *Pneumocystic Jiroveci,* and chronic cryptosporidia diarrhea occur when the CD_4 count is <200 cells/uL. Toxoplasmosis, cytomegalovirus (CMV), and mycobacterium avium complex (MAC) infections can occur when the CD_4 is <100 cells/uL.

AIDS Defining Conditions (ADC) That Occur in the Symptomatic Stage

The following are ADC conditions:

- Recurrent bacterial infections.
- Candida infection affecting the esophagus, trachea, bronchi.
- Disseminated coccidiomycosis, histoplasmosis.
- Extrapulmonary cryptococcosis.
- Chronic cryptosporidiosis.
- Cytomegalovirus (CMV).
- More advanced cases present with persistent mucocutaneous herpes simplex infection (HSV), HIV encephalopathy, Kaposi's sarcoma, primary lymphoma of the brain, non-Hodgkin's B-cell lymphoma, MAC, extrapulmonary TB (dissem TB), pneumocystic Jeroveci pneumonia, progressive multifocal leucoencephalopathy, recurrent salmonella infection, and toxoplasmosis of the brain.
- Cytomegalovirus (CMV) can affect the eyes, the brain, and the adrenal glands.
- Papilloma virus that causes warty cauliflower type of lesions on the gums.
- Mycobacterium avium complex (MAC) and mycobacterium Kansassi (MK) occur only in the immune-compromised patients and not in healthy, immune-competent patients.
- Kaposi's sarcoma begins as a pink pinhead-sized lesion that gradually enlarges and changes color from pink to purple to black. Kaposi's is usually multifocal involving the trunk, upper extremities, and the head and neck region.

HIV and AIDS Criteria Summary

HIV

The patient is said to have HIV when there is evidence that confirms presence of HIV. There is ongoing viral replication and progressive immune system decline.

AIDS

The patient is said to have AIDS when there is HIV infection and ADCs or the patient has CD_4 <200 cells/uL. There is ongoing viral replication and progressive immune system decline.

General Overview of HIV/AIDS in the U.S.

HIV is now one of the top 10 causes of death in the U.S. People are now living longer with HIV and the death rate is decreasing. The numbers of HIV cases among Blacks and Hispanics have increased; the numbers among Whites have declined. The numbers among Asians has stayed low throughout. Transmission by intravenous drug use (IVDU) increased and unprotected heterosexual contacts recorded the steepest rise. The numbers decreased for men having sex with men (MSM) and MSM IV drug users.

HIV/AIDS TESTS

The HIV tests detect the presence of the human immunodeficiency (HIV) antibodies, antigens, or RNA in the serum or saliva. The three sets of tests associated with HIV/ AIDS are:

1. Diagnostic tests
2. Quantitative tests
3. Organ assessment tests with medication intake

DIAGNOSTIC TESTS

The average window period (the time from infection until antibodies develop) with the antibody tests is about 22 days. Occasionally a patient may have a delay in forming antibodies for about 3–6 months. The two sets of diagnostic tests that help with the diagnosis of infection are:

1. Non-Rapid diagnostic tests
2. Rapid diagnostic tests

The Non-Rapid Diagnostic Tests

It takes about 7–10 days to obtain the results. The two non-rapid diagnostic tests are:

1. The Enzyme Linked Immune Absorbent Assay (ELISA) Test
2. The Western Blot Test

The ELISA Test

The ELISA Test is said to be reactive when it detects antibodies to HIV-1. Once positive, the blood is tested again to confirm that indeed the ELISA Test is positive. The ELISA Test is reported as a number and is 99% sensitive.

The Western Blot Test

The Western Blot Test is a more specific test and it is 99.5% sensitive. The Western Blot Test determines the size of the antigens in the test kit binding to the antibodies. Blood showing a positive ELISA is subjected to the Western Blot Test. Thus, the Western Blot Test is a confirmatory testing for HIV infection. A positive Western Blot Test confirms that the patient has the HIV infection.

The Rapid Diagnostic Tests

These tests provide results immediately or within 20 min. The two Rapid Diagnostic Tests are

1. The OraQuick Rapid-HIV Antibody Test
2. The Reveal Rapid-HIV Antibody Test

The OraQuick Rapid HIV-1 Antibody Test

This test detects antibodies and is approved for use with a finger-stick or anticoagulated whole blood or serum or oral fluid specimens. Results are obtained within 20 min from the testing. The test is 99.6% sensitive and 100% specific. The specificity of the OraQuick assay is *higher* than the Reveal Rapid assay.

The Reveal Rapid HIV-1 Antibody Test

This test requires the use of a serum or plasma specimen that is added to the test cartridge. The result is read immediately after the solution is absorbed. If a serum sample is used, the Reveal Rapid assay is 99.8% sensitive and 99.1% specific. If a plasma sample is used, the test is 98.6% specific.

THE QUANTITATIVE TESTS

There are two tests:

1. The CD_4 Count
2. The Viral Load

The Role of Quantitative Virology and Antiretroviral Therapy

CD_4 counts and HIV/RNA assays are of greatest clinical significance for efficient monitoring of the HIV infection. The CD_4 count provides an estimate of the patient's immune system status. CD_4 counts also are used to determine a patient's response to therapy.

The CD_4 count should be repeated every 3–6 months and the normal CD_4 count fluctuates between 500–1,500 cells/μL.

Correlation of CD_4 Count and Lymphocyte Percentage Reported on Laboratory Tests

Lymphocyte percentage reported on laboratory tests can be correlated to the appropriate CD_4 count to get a better understanding of the patient's immunity status.

Lymphocyte Percentage to CD_4 Count Conversion

- 29% lymphocytes = CD_4 count >500 cells/μL
- 14–28% lymphocytes = CD_4 200–500 cells/μL
- <14% lymphocytes = CD_4 count <200 cells/μL

HIV RNA or Viral Load

HIV RNA/Viral Load assays permit the detection of minute quantities of HIV RNA in the blood and tissues of the patient, in all stages of the disease. It is a strong predictor of disease progression. A threefold change with successive tests is said to be significant. If HIV RNA levels are repeatedly <10,000 copies/mL, therapy may be deferred. HIV RNA levels <75 copies/mL indicate an "undetectable viral load."

Serial HIV RNA assays must be repeated every 3–4 months. Longevity is increased if viral loads are kept constantly at negligible levels.

ORGAN ASSESSMENT TESTS WITH MEDICATION INTAKE

The following tests are required when the patient is on HIV/AIDS medications to detect adverse side effects with the medications:

1. **The CBC:** The CBC must be repeated every 3–6 months or sooner, if indicated. AZT and d4T cause macrocytic anemia.
2. **Liver Function Tests (LFTs):** LFTs are done to monitor the liver enzymes that may be affected with the HIV/AIDS medications.
3. **Renal Function Tests:** Urinalysis and serum creatinine are monitored while the patient is on the HIV/AIDS medications.
4. **Fasting Blood Sugar (FBS):** The FBS is monitored for patients on Highly Active Antiretroviral Therapy (HAART) because HAART can raise the blood sugar levels. The FBS must be repeated at 3–4 months.
5. **Lipid Profile:** The lipid profile is monitored for patients on HAART because the lipid levels can be affected with HAART. The lipid profile must be repeated at 3–4 months.

Table 47.1 provides a summary of HIV/AIDS Medications.

Highly Active Antiretroviral Therapy (HAART)

HAART has been able to suppress the virus such that HIV is now considered a chronic disease. Once started, HAART has to continue for life, so the question is when to start the treatment.

The physician and the patient have to weigh the short- and long-term risks or toxicities associated with HAART. The biggest benefit has been a 50% reduction in mortality. The drawbacks have been lipodystrophy and metabolic abnormalities increasing the risks for cardiovascular disease.

Not all HIV-associated conditions are reduced with HAART. Suppression of HIV does not mean that there will be associated decline in the replication of hepatitis C virus. In fact, it may worsen the hepatitis C coinfection.

Incidence of Kaposi's sarcoma is decreasing, but the incidence of immunoblastic lymphoma, Hodgkin's lymphoma, invasive cervical cancer, and Burkitt's lymphoma are not.

HAART-Associated Lipodystrophy Syndrome and Metabolic Abnormalities

The resultant lipodystrophy syndrome is associated with abnormal fat accumulation causing central, intraabdominal obesity and fat buildup around the back of the neck known as a "buffalo hump." Subcutaneous fat atrophy between the skin and the muscles mostly affecting the face, arms and legs also occurs.

Table 47.1. HIV/AIDS medications

All drugs listed use the following sequence:
Generic Name: Drug Abbreviation: Trade Name

Drug Category	Medications	Side Effects
I. Nucleoside Reverse Transcriptase Inhibitors (NRTI)	1. Abacavir: ABC (Ziagen) 2. ABC + ZDV + 3TC: (Trizivir) 3. Combivir: CBV (AZT + 3TC) 4. Didanosine: ddl (Videx; Videx-EC) 5. Emtricitabine: FTC (Emtriva) 6. Epzicom: (ABC + 3TC) 7. Lamivudine: 3TC (Epivir) 8. Stavudine: d4T (Zerit) 9. Tenofovir: TDF (Viread) 10. Trizivir: (AZT + 3TC + ABC) 11. Truvada: (TDF + FTC) 12. Zalcitabine: ddC (Hivid) 13. Zidovudine: (Retrovir, AZT)	Lactic acidosis with steatosis is an adverse reaction associated with this class of drugs.
II. Non-Nucleoside Reverse Transcriptase Inhibitors (NNRTI)	1. Delaviridine: DLV (Rescriptor) 2. Efavirenz: EFV (Sustiva) 3. Nevirapine: NVP (Viramune)	
III. Protease Inhibitors (PI)	1. Atazanavir: ATV (Reyataz) 2. Fosamprenavir: FPV (Lexiva) 3. Indinavir: IDV (Crixivan) 4. lopinavir: (Crixivan, IDV) 5. Lopinavir + Ritonavir: LPV/r (Kaletra) 6. Nelfinavir: NFV (Viracept) 7. Ritonavir: RTV (Norvir) 8. Saquinavir: SQV (Invirase) 9. Tipranavir: TPV (Aptivus)	Hyperglycemia Hyperlipidemia Lipodystrophy Hepatitis 26% increased incidence of MI
IV. Cellular Inhibitors	Hydroxyurea: HU (Droxia/Hydrea)	
V. Immune-Based Therapy	1. Aldesleukin: (Proleukin) 2. Interleukin-2: (Proleukin) 3. HIV Immunogen: (Salk vaccine/Remune) 4. Intravenous immune globulin: IVIG	
VI. Fusion Inhibitors: Prevent the fusion of HIV-1 with CD_4 cells.	Enfurvitide: ENF (T-20, Fuzeon)	
VII. Once-Daily 3-Drug Combination Pill: Atripla	Tenofovir: TDF (Viread) + Emtricitabine: FTC (Emtriva) + Efavirenz: EFV (Sustiva): (Atripla)	
VIII. Newer Drugs to Be FDA Approved: CCR5 Receptor Blocker	Maraviroc **Drug Facts:** It is postulated that the HIV virus first attacks human cells by hooking onto a receptor on the white blood cells. CCR5 is a defective version of this cell receptor. Maraviroc works by binding to the CCR5 receptor preventing the virus from entering and infecting the human cells. Maraviroc is expected to benefit those patients resistant to the current 3-drug therapy.	

HAART is also associated with lipid metabolism changes demonstrating a low HDL and high triglycerides.

Glucose metabolism changes showing insulin resistance and glucose intolerance is another side effects of HAART.

Cumulative Side Effects of HIV/AIDS Medications

The side effects associated with HIV/AIDS medications must be assessed and appropriately treated where possible by the dentist prior to the start of dentistry.

The side effects that can occur are heart disease, liver disease demonstrating elevated ALT levels and hepatic necrosis, xerostomia, change in prevalence and incidence of oral lesions, Steven-Johnson syndrome, lactic acidosis, pancreatitis, nephrotoxicity, marrow suppression, gastrointestinal intolerance, peripheral neuropathy, rash, CNS toxicity, insulin resistance, hyperlipidemia, fat atrophy, and fat accumulation.

PROPHYLAXIS AND TREATMENT OF OPPORTUNISTIC INFECTIONS (OIS)

PCP occurs within 1 year in 60% of patients with HIV and CD_4 <200 cells/uL. Thus, prophylaxis against PCP is a must as a preventative therapy.

Primary and Secondary Opportunistic Infections Prophylaxis

Primary Prophylaxis

Primary prophylaxis is provided when there is no evidence of the disease against which the prophylaxis is being given. PCP prophylaxis is an example of primary prophylaxis. PCP prophylaxis is inexpensive and effective. Trimethoprim-sulfamethoxazole (Bactrim) is the recommended regimen for PCP prophylaxis.

Bactrim also protects the patient from toxoplasmosis, salmonellosis, or any staphylococcal infection. Bactrim does not protect the patient against shigella, pneumococcal or pneumococcal strep, klepsiella, or pseudomonas.

All adults and adolescents regardless of HAART are given prophylaxis when any one of the listed states occurs:

- The patient has CD_4 <200 cells/uL.
- When there is a history of oral candidiasis.
- When the CD_4 cells account for <14% of the lymphocyte count.
- If there is a history of AIDS but without CD_4 <200/uL.

Secondary Prophylaxis

Secondary prophylaxis is provided *after* the disease against which the prophylaxis is being given has occurred. The patient gets treated for the disease *first* and the prophylaxis is given after recovery to prevent any future attacks with the disease. Prophylaxis against CMV is secondary prophylaxis. It is expensive and its effectiveness is questionable.

INITIATION OF HIV/AIDS TREATMENT

The following should be evaluated in a newly positive patient:

- The patient's readiness to begin treatment
- The viral serology
- Primary and secondary prophylaxis
- Vaccinations

HAART therapy should be started if the patient is symptomatic, regardless of the CD$_4$ count, or if the patient is asymptomatic but the CD$_4$ <200 cells/uL.

Treatment should be based on at least two consistent determinations of the CD$_4$ count and viral load. The treatment should be individualized and be deferred when the viral load is low and the CD$_4$ is stable. Treatment should be considered when the viral load shows RNA >100 K copies/uL.

Preferred HAART Regimens

Three drugs are the preferred regimens for HAART. The two sets of options are:

Option A: Protease inhibitor + 2 nucleoside reverse transcriptase inhibitors: Lopinavir/ritonavir (Kaletra) + (3TC or FTC) + ZDV

Option B: Non-nucleoside reverse transcriptase inhibitor and 2 nucleoside reverse transcriptase inhibitors: Efavirenz + (3TC or FTC) + (ZDV or TDF).

Tables 47.2 and 47.3 show a summary of the 2004 DHHS and IAS-USA guidelines for HIV/AIDS treatment initiation.

PREGNANCY AND HIV/AIDS

HAART can begin at the end of the first trimester. Efavirenz and a combination of D4T are avoided during pregnancy. Drug adherence is an issue since it has to be taken every day for the rest of the patient's life.

The treatment goal is to obtain maximum and durable suppression of the viral load, restoration and preservation of immunological function, improvement of quality of life, and reduction of HIV-related morbidity and mortality.

A C-section is done beyond 36 weeks if the pregnant patient has received no HIV treatment to prevent vertical transmission from mother to child. A C-section is done at 38 weeks if the patient has received HIV treatment.

The 2005 U.S. Public Health Service Recommendations for Antiretroviral Therapy (ART) During Pregnancy consists of any one of the following:

Table 47.2. 2004 Department of Health and Human Services (DHHS) guidelines for the indications for Antiretroviral Therapy (ART) in adult patients

Clinical Status	CD$_4$ Count	Viral Load	Suggestion
Symptomatic Patient with or without AIDS	Any count	Any Viral Load	Start treatment (Rx).
Asymptomatic AIDS	<200 cells/μL	Any Viral Load	Start treatment.
Asymptomatic Patient	CD$_4$: 200–350 cells/μL	Any Viral Load	Rx may be suggested.
Asymptomatic	CD$_4$: >350 cells/μL	>100,000 c/mL	Rx may/may not be considered.
Asymptomatic	CD$_4$: >350 cells/μL	<100,000 c/mL	Defer Rx and observe.

Table 47.3. 2004 International AIDS Society (IAS)-USA guidelines for the indication for Antiretroviral Therapy (ART) in adult patients

Clinical Status	CD$_4$ Count	Viral Load
Symptomatic patient with/without AIDS	Treat.	—
CD4: <200 cells/μL	Treat.	—
CD4: 200–350 cells/μL	Consider treatment.	Especially if the Viral Load is >50,000–100,000 c/mL and the CD$_4$ is closer to 200 cells or the CD$_4$ has declined by more than 100 cells/year.
CD4: 350–500 cells/μL	Monitor.	Consider treatment if the Viral Load is >100,000 c/mL or the CD$_4$ has declined by more than 100 cells/year.
CD4: >500 cells/μL	Monitor.	—

Table 47.4. Appropriate Drugs for the management of opportunistic infections in the HIV/AIDS pregnant patient

Medication	Drug Category	Suggestion
Acyclovir	Category B	Safe: Follow standard prescription guidelines.
Amphotericin B	Category B	Safe: Follow standard prescription guidelines.
Azithromycin	Category B	Safe: Follow standard prescription guidelines.
Clindamycin	Category B	Safe: Follow standard prescription guidelines.
Metronidazole	Category B	Safe: Follow standard prescription guidelines.
Valacyclovir	Category B	Safe: Follow standard prescription guidelines.
Famciclovir	Category B	Limited data on the drug, ***reserve*** for ***severe*** herpes only.
Clarithromycin	Category C	Contraindicated.
Doxycycline	Category D	Contraindicated.
Fluconazole	Category C	Avoid. Use Amphotericin B instead.
Ganciclovir	Category C	Avoid.
Itraconazole	Category C	Avoid.

1. AZT and 3TC (Nucleoside and Nucleotide)
2. NVP (NNRTI) or NFP (PI)
3. Any of the fusion inhibitors.

Tables 47.4 and 47.5 present drugs for managing opportunistic infections in pregnant patients and a summary of opportunistic infections treatment options, respectively.

HIV/AIDS DENTAL ASPECTS AND SUGGESTED DENTAL GUIDELINES

Always obtain the following laboratory tests from the patient's M.D. using a signed consent form:

Table 47.5. Summary of opportunistic infections (OIs) standard treatment options

Opportunistic Infection	Standard Preferred Treatment
Pneumocystis Jiroveci (Formerly PCP)	Trimethoprim-Sulphamethoxazole (TMP-SMX)
Toxoplasmosis	Trimethoprim-Sulphamethoxazole (TMP-SMX)
Mycobacterium avium complex (MAC)	Azithromycin 1200 mg/week and Clarithromycin 500 mg bid
Oral Candida	**Prescribe any one of the following:** 1. Clotrimazole troches 10 mg PO 5×/d 2. Nystatin suspension 5 mL qid 3. Nystatin pastilles 4–5×/d 4. Fluconazole 100 mg qd PO 5. Itraconazole oral suspension 200 mg qd
Esophageal Candida	**Prescribe any one of the following:** 1. Fluconazole 100 mg qd, (maximum 400 mg qd), PO × 14–21 d 2. Itraconazole oral suspension 200 mg qd PO
Cryptococcus	Amphotericin B + Flucytosine
Cytomegalovirus (CMV)	Ganciclovir + Valganciclovir
Herpes Simplex	Acyclovir 400 mg 4–5×/d PO, continue until vesicles heal. Provide maintenance with Acyclovir in relapse cases.

1. **The CBC with Platelet Count:** Megaloblastic anemia, neutropenia, and peripheral neuropathy (due to folic acid deficiency) are frequent side effects of anti-HIV medications. The use of opioids and block anesthesia are contraindicated when the hemoglobin is <10 g/dL.
2. The CD_4 count
3. The viral load
4. The PT/INR because the liver is frequently affected
5. The LFTs
6. Serum creatinine
7. The FBS, PPBS, and HbA_1C

The following are dental guidelines:

1. Use a nonalcoholic mouth rinse **prior** to every appointment to degerm the oral cavity. Have the patient also use the mouth rinse daily as home care, once a day. Follow this pretreatment mouth rinse protocol for all your patients.
2. When making a decision on which antibiotic to prescribe always *first* determine *which* other antibiotic the HIV patient is taking currently for some other infection or as part of opportunistic infection (OI) prophylaxis.

    Determine whether the antibiotic already in use is a cidal or a static antibiotic. To treat a dental infection in one such patient you need to match the cidal or static criteria for the antibiotics to work. A cidal OI antibiotic works best with a cidal oral infection management antibiotic, and a static OI antibiotic works best with a static oral infection management antibiotic.

3. Prior to treatment assess the current CD_4 count and the WBC count. If the CD_4 count is ≤200 cells/μL and the WBC count is normal (3.5–11 K/mm^3), proceed with the dental management as in a normal patient.

4. In patients with a decreased WBC count (≤3,500 cells/mm^3) calculate the absolute neutrophil count (ANC).

ANC = total WBC × [neutrophils% + bands%]. The average ANC is 1,500–7,200/μL.

Follow the ANC guidelines as discussed in Chapter 11, "Complete Blood Count (CBC): Assessment, Analysis, and Dental Management Guidelines," and summarized in Table 11.2.

Drugs Contraindicated with HIV/AIDS Medications

The following drugs are contraindicated:

1. **Protease inhibitors** should not be combined with the following drugs due to DDIs associated with **the CYP3A4 enzyme:** Demerol, Darvon, clarithromycin, tetracycline, doxycycline, metronidazole, diazepam, lorazepam (diazepam and lorazepam may be used with caution as a single dose prior to a procedure), and azole antifungals: clotrimazole, fluconazole, ketoconazole.

2. **Antihistamines: Avoid** asternizole and terfenadine.

3. **Psychotropics: Avoid** midazolam (Versed) (may be used with caution as a single dose prior to a procedure), triazolam (Halcion), alprazolam (Xanax).

4. **Antifungals: Avoid** itraconazole, ketoconazole, voriconazole.

5. **Anticonvulsants: Avoid** phenobarbital.

6. **Antibiotics: Avoid** clarithromycin (Table 47.6).

7. **H_2 Blockers: Avoid with H_2 blockers.** Keep a 2-hr interval between the HIV medications and the H_2 blocker.

SEXUALLY TRANSMITTED DISEASES (STDS)

Sexually Transmitted Diseases Overview

STDs discussed in this section are chlamydia, genital herpes, gonorrhea, and syphilis.

The occurrence of STDs in the past must always be confirmed during patient assessment. Always confirm what STDs were diagnosed in the patient. Is there a history of **completion** of treatment in a patient presenting with a positive history of STDs? STDs when left untreated or incompletely treated can lead to pelvic inflammatory disease (PID) in the female patient and consequent infertility.

An astute dental provider could recognize STD lesions in the oral cavity and refer the patient to the medical side for thorough evaluation and treatment.

CHLAMYDIA

Chlamydia Facts

Chlamydia is caused by the bacterium, Chlamydia trachomatis. Chlamydia can infect both males and females. An untreated infection causes irreversible damage and infertility. It is considered a relatively silent disease because symptoms caused by the infection are usually mild or absent. Symptoms when present occur within 1–3 weeks of the start of the infection. The patient usually experiences a vaginal discharge or burning on urination.

Table 47.6. Suggested anesthetic, analgesic, and antibiotic guidelines for patients on HIV/AIDS medications

Drug Category	Drug: Generic (Trade)	Suggested Guideline
Anesthetics	2% Lidocaine **(Xylocaine)**	Safe: Use maximum 2 carpules.
	4% Prilocaine HCL **(Citanest Forte)**	Avoid with anemia.
	0.5% Bupivacaine **(Marcaine)**	Safe: Use maximum 2 carpules.
	4% Septocaine **(Articaine)**	Avoid with anemia.
	3% Mepivacaine HCL **(Carbocaine)** **OR**	Safe: Use maximum 2 carpules.
	2% Mepivacaine HCL (Carbocaine) **with Levonordefrin (NeoCobefrin)**	
	4% Prilocaine HCL **(Citanest Plain)**	Avoid with anemia.
Analgesics	Codeine + Acetaminophen: **Tylenol #1–4**	Safe: Use standard dose.
	Oxycodone + Acetaminophen **(Percocet)**	Safe: Use standard dose.
	Hydrocodone + Acetaminophen **(Vicodin)**	Safe: Use standard dose.
	Meperidine **(Demerol)**	Avoid.
	Propoxyphene **(Darvon)**	Avoid.
Antibiotics	Penicillin **(Pen. VK)**	Safe: Use standard dose.
	Amoxicillin **(Amoxil)**	Safe: Use standard dose.
	Amoxicillin + Clavulanic acid **(Augmentin)**	Safe: Use standard dose.
	Cephalexin **(Keflex)**	Safe: Use standard dose.
	Cefadroxil **(Duricef)**	Safe: Use standard dose.
	Azithromycin **(Zithromax)**	Safe: Use standard dose.
	Clarithromycin **(Biaxin)**	Avoid.
	Clindamycin **(Cleocin)**	Safe: Use standard dose.
	Tetracycline HCL	Avoid.
	Doxycycline **(Vibramycin)**	Avoid with Protease Inhibitors; safe with other HIV drugs.
	Metronidazole **(Flagyl)**	Avoid with Protease Inhibitors; safe with other HIV drugs.
Antivirals	Acyclovir **(Zovirax)**	Safe: Use standard dose.
	Valacyclovir **(Valtrex)**	Safe: Use standard dose.
Antifungals	Clotrimazole **(Mycelex)**	Avoid with Protease Inhibitors, use Nystatin instead. Safe with other HIV drugs.
	Mycostatin **(Nystatin)**	Safe: Use standard dose.
	Fluconazole **(Diflucan)**	May be used with caution with Protease inhibitors, safe with other drugs.
	Ketoconazole **(Nizoral)**	Avoid.
Benzodiazepines	Diazepam **(Valium)**	Restrict. Use lowest dose if required after M.D. consult.
	Lorazepam **(Ativan)**	Restrict. Use lowest dose if required after M.D. consult.

Chlamydia infection has gained much prominence and concern because it is now being considered an important etiological factor for periodontal and coronary artery diseases.

Chlamydia Treatment

Chlamydia infection is treated with a **single dose** of 500 mg azithromycin (Zithromax) or doxycycline (Vibramycin) 100 mg bid for 7 days.

To completely eradicate the infection, all sex partners of the patient must be tested and treated accordingly.

GENITAL HERPES

Genital Herpes Facts

Genital herpes can be caused by the herpes simplex viruses type 1 (HSV-1) and type 2 (HSV-2). However, most genital herpes is caused by HSV-2.

With the initial genital herpes outbreak, the patient experiences vesicles or blisters around the genitals or the rectum. The initial infection is painful and ulcerative and lasts for 2–4 weeks. Subsequent outbreaks are less severe and can reoccur with variable frequency. The virus is present in the secretion from the vesicles and can be transmitted by sexual contact.

Genital Herpes Treatment

Genital herpes cannot be cured, but the outbreaks can be attenuated with antiviral medications. The patient is typically on chronic suppressive therapy to reduce symptoms and transmission of the disease.

GONORRHEA

Gonorrhea Facts

Gonorrhea is caused by the bacterium Neisseria gonorrhoeae. The bacterium grows in warm, moist areas of the reproductive system, rectum, anus, mouth, throat, and eyes.

Men are usually more symptomatic than women and experience clear to purulent discharge, painful urination, or soreness of the genitals. Symptoms are usually minimal in women and often simulate a urinary tract infection.

Gonorrhea Treatment

The patient with nonresistant bacteria is usually treated with Ceftriaxone 125 mg IM in a single dose **or** Cefixime 400 mg is given orally in a single dose or 400 mg by suspension (200 mg/5 ml).

SYPHILIS

Syphilis Facts

Syphilis is caused by the bacterium Treponema pallidum. Syphilis infection can manifest in three ways: primary, secondary, or tertiary. An observant dental provider could occasionally encounter a primary syphilis chancre sore in the oral cavity. Immediate treatment at this point will prevent the progression to the secondary and tertiary stages.

Primary Stage

The primary stage of syphilis is usually characterized by the appearance of a single chancre or sore on the genitalia within 2–12 weeks of infection. The chancre is painless and can heal in 3–6 weeks without treatment. When left untreated, the infection will progress to the secondary stage.

Secondary Stage

The secondary stage is characterized with the appearance of a nonitchy skin rash on the palms of the hands and soles of the feet. Additionally, the patient also presents with mucous membrane lesions, fever, lymphadenopathy, sore throat, weight loss, and flulike symptoms. The secondary stage manifests soon after the primary stage, when left untreated.

Tertiary Syphilis

Tertiary syphilis occurs many years after the disappearance of the symptoms and signs experienced in the secondary stage. The infection ultimately causes neurological, cardiac, and musculoskeletal damage leading to dementia, paralysis, and blindness.

Syphilis Treatment

Syphilis should be treated immediately, in the primary stage, to prevent progression to the secondary and tertiary stages. A single intramuscular injection of penicillin, results in complete cure.

Oral Lesions and Dentistry

48

Therapeutic Management of Oral Lesions in the Immune-Competent and the Immune-Compromised Patient in the Dental Setting

OVERVIEW (TABLE 48.1)

The common oral lesions seen in the immune-competent and the immune-compromised patient will be collectively discussed because many of the lesions overlap in the two populations. The severity and duration, however, often differ.

The immunity can be compromised because of HIV/AIDS, chemotherapy, radiotherapy, leukemias, lymphomas, connective tissue disorders, and poorly controlled diabetes, to name a few. Stress, chronic corticosteroid therapy, severe sun exposure, and broad-spectrum antibiotic use are often the cause of oral lesions in the immune-competent patient. Thus, presence of oral lesions, by themselves, are not diagnostic of HIV infection or other causes of decreased immunity.

With the presence of oral lesions, the clinician must assess the medical history and decide whether appropriate laboratory tests need evaluation to confirm the presence or absence of all causes of decreased immunity, including HIV infection. Once confirmed, however, the underlying cause or disease state should be addressed and appropriately managed *along* with the care of the oral lesions.

When treating an HIV patient, the dentist must refer a formerly asymptomatic, untreated, known HIV patient to the physician on discovery of new oral lesions. The physician will evaluate the patient's CD_4 count and the viral load to determine whether antiretroviral treatment needs to be started. The oral lesions can resolve with improvement of the patient's immunity following antiretroviral treatment. Recurrence of oral lesions following resolution in the HIV/AIDS patient can indicate failure of therapy or galloping HIV infection.

In spite of tremendous advances in antiretroviral therapy, oral lesions do occur and they must be appropriately managed.

The oral lesions have a tendency to recur more often with reduction of immunity, and in the HIV patient it can herald the start of the symptomatic phase. Oral herpes simplex or zoster, oral and/or esophageal candidiasis, angular chilities, xerostomia, and aphthous ulcers can affect the immune-competent or the immune-compromised patient.

Oral viral leukoplakia (OVL) or hairy leukoplakia (HL), HIV-gingivitis, HIV-periodontitis, HIV necrotizing stomatitis, Kaposi's sarcoma, cytomegalovirus, or papilloma virus infections are found only in the HIV/AIDS patient.

Table 48.1. Prescriptions: Management of oral lesions in the immune-competent and the immune-compromised patient

Infection/Lesion, Medication(s), Drug Category	Prescription/Treatment Guidelines
HERPES SIMPLEX	
Valacyclovir (Valtrex): Drug Category B	1. **Rx: Valtrex caplet,** 1 g/caplet Disp: 4 caplets Sig: Take 2 g q12h for 1 day only. 2. **Therapy for first Herpes infection:** Rx: Valtrex 1 g bid × 10 days 3. **Therapy for recurrent Herpes infection:** Rx: 500 mg bid × 5 days
Acyclovir (Zovirax): Drug Category B	1. **5-Day Rx:** Zovirax capsules, 200 mg/cap Disp: 25 capsules Sig: 1 capsule q4h while awake or take 5 capsules per day. Start when symptoms begin. 2. **5-day therapy with kidney disease:** GFR < 10 mL/min or dialysis: 200 mg q12h for 5 days
Acyclovir (Zovirax) capsules: Drug Category B	1. **14-Day Rx:** Zovirax capsules, 200 mg/capsule Disp: 70 capsules Sig.: 1 capsule 5 times/day × 2 weeks 2. **14-day Rx. with kidney disease:** GFR < 10 mL/min or dialysis: Dose 200 mg q12h
Acyclovir (Zovirax) ointment: Drug Category B	**Rx: 5% Zovirax ointment for recurrent Herpes:** Disp: 15 g tube Sig: Apply to sores 5–6 times daily. Zovirax ointment is most effective when used with Zovirax capsules.
HERPES ZOSTER	
Valacyclovir (Valtrex): Drug Category B	1. **Rx: Valtrex caplet,** 1 g/caplet Disp: 21 caplets Sig: Take 1 g tid for 7 days. 2. **Kidney disease dose**: GFR < 30 mL/min or s.creatinine > 3 mg/dL to predialysis: 1 g q24h
Acyclovir (Zovirax): Drug Category B	1. **Rx: Zovirax capsules,** 200 mg/capsule Disp: 140 capsules Sig: 800 mg 5 times/day × 7 days 2. **Kidney disease dose:** **a.** GFR 10–25 mL/min or s.creatinine > 3 mg/dL to predialysis: Rx: Dose 800 mg q8h **b.** GFR < 10 mL/min or dialysis: Rx: Dose 800 mg q12h

Table 48.1. *Continued*

Infection/Lesion, Medication(s), Drug Category	Prescription/Treatment Guidelines

HERPES CHRONIC SUPPRESSIVE THERAPY

Valacyclovir (Valtrex):
Drug Category B

Rx: Valtrex caplet, 500 mg/caplet
Disp: Dispense for 6 months to 1 year according to the patient's immunity.
Sig: 500 mg OD (once a day) or bid

Acyclovir (Zovirax):
Drug Category B

1. **Rx: Zovirax capsules,** 200 mg/capsule
   Disp: Variable
   Sig: 200 mg tid for up to 6 months or 400 mg bid/tid, for up to 3 years
2. **Chronic suppressive Rx with kidney disease:** GFR < 10 mL/min or dialysis: Dose 400 mg q12h or 200 mg q12h

HIV-GINGIVITIS

0.12% Chlorhexidine Gluconate (Peridex)

Oral hygiene and scaling with Betadine irrigation
Rx: Chlorhexidine (Peridex):
Disp: 3 × 16 oz bottles
Sig: Rinse with 1/2 oz for 30 sec bid after oral hygiene.

HIV-PERIODOTITIS

Treat with 0.12% Chlorhexidine Gluconate (Peridex) AND
Antibiotics:
1st Choice: Metronidazole
2nd Choice: Clindamycin, Cephalexin (Keflex) or Amoxicillin with Clavulanate potassium or Ciproflaxin

Oral hygiene and scaling with Betadine irrigation.
Rx: Chlorhexidine (Peridex):
Disp: 3 × 16 oz bottles
Sig: Rinse with 1/2 oz for 30 sec bid after oral hygiene.
Rx: Metronidazole (Flagyl): 250 mg/tablet
Disp: 20 tablets × 5 days
Sig: 1 tab qid
Clindamycin:
150/300 mg qid × 5 days
Cephalexin (Keflex):
250/500 mg bid/tid × 5 days
Amoxicillin with Clavulanate potassium (Augmentin):
250/500 mg tid × 5 days
Ciproflaxin (Cipro):
500 mg bid × 5 days. Use in refractory cases only.

ORAL CANDIDIASIS: PSEUDOMEMBRANOUS or HYPERTROPHIC or ERYTHEMATOUS

As First Choice: Use topicals.
Refractory/Severe Cases: Use systemic antifungals.

Clotrimazole (Mycelex) Troche:
Category B/C
Topical Azole antifungal

Rx: Clotrimazole (Mycelex)
Troches, 10 mg/troche
Disp: 70 troches
Sig: Use 1 troche 5×/day, *swallow saliva*. No eating/drinking for 30 min after use.
Also dispense: Chlorhexidine for all patients.

Table 48.1. *Continued*

Infection/Lesion, Medication(s), Drug Category	Prescription/Treatment Guidelines
Nystatin (Mycostatin) Prescriptions: Topical Polyene antifungal Drug Category B	**a. Rx: Nystatin (Mycostatin)** Lozenge 200,000 units/lozenge Disp: 70 lozenges (14-day supply) Sig: Dissolve 1 lozenge in the mouth 5 times daily. There should be **no** eating or drinking for 30 min after use. **b. Rx: Nystatin oral suspension 100,000 units/ml** Disp: 473 mL (1 pint) bottle (14-day supply) Sig: Use 1 tsp or 5 ml, qid. Rinse and hold in the mouth as long as possible before swallowing. There should be **no** eating or drinking for 30 min after use. **c. Rx: Nystatin oral suspension 100,000 units/ml for dentures** Disp: 473 mL (1 pint) bottle Sig: Add 5–10 mL of 1:100,000 units Nystatin to 1/2 cup of water and soak the dentures overnight daily, for 14 days. Rinse the dentures before use. **d. Rx: Nystatin pastille 200,000 units/pastille** Disp: 70 pastilles Sig: Dissolve 1 pastille in the mouth 4–5 times/day for 14 days. **e. Nystatin (Mycostatin) cream:** The cream can be applied to dentures before insertion or can be used for angular cheilitis. Rx: 100,000 units/g Disp: 15 or 30 g tube Sig: Apply to the affected area 4–5 times/day. Do **not** eat or drink for 30 min after use.
Amphotericin B: Topical Polyene antifungal Drug Category B	**a. Rx: 3% Topical Amphotericin B cream** Disp: 20 g tube Sig: Apply to the affected area 3–4 times/day for 2–4 weeks. **b. Oral Amphotericin B:** Oral Amphotericin B is dispensed as a capsule or a suspension. The oral forms are poorly absorbed. **i. Rx: Amphotericin B 500 mg/capsule** Disp: 56 capsules Sig: Take 500 mg capsule PO qid for 2 weeks. **ii. Rx: Amphotericin B suspension: 500 mg/mL** Disp: 56 mL suspension Sig: Use 1 mL of the suspension, swish and swallow qid for 2 weeks.

Table 48.1. *Continued*

Infection/Lesion, Medication(s), Drug Category	Prescription/Treatment Guidelines

REFRACTORY ORAL/SYSTEMIC CANDIDIASIS

Fluconazole (Diflucan):
Systemic Azole antifungal
Drug Category C

Rx: Fluconazole (Diflucan) 100 mg/capsule
Disp: 15 capsules
Sig: Day 1: Take 2 capsules. Days 2–14: Take 1 capsule daily.

ESOPHAGEAL CANDIDIASIS

Fluconazole (Diflucan):
Systemic Azole antifungal
Drug Category C

Rx: Fluconazole (Diflucan) 100 mg/capsule
Disp: Variable
Sig: 100 mg qd (maximum 400 mg qd) for 14–21 days

Itraconazole (Sporanox):
Triazole antifungal
Drug Category C

Rx: Itraconazole oral cuspension
Sig: 200 mg qd PO × 10–21 days

ANGULAR CHEILITIS

Clotrimazole (Mycelex) Cream:
Drug Category B/C

Rx: Clotrimazole (Mycelex) Cream
Disp: 15 g tube
Sig: Rub on lesions 2–3 times daily.

Nystatin (Mycolog) Ointment:
Drug Category B

Rx: Mycolog cream (Nystatin)
Disp: 15 g tube
Sig: Rub on lesions 2–3 times daily.

Clioquinol and Hydrocortisone (Corque Topical):
Drug Category C

Rx: Clioquinol and Hydrocortisone (Corque Topical)
Disp: 15 g tube
Sig: Rub into affected area 2–3 times daily.

RECURRENT APHTHOUS ULCERS

Tetracycline Capsules
Drug Category D

Tetracycline capsules: Dissolve a 250-mg tetracycline capsule in 180 mL water. Swish and spit qid for several days till ulcers heal. Do not eat or drink for 30 min. Avoid in kids and during pregnancy.

Tetracycline Suspension:
Drug Category D

Tetracycline suspension: Dispense 250 mg tetracycline/5 ml. Swish and expectorate qid till ulcers heal. Do not eat or drink for 30 min. Avoid in children and pregnant women.

Triamcinolone 0.1% (Kenalog in Orabase):
Topical steroid; use sparingly for pain relief.

Triamcinolone 0.1% (Kenalog in Orabase):
Apply the paste to ulcers bid/qid until the ulcers heal.
Disp: 5 g tube
Sig: Apply a thin film *without rubbing*, on affected areas up to 3 times daily.

0.05% Flucinonide (Lidex) Ointment Mixed 50/50 with Orabase

Rx: 0.05% Lidex ointment mixed 50/50 with Orabase
Disp: 30 g total
Sig: Apply a thin layer on the lesions 4–6 times daily.

Table 48.1. *Continued*

Infection/Lesion, Medication(s), Drug Category	Prescription/Treatment Guidelines
Dexamethasone Elixir	**Rx: Dexamethasone Elixir,** 0.5 mg/5 mL Disp: 250 ml Sig: Rinse with 1 tsp solution in the mouth for 1 min 4–5 times daily and *expectorate.*
Thalidomide (Thalomid): Drug Category X	**Thalidomide (Thalomid),** 200 mg OD/bid × 3–8 weeks is reserved for HIV/AIDS or refractory patients
Xylocaine 2% Viscous	**Rx: Xylocaine 2% Viscous** Disp: 100 ml or 450 ml Sig: Use 2 tsp to rinse the oral cavity, as needed, and *expectorate.*
Diphenhydramine (Benadryl) Syrup with Liquid Bismuth Subsalicylate (Kaopectate)	**Rx: Diphenhydramine (Benadryl) syrup (5 mg/mL) with Liquid Bismuth Subsalicylate (Kaopectate), mix 50/50** Disp: 8 oz. total Sig: Rinse with 2 tsp, as needed for pain relief; *expectorate.*
Diphenhydramine (Benadryl) Syrup with Magnesium Hydroxide Antacid	**Rx: Diphenhydramine (Benadryl) syrup (5 mg/mL) with Magnesium Hydroxide antacid, mixed 50–50** Disp: 8 oz total Sig: Rinse with 2 tsp, as needed for pain relief; *expectorate.*
Topical 0.15 Benzydamine (Difflam or Tantum) Oral Rinse	**Rx: Topical 0.15 Benzydamine (Difflam/ Tantum) oral rinse:** Apply to the ulcers four times/day for 2 weeks or until the ulcers heal. Treats mild disease.
Topical Carellose: (Orabase: Pectin plus Gelatin)	**Rx: Topical Carellose (Orabase: Pectin plus Gelatin):** Apply to the ulcers qid for 2 weeks or until the ulcers heal. A protective bioadhesive preparation for mild disease.
Topical Corticosteroids: Spray/cream/pellet For mild disease	a. **Rx: 1% Triamcinalone dental paste (Adrortyl or Kenolog in Orabase):** b. **Rx: Hydrocortisone, 2.5 mg pellets (Corlan)** c. **Rx: 0.12% or 0.2% Chlorhexidine gluconate aqueous mouthwash (Peridex) or 1% Chlorhexidine gluconate gel.** Apply to the ulcers qid with **all 3** preparations for 2 weeks/ until the ulcers heal.
Rx: Systemic Corticosteroids: For severe disease	**Rx: 30–60 mg prednisone** PO daily for 1 week, followed by a 1-week dose taper.

Table 48.1. *Continued*

Infection/Lesion, Medication(s), Drug Category	Prescription/Treatment Guidelines
XEROSTOMIA	
	Xerostomia Treatment Options: Daily oral hygiene; 3–6-month recall; nonalcoholic Peridex mouth rinse; topical Fluorides; saliva substitutes; saliva stimulants.
Saliva Substitutes	The combined use of Biotene and Oralbalance is very effective in the management of xerostomia.
Biotene® Products	**Biotene®:** Available as sugar-free gum, alcohol-free mouthwash, and toothpaste. **Biotene® mouthwash:** Use 1 Tbsp PRN, swish, and expectorate. It works best when used with Biotene® toothpaste. **Biotene® toothpaste:** The toothpaste is nonirritating and it contains the protective enzyme systems needed for optimal oral health. The toothpaste should be used postmeals and at bedtime.
Oralbalance®	**Oralbalance®** is available as a moisturizing gel.
Saliva Stimulant **Pilocarpine HCL (Salagen):** Increases saliva secretion by systemic cholinergic stimulation	**Pilocarpine HCL (Salagen),** 5 mg/tab Disp: Variable Sig: 1–2 tablets tid/qid per day taken 30 min **prior** to meals
CHEMOTHERAPY-/ RADIOTHERAPY- ASSOCIATED SIDE EFFECTS	Refer to Table 51.2 for chemotherapy- or radiotherapy-associated oral lesions or side effects and suggested management guidelines.

The treatment guidelines for oral herpes, oral candidiasis, xerostomia, and aphthous ulcers in the HIV/AIDS and the non-HIV/AIDS patient are the same.

The viral infections in the HIV/AIDS patients are generally treated for a longer duration when compared with the non-HIV/AIDS patient. The HIV/AIDS patients also often need chronic suppressive therapy.

COMMON ORAL LESIONS

The following are common oral lesions that are encountered in dentistry:

1. **Viral Infections:** Viral infections encountered in the immune-competent or immune-compromised patients are herpes simplex and herpes zoster. Cytomegalovirus infection occurs in the immune-compromised patient only.
2. **Oral Viral Leukoplakia (OVL) or Hairy Leukoplakia (HL):** OVL or HL is specific for HIV/AIDS.
3. **Fungal Infections:** Oral and/or esophageal candidiasis and angular cheilitis are seen in both populations.

4. **HIV-Gingivitis (HIV-G):** HIV-G is specific for HIV/AIDS.
5. **HIV-Periodontitis (HIV-P):** HIV-P is specific for HIV/AIDS.
6. **HIV Necrotizing Stomatitis:** This lesion is also specific for HIV/AIDS.
7. **Kaposi's Sarcoma:** Kaposi's sarcoma is specific for HIV/AIDS.
8. **Oral Warts:** Oral warts are caused by the papilloma virus and occur specifically in the HIV/AIDS patient.
9. **Aphthous Ulcers:** These ulcers occur in both populations.
10. **Xerostomia:** This occurs in both populations.
11. **Petechiae and Ecchymosis:** These occur in both populations.

DETAILED DISCUSSION OF COMMON VIRAL INFECTIONS

Herpes Simplex, Herpes Zoster, and Cytomegalovirus

Herpes Simplex (HSV)

HSV lesions may be solitary, multiple, or confluent, and they may be vesicular or keratinized. There is no erythematous halo associated with the vesicles, but the margins are round to slightly irregular.

The lesions may be in the periodontal region, dorsum of the tongue, hard palate, or attached gingiva.

The lesions resolve in less than a week in the immune-competent patient, but HSV outbreaks in the HIV patients usually last longer.

Herpes Zoster

Herpes zoster consists of unilateral vesicular erosive eruptions of the skin and oral mucosa along the distribution of the trigeminal nerve. It is often preceded or accompanied by **pain.**

Cytomegalovirus (CMV)

CMV presents as oral ulcers from which cytomegalovirus can be isolated.

VIRAL INFECTION TREATMENTS

Drugs commonly prescribed for recurrent herpetic infections are:

- Valacyclovir HCL (Valtrex)
- Acyclovir (Zovirax)

VALACYCLOVIR HCL (VALTREX)

Valtrex Facts

Valtrex is a category B drug and it rapidly converts to acyclovir on ingestion. It acts on HSV-1, HSV-2, and the varicella zoster virus (VZV). Valtrex is recommended for the treatment of herpes zoster, genital herpes, and herpes labialis (cold sore). A 50–75% dose reduction is recommended in patients with end-stage renal disease (ESRD). Patients on hemodialysis should get Valtrex after the dialysis. No dose adjustments are needed in patients with cirrhosis.

Valtrex is a better choice than acyclovir (Zovirax) because of its efficacy and shorter duration of treatment time. Valtrex strength per caplet is 500 mg or 1 g per caplet.

Valacyclovir (Valtrex) Prescriptions

1. **Valacyclovir (Valtrex) Therapy for Herpes Simplex (Cold Sore):**
   Rx: Valtrex caplet, 1 g/caplet
   Disp: 4 caplets
   Sig: Take 2 g q12h for 1 day only.
2. **Valacyclovir (Valtrex) Therapy for First Herpes Infection:**
   Rx: Valtrex 1 g bid × 10 days
3. **Valacyclovir (Valtrex) Therapy for Recurrent Herpes Infection:**
   Rx: 500 mg bid × 5 days
4a. **Valacyclovir (Valtrex) Therapy for Herpes Zoster:**
   Rx: Valtex caplet, 1 g/caplet
   Disp: 21 caplets
   Sig: Take 1 g tid for 7 days. Begin the drug with the start of symptoms or within 48 hr of the rash.
4b. **Valacyclovir (Valtrex) Therapy for Herpes Zoster with Kidney Disease**:
   GFR <30 mL/min or s. creatinine >3 mg/dL to predialysis:
   Rx: 1 g q24h
5. **Valacyclovir (Valtrex) Chronic Suppressive Therapy:**
   The chronic suppressive therapy should be dispensed for any type of herpes recurrences.
   Rx: Valtrex caplet, 500 mg/caplet
   Disp: Dispensed for 6 months to 1 year according to the patient's immunity.
   Sig: 500 mg OD (once a day) or bid

ACYCLOVIR (ZOVIRAX) PRESCRIPTIONS

Acyclovir is a Category B drug and is safe to use during pregnancy:

1. **Acyclovir (Zovirax) for Recurrent Herpes:**
   Rx: 5% Zovirax ointment
   Disp: 15 g tube
   Sig: Apply to lip sores 5–6 times daily.
       Zovirax ointment is most effective when used in conjunction with Zovirax capsules.
2a. **5-Day Duration, Acute Acyclovir (Zovirax) Therapy:** The 5-day therapy is usually given if the cold sores last for less than 1 week. This is less likely in an immune-compromised patient and more likely in an immune-competent patient.
   Rx: Zovirax capsules, 200 mg/capsule
   Disp: 25 capsules
   Sig: 1 capsule q4h while awake or total of 5 capsules/day. Start the intake as soon as the symptoms begin.
2b. **5-Day Acute Acyclovir (Zovirax) Therapy with Kidney Disease:**
   GFR <10 mL/min or dialysis:
   Rx: 200 mg q12h for 5 days
3a. **14-Day duration, Acute Acyclovir (Zovirax) Therapy:**
   The 14-day therapy is usually given if the cold sores last for 1–2 weeks. This is more likely to happen in an immune-compromised patient.
   Rx: Zovirax capsules, 200 mg/capsule

Disp: 70 capsules
Sig: Take 1 capsule 5 times/day × 2 weeks

3b. **14-Day Acute Acyclovir (Zovirax) Therapy with Kidney Disease:**
GFR <10 mL/min or dialysis:
Rx: Dose 200 mg q12h

4a. **Acyclovir (Zovirax) Chronic Suppressive Therapy:**
Rx: Zovirax capsules, 200 mg/capsule
Disp: Variable
Sig: 200 mg tid or 400 mg bid/tid for up to 1 year and then reevaluate

4b. **Acyclovir (Zovirax) Chronic Suppressive Therapy with Kidney Disease:**
GFR <10 mL/min or dialysis:
Rx: Dose 400 mg q12h or 200 mg q12h

5a. **Acyclovir (Zovirax) Normal Dose for Herpes Zoster Therapy:**
Rx: Zovirax capsules, 200 mg/capsule
Disp: 200 capsules
Sig: 800 mg (4 capsules) 5 times/day × 10 days

5b. **Kidney Disease and Acyclovir (Zovirax) Dose for Herpes Zoster Therapy:**
GFR 10–25 mL/min or s. creatinine >3 mg/dL to predialysis:
Rx: Dose 800 mg q8h
GFR <10 mL/min or dialysis:
Rx: Dose 800 mg q12h

ORAL VIRAL LEUKOPLAKIA (OVL) OR HAIRY LEUKOPLAKIA (HL)

OVL or HL is specific for HIV/AIDS. Oral viral leukoplakia (OVL) or hairy leukoplakia (HL) consists of vertically corrugated, slightly elevated white surface alterations of the lateral or ventral tongue margin that do not wipe off.

Hairy leukoplakia is caused by the Epstein-Barr virus. No definitive therapy has proven to be effective in the treatment of OVL. Several antiviral drugs including acyclovir have been investigated as potential treatments for OVL. Further studies are necessary in order to determine the treatment effectiveness of these agents.

Antifungal therapy should be implemented if candida is found to superinfect the OVL lesion.

If the lesion is traumatized or not esthetic to look at, OVL may be treated with Zovirax at doses greater than 1 g/day till the lesion resolves. Usually, however, no treatment is necessary.

HIV-GINGIVITIS (HIV-G)

HIV-gingivitis is specific for HIV/AIDS. HIV-G consists of an erythematous gingival band along the gingival margin and it extends into the adjacent attached and alveolar mucosa. HIV-G does not respond to calculus and plaque removal. It also does not respond to all measures used for oral hygiene.

HIV-Gingivitis General Guidelines of Care

The general guidelines of care consist of the following:

1. The patient must be given intensive oral hygiene instructions. Scaling and root planing should be done with 10% povidone-iodine (Betadine) irrigation. 0.12% chlorhexidine gluconate (Peridex) home rinses should be prescribed:

Rx: 0.12% chlorhexidine gluconate (Peridex)
Disp: 3 × 16 oz bottles
Sig: Rinse with 1/2 oz for 30 sec bid after completion of oral hygiene.

2. There should be careful follow-up and maintenance and use Peridex short term as it stains the oral mucosa. Use any non-alcoholic mouth rinse in all medically compromised patients to minimize alcohol related xerostomia.

HIV-PERIODONTITIS (HIV-P)

HIV-periodontitis is specific for HIV/AIDS. The HIV-P lesions are severely destructive. They are characterized by soft tissue ulceration and necrosis. There is rapid progressive loss of bone and periodontal attachment.

HIV-P is frequently associated with deep pain and spontaneous bleeding. The tissue loss, which is so rapid, may occur within a period of 4 weeks. Without treatment, HIV-periodontitis may progress to necrotizing stomatitis.

HIV-P Treatment

Treatment is as follows:

1. Initial debridement with 10% betadine irrigation should be done. In cases of severe necrosis, pain, and fever, antibiotics and analgesics may become necessary.
2. 0.12% chlorhexidine gluconate (Peridex) home rinses should be prescribed. Intensive oral hygiene instructions should be provided and the patient must be reevaluated in 1 week.
3. Follow-up should consist of scaling and root planing by quadrants, using 10% betadine irrigation, and the Peridex home rinses, as prescribed above, should be continued.
4. Oral hygiene instructions should be reenforced. There should be careful follow-up and maintenance.
5. The patient should be recalled every 4 weeks till stable. Thereafter, 3-month recalls should be scheduled.

HIV-Periodontitis Recommended Antibiotic Therapy

1. **First Drug of Choice:**
   Rx: Metronidazole (Flagyl) 250 mg/tablet
   Disp: 20 tabs for 5 days
   Sig: 1 tab qid until gone
   Metronidazole, a Category B drug is safe during pregnancy.
2. **Alternate Antibiotic Choices:** Dispense any one of the following anaerobic complex organism effective antibiotics if metronidazole is contraindicated due to liver disease or alcoholism. All the antibiotics listed below with the exception of Cipro (Category B/C), are Category B drugs and safe for use during pregnancy.
   2a. **Clindamycin:** 150/300 mg qid × 5 days
   2b. **Cephalexin (Keflex):** 250/500mg bid/tid × 5 days
   2c. **Amoxicillin with Clavulanate potassium (Augmentin):** 250/500 mg tid × 5 days
   2d. **Ciproflaxim (Cipro):** 500 mg bid × 5 days, in refractory cases

It is best to use the lower dose of the antibiotics to prevent candida-associated superinfection.

HIV-NECROTIZING STOMATITIS

HIV-necrotizing stomatitis is specific for HIV/AIDS. It is an acute, localized, painful, necrotizing, ulcerated lesion of the oral mucosa. It results in exposure of the underlying bone. The lesion may extend into contiguous tissues. The margins are undermined and sharply defined.

The exact etiology cannot be identified even by biopsy. Without treatment, HIV-G may progress from a mild gingivitis to a destructive periodontitis, and this progression may take place within weeks.

HIV-Necrotizing Stomatitis Treatment

Treatment of necrotizing stomatitis is essentially the same as that recommended for HIV-periodontitis. Initial debridement should be done with 10% betadine irrigation. Antibiotics are necessary in cases of severe necrosis, pain, and fever. Antibiotic suggestions are the same as with HIV-periodontitis. 0.12% chlorhexidine gluconate (Peridex) home rinses should be prescribed. Intensive oral hygiene home instructions should be provided. The patient must be reevaluated 1 week later.

This should then be followed by scaling and root planing by quadrant using 10% Betadine irrigation. Continue Peridex home rinses after the scaling and root planing and reinforce oral hygiene instructions. Also reenforce careful follow-up and maintenance. Recall the patient every 4 weeks until stable and then schedule 3-month recalls.

ORAL AND ESOPHAGEAL CANDIDIASIS

Oral candidiasis can occur in either the immune-competent or the immune-compromised patient. Long-term or high-dose antibiotic use, chronic corticosteroid therapy, xerostomia anemia, stress, and ill-fitting dentures are some of the causes for candidiasis in the immune-competent patient. The underlying cause must always be addressed and treated to completely eradicate the fungus, along with antifungal prescriptions for local or systemic use.

In either population oral candidiasis can present as pseudomembranous candidiasis or as hypertrophic or erythematous candidiasis. Oral candidiasis can extend down toward the esophagus causing the patient to experience dysphagia (difficulty swallowing) and/or odynophagia (painful swallowing).

All fungal infections must be treated for 14 days and significant esophageal candidiasis is treated for at least 21 days. In addition to the antifungal prescription, the dentist must also prescribe an antifungal soaking solution, for all removable oral appliances that must be soaked daily, for 14 days to completely eradicate the fungus.

The suggested guidelines for treatment of pseudomembranous candidiasis or hypertrophic or erythematous candidiasis are all the same: antifungals plus chlorhexidine mouth rinse. Always start with topical antifungals and avoid the azole antifungals in HIV/AIDS patients taking protease inhibitors. Use systemic antifungals in refractory cases or in patients with systemic fungal infections.

Dispense chlorhexidine or nonalcoholic mouth rinses for use after oral hygiene for all types of candidiasis:

Rx: Chlorhexidine (Peridex)
Disp: 3×16 oz bottles
Sig: Rinse with half-oz for 30 sec twice/day after oral hygiene.

ANTIFUNGAL DRUGS

Antifungal Drugs Classification

Refer to Chapter 7, "Antifungals Commonly Used in Dentistry: Assessment, Analysis, and Associated Dental Management Guidelines," for a complete discussion on antifungal classification and facts.

CLOTRIMAZOLE (MYCELEX) TROCHES

Clotrimazole (Mycelex) Troches Facts

Clotrimazole is more popular because it is very convenient to use, but it is costly. It looks more like a peppermint candy and less like a medication so the patient compliance rate is higher. The troches contain sucrose so the risk of caries exists if the drug is used for more than 3 months. Do not prescribe Clotrimazole troches if the HIV patient is on protease inhibitors or there is significant xerostomia.

Clotrimazole Prescription

Rx: Clotrimazole (Mycelex) Troches, 10 mg/troche
Disp: 70 troches (14-day supply)
Sig: Dissolve 1 troche in the mouth 5 times daily and *swallow the saliva.* There should be **no** eating or drinking for 30 min after use.

NYSTATIN (MYCOSTATIN)

Nystatin (Mycostatin) Overview

Nystatin (Mycostatin) is available as a lozenge, pastille, cream, or oral suspension. The nystatin oral suspension contains alcohol and sucrose. In patients with removable appliances, the suspension should be dispensed, along with the oral antifungal agent, for 14 days.

Oral nystatin suspension is the preferred antifungal preparation over Clotrimazole troches or nystatin lozenges for patients with xerostomia. Lack of saliva makes it difficult for the patient to suck on the troche or lozenge. Nystatin is *the* topical agent for an HIV patient on protease inhibitors.

Nystatin (Mycostatin) Prescriptions

1. **Nystatin (Mycostatin) Lozenge**:
   Rx: Nystatin (Mycostatin) Lozenge 200,000 units/lozenge
   Disp: 70 lozenges (14-day supply)
   Sig: Dissolve 1 lozenge in the mouth 5 times daily.
   There should be **no** eating or drinking for 30 min after use.
2. **Nystatin Oral Suspension:**
   Rx: Nystatin Oral Suspension 100,000 units/mL
   Disp: 473 mL (1 pint) bottle (14-day supply)
   Sig: Use 1 tsp or 5 ml, qid.
   Rinse and hold in the mouth as long as possible before swallowing. There should be **no** eating or drinking for 30 min after use.
   Note: Nystatin oral suspension also comes in a 60 mL bottle.

3. **Nystatin Oral Suspension for Dentures:**
   Rx: Nystatin Oral Suspension 100,000 units/ml
   Disp: 473 mL (1 pint) bottle
   Sig: Add 5–10 mL of 1:100,000 units nystatin to half a cup of water and soak the dentures overnight daily, for 14 days. Rinse the dentures before use.
4. **Nystatin Pastille:**
   Rx: Nystatin Pastille 200,000 units/pastille
   Disp: 70 pastilles
   Sig: Dissolve 1 pastille in the mouth 4–5 times/day, for 14 days.
5. **Nystatin (Mycostatin) Cream:**
   The cream can be applied to dentures before insertion or can be used for angular cheilitis.
   Rx: Nystatin (Mycostatin) cream 100,000 units/g
   Disp: 15 or 30 g tube
   Sig: Apply to the affected area 4–5 times/day.
   Do **not** eat or drink for 30 min after use.

AMPHOTERICIN B

Amphotericin B Facts

Amphotericin B can be used in the pregnant patient because it is a category B drug. It can also be used in HIV patients on protease inhibitors. It is minimally absorbed and relatively nontoxic.

Amphotericin B Prescriptions

1. **Topical Amphotericin B:**
   Rx: 3% Topical Amphotericin B Cream
   Disp: 20 g tube
   Sig: Apply to the affected area 3–4 times/day, for 2–4 weeks.
2. **Oral Amphotericin B:**
   Oral Amphotericin B is dispensed as a capsule or a suspension. The oral forms are poorly absorbed.
   2a. **Rx: Amphotericin B 500 mg/capsule**
      Disp: 56 capsules
      Sig: Take 500 mg capsule PO qid for 2 weeks.
   2b. **Rx: Amphotericin B suspension: 500 mg/mL**
      Disp: 56 mL suspension
      Sig: Use 1 mL of the suspension, swish and swallow qid for 2 weeks.

FLUCONAZOLE (DIFLUCAN)

Fluconazole (Diflucan) Facts

Fluconazole (Diflucan) is prescribed if the patient fails to respond to topical antifungal treatments, and it is also prescribed for esophageal candidiasis. Diflucan is the drug of choice for systemic antifungal treatment. Diflucan is a Category **C** drug. It should be avoided in the pregnant patient and Amphotericin B should be prescribed instead.

Fluconazole (Diflucan) Prescriptions

1. **Treatment for Refractory Oral or Systemic candidiasis:**
   Rx: Fluconazole (Diflucan) 100 mg/capsule
   Disp: 15 capsules
   Sig: Day 1: Take 2 capsules. **Days 2–14:** Take 1 capsule daily.
2. **Fluconazole (Diflucan) Treatment for Esophageal Candidiasis:**
   Rx: Fluconazole (Diflucan) 100 mg/capsule
   Disp: Variable
   Sig: 100 mg qid (maximum 400 mg qid) for 14–21 days

ANGULAR CHEILITIS

Angular Cheilitis Facts

Angular cheilitis can occur in the immune-competent or the immune-compromised patient. The common etiological factors are stress, flu, ill-fitting dentures, malnutrition, and anemia. The underlying cause must be simultaneously eradicated while treating the angular cheilitis with topical creams.

Candidiasis is a frequent superinfection of angular cheilitis and the candidiasis must also be treated with appropriate antifungal therapy. Clotrimazole (Mycelex) or nystatin (Mycolog) creams are more commonly dispensed for angular cheilitis. Clioquinol-hydrocortisone (HC) (Vioform-HC) cream is reserved for the refractory or very severe cases experiencing profound cracking and pain.

Angular Cheilitis Prescriptions

1. **Clotrimazole (Mycelex) Cream:**
   Rx: Clotrimazole (Mycelex) cream
   Disp: 15 g tube
   Sig: Rub into the affected area 2–3 times daily for 2 weeks.
2. **Nystatin (Mycolog) Cream:**
   Rx: Nystatin (Mycolog) Cream
   Disp: 15 g tube
   Sig: Rub into the affected area 2–3 times daily.
3. **Clioquinol-Hydrocortisone (HC) (Vioform-HC) Cream:**
   Rx: Clioquinol-Hydrocortisone (HC) (Vioform-HC) Cream
   Disp: 15 g tube
   Sig: Rub into affected area 2–3 times daily.

ORAL KAPOSI'S SARCOMA (KS)

Oral Kaposi's sarcoma is specific for HIV/AIDS. Kaposi's sarcoma in the oral cavity presents as a brown, red, blue, or purple macule, papule, or nodule. Kaposi's sarcoma has a predilection for the hard palate and the attached gingiva, but KS can appear on other mucosal sites as well. Patients with AIDS-associated Kaposi's sarcoma usually die not because of the sarcoma but as a result of an opportunistic infection. Many asymptomatic patients do not require treatment. Treatment modalities include surgery, radiation, and chemotherapy.

ORAL WARTS

Oral warts are specific for HIV/AIDS. They are papillary outgrowths of the oral mucosa and are caused by the papilloma virus. The diagnosis is confirmed by routine histo-pathologic analysis. Oral warts tend to be troublesome and frequently recur after removal.

Treatment for oral warts usually consists of simple surgical excision. This form of treatment is used alone or in conjunction with cryotherapy.

RECURRENT APHTHOUS ULCERS (RAU)

Aphthous ulcers frequently affect young adults and their occurrence can also be familial. The exact etiology is not known but stress, localized trauma, food allergy, or infection (HSV or Helicobacter pylori) are frequently implicated as etiological factors. Patients with aphthous ulcers may have associated cell-mediated immunity problems along with systemic B and T cell–mediated immunity concerns.

Aphthous Ulcer Classification

Aphthous ulcers can be classified into three categories:

1. Minor aphthous ulcers
2. Major aphthous ulcers
3. Herpetiform aphthous ulcers

Minor Aphthous Ulcerations

Minor ulcers are benign aphthae. They tend to be small, shallow, single, or multiple lesions. They are highly recurrent, well-circumscribed, painful lesions, occur on nonkeratinized tissue, and measure 0.2–0.5 cm in diameter. They are usually located on labial or buccal mucosa, the soft palate, or floor of the mouth. Minor ulcers have no systemic symptoms and signs.

Major Aphthous Ulcerations

Major Aphthous Ulcerations Overview

The major aphthous ulcers measure more than 0.5 cm in diameter and are extremely painful and recurrent. They are larger and deeper ulcerations that tend to scar on healing and are serious aphthae. These ulcers are associated with systemic symptoms and signs: uveitis, conjunctivitis, arthritis, genital ulcerations, fever, or adenopathy.

Major Aphthae Etiological Factors

Major aphthae can be due to infections, autoimmune conditions, or hematological causes:

1. **Infections:** Human immunodeficiency virus (HIV) infection, herpes, CMV, bacteria, fungus (cryptosporidium, mucormycosis, histoplasma), and syphilis can be associated with major aphthae.
2. **Autoimmune conditions:** lupus erythematosus, Behçet's syndrome, Reiter's syndrome, bullous pemphigoid, Pemphigus vulgaris, and Crohn's disease patients often suffer from major aphthae.

    a. **Behçet's syndrome:** Behçet's syndrome is an autoimmune vasculitis that causes recurrent oral and genital ulcerations, uveitis, and retinitis.

    b. **Reiter's syndrome:** Reiter's syndrome is associated with oral ulcers, uveitis, conjunctivitis, and HLA B27-positive arthritis following nongonococcal urethritis or bacillary dysentery.

    c. **Crohn's disease:** These patients may present with associated oral ulcerations.

    d. **Lupus erythematosus, bullous pemphigoid, and pemphigus vulgaris:** Always determine the associated symptoms to make a differentiation from benign recurrent aphthae.

3. **Hematological cause:** Patients with cyclic neutropenia can suffer from major aphthae. Cyclic neutropenia should be considered when the patient has oral ulcers with fever and this happens during the neutropenic period.

Herpetiform Ulcerations

The herpetiform ulcers are less than 0.2 cm in diameter and are also painful lesions. They tend to be more numerous in number and vesicular in nature.

Recurrent Aphthous Ulcerations Treatment Options and Prescriptions

Aphthous ulcers can be treated with any of the following medications:

1. Antibiotics
2. Antiinflammatory medications
3. Immune modulators
4. Topical anesthetics
5. Other Agents

Antibiotic Therapy Prescriptions

Tetracycline and minocycline antibiotics are used because infectious agents are postulated to be one of the causes for aphthous ulcers.

1. **Tetracycline Capsules:**
   Rx: Dissolve a 250 mg tetracycline capsule in 180 mL water.
   Sig: Swish and expectorate, qid for several days till ulcers heal.
       Reduction of pain and reduction of duration of ulcerations may result. Do not eat or drink for 30 min afterward.

2. **Tetracycline Suspension:**
   Rx: Dispense 250 mg tetracycline/5 ml
   Sig: Swish and expectorate, qid till ulcers heal.
       Do not eat or drink for 30 min afterward. Avoid in children and pregnant women.

Antiinflammatory Agents Prescriptions

Local Antiinflammatory Agents

Topical agents provide quick relief and can attenuate the duration of the ulcers.

    Triamcinolone 0.1% (Kenalog in Orabase) is a topical corticosteroid that should be used sparingly to gain temporary pain relief associated with oral ulcerations.

1. **Triamcinolone 0.1% (Kenalog in Orabase):**
   Rx: Triamcinolone 0.1% (Kenalog in Orabase):
   Disp: 5 g tube
   Sig: Apply a thin film, *without rubbing*, on affected areas up to 3 times daily until the ulcers heal.
2. **Flucinonide (Lidex):**
   Rx: 0.05% Lidex ointment mixed 50/50 with Orabase
   Disp: 30 g total
   Sig: Apply a thin layer on the lesions 4–6 times daily.
3. **Dexamethasone (Decadrone) Elixir:** Use dexamethasone (Decadron) elixir for severe ulcers as a rinse and expectorate. A secondary fungal infection could develop.
   Rx: Dexamethasone Elixir, 0.5 mg/5mL
   Disp: 250 ml
   Sig: Rinse with 1 tsp solution in the mouth for 1 min 4–5 times daily and *expectorate.*

Immune Modulators Prescription

Rx: Thalidomide (Thalomid) 200 mg OD/bid × 3–8 weeks

Thalidomide is a Category X drug and it is reserved for HIV-infected patients only.

Topical Anesthetics Prescription

Rx: Xylocaine 2% Viscous
Disp: 100 mL or 450 mL
Sig: Use 2 tsp to rinse the oral cavity, as needed to relieve pain, and *expectorate.*

Prescription of Other Agents for Recurrent Aphthous Ulcerations

1. **Diphenhydramine (Benadryl) Syrup (5 mg/mL) with Liquid Bismuth Subsalicylate (Kaopectate):**
   Rx: Diphenhydramine (Benadryl) syrup (5 mg/mL) with liquid bismuth subsalicylate (Kaopectate), mix 50/50
   Disp: 8 oz total
   Sig: Rinse with 2 tsp, as needed to relieve pain or burning, and *expectorate*.
   Expectoration will prevent constipation because Kaopectate is an antidiarrhea preparation. You may have to suggest the patient take Maalox if the patient swallows the mixture and constipation occurs.
2. **Diphenhydramine (Benadryl) Syrup (5 mg/mL) with Magnesium Hydroxide Antacid:**
   Rx: Diphenhydramine (Benadryl) syrup (5 mg/mL) with magnesium hydroxide antacid, mixed 50/50
   Sig: Rinse with 2 tsp, as needed to relieve pain or burning, and *expectorate.*

XEROSTOMIA (DRY MOUTH)

Xerostomia is a condition associated with decreased saliva production and an alteration in the saliva composition such that the saliva gets thickened and viscous. Xerostomia causes a reduction of the protective proteolytic enzymes and antibodies in the saliva, thus increasing the incidence of oral infections, candidiasis and caries.

Xerostomia is associated with impaired chewing, speech impairment, decreased taste sensation, halitosis, and an increased incidence of oral infections.

Xerostomia Etiology

Xerostomia can be caused by:

1. **Medications:** Medications with anticholinergic effects: antipsychotics, antidepressants, antiretroviral drugs, sedatives, hypnotics, antihistamines, anticonvulsants, and muscle relaxants can cause xerostomia.
2. **Age:** Xerostomia is more common in the elderly.
3. **Sjögren's syndrome:** Sjögren's syndrome is an autoimmune condition that is associated with lymphocytic infiltration of the salivary glands. It is more common in women than in men.

   Primary Sjögren's syndrome is associated with xerostomia and keratoconjunctivitis. Secondary Sjögren's syndrome is associated with systemic lupus erythematosus, scleroderma, and other connective tissue disorders.

   Presence of Anti-Ro/SSA or Anti-La/SSB on blood tests are very suggestive of Sjögren's syndrome.
4. **Diabetes:** Uncontrolled diabetes is often associated with xerostomia.
5. **Head and Neck Radiation Therapy:** The amount of salivary gland destruction depends on the amount of radiation dose given during radiation therapy. The destruction is often permanent with higher doses, but with lower doses the glands may bounce back in 6–12 months. Doses greater than 30 Gy can cause permanent damage of the salivary glands.

Xerostomia Manifestations

Xerostomia can be associated with dental caries, erythematous oral mucosa, oral and/or esophageal candidiasis, angular cheilitis, mucositis, and oral ulcerations.

Xerostomia Treatment Options

Treatment options for xerostomia are

1. Daily, good oral hygiene.
2. Frequent dental care and hygiene recall every 3–6 months.
3. Nonalcoholic chlorhexidine or any other nonalcoholic mouth rinse to assist with the care of gingivitis and plaque formation.
4. **Saliva substitutes:** The use of saliva substitutes Biotene products, Salivart, or Xerolube is highly advocated.
5. **Saliva stimulants:** Pilocarpine, a saliva stimulant, is reserved for refractory cases.
6. **Topical fluorides:** Applying regularly along with 0.05% fluoride rinse is highly recommended. Patients with severe xerostomia should get 1.23% acidulated phosphate fluoride gel for 4 min, 4 times per year.

Saliva Substitutes Detailed Discussion

Common saliva substitutes are

1. **Water:** Water intake should be frequent throughout the day.
2. **Milk:** Milk buffers oral acids and provides calcium and phosphate.
3. **Biotene® and Oralbalance®:** These products contain three enzyme systems and a protein, similar to those found in natural saliva. These enzyme systems penetrate the plaque-forming bacterial cell walls and thus maintain a healthy oral flora. The combined use of Biotene and Oralbalance has been found to be very effective in the management of xerostomia. Oralbalance is available as a moisturizing gel. Biotene is available as a sugar-free gum, alcohol-free mouthwash, and toothpaste:
   a. **Biotene mouthwash:** Use 1 Tbsp PRN, swish, and expectorate. It works best when used with Biotene toothpaste.
   b. **Biotene toothpaste:** The toothpaste is nonirritating and it contains the protective enzyme systems needed for optimal oral health. The toothpaste should be used postmeals and at bedtime.

Saliva Stimulants Detailed Discussion

Parasympathetic nervous system stimulation causes salivary secretion and this can be achieved by the simple process of chewing or sucking on sugar-free candy and with the use of pilocarpine HCL (Salagen).

Pilocarpine HCL (Salagen) Overview

Pilocarpine increases saliva secretion by systemic cholinergic stimulation. Pilocarpine's effectiveness relies on the presence of intact salivary gland tissue and nerve supply. In the case of the irradiated patient, it would be the intact tissue outside the area of radiation.

Pilocarpine HCL should be reserved for radiation, drug-induced or Sjögren's syndrome–associated xerostomia.

Increased frequency of cardiovascular and pulmonary side effects contraindicates the use of pilocarpine HCL (Salagen) in patients with moderate to severe asthma, COPD, and cardiac arrythmias. It is also contraindicated in patients with a history of renal stones and gallstones and narrow angle glaucoma.

Pilocarpine HCL Side Effects

Common side effects experienced are perspiration (earliest side effect), nausea, dizziness, lacrimation, headaches, tachycardia, tremors, dysphagia, and heartburn.

Pilocarpine HCL (Salagen) Prescription

Rx: Salagen, 5 mg/tablet
Disp: Variable
Sig: 1–2 tablets tid/qid per day *taken 30 min prior to meals.*

The patient should be treated for a minimum of 90 days for optimal effect. Pilocarpine effect begins in 15 min and lasts for 2–3 hr. The patient should drink 2 L of water daily when taking pilocarpine HCL.

XVI

The Female Patient: Pregnancy, Lactation, and Contraception

49

Pregnancy and Lactation: Assessment and Associated Dental Management Guidelines

PREGNANCY, LACTATION, AND CONTRACEPTION GENERAL OVERVIEW

Many providers in the past were hesitant about providing care during pregnancy out of fear for the safety of the fetus and the mother and the uncertainty of the safety of local anesthetics, analgesics, and antibiotics. We now know that pregnancy does not contraindicate dentistry and dentistry can occur throughout the pregnancy, give or take a few weeks.

A knowledgeable provider today is a more confident provider. The goal of this section is to provide you with the knowledge of the current concepts associated with pregnancy, lactation, and contraception so you can proceed with confidence in the dental setting.

Pregnancy Overview

In order to know how and when to proceed with dentistry one needs to understand the symptoms, signs, and tests associated with pregnancy. The practitioner should be aware of the medications that can and cannot be used during pregnancy as well as facts regarding radiation exposure during pregnancy.

Pregnancy and Trimesters

The 40 weeks of pregnancy are divided into 3 trimesters:

The First Trimester: from 1–14 weeks
The Second Trimester: from 14–28 weeks
The Third Trimester: from 28–40 weeks

Pregnant Patient Assessment During Initial Dental Visit

During the pregnant patient's first dental visit, determine the stage of her pregnancy. Determine whether she is experiencing any pregnancy-associated symptoms, as discussed below, that need to be accommodated.

Assess whether she is presenting with acute dental problems or is in for routine dental care. All emergency and routine care can continue during pregnancy.

You must make provisions for, and confirm, her comfort in the dental chair through the duration of the dental appointment.

Pregnancy-Associated Symptoms and Signs

The early symptoms and signs of pregnancy are described in the following sections.

Amenorrhea

Conception occurs 14 days after the first day of the previous menstrual cycle. A patient having regular menstrual periods will know when her cycle is delayed and whether she is pregnant. It is always important to ask your patient if she could be pregnant and when was the last menstrual period (LMP).

Nausea and Vomiting

"Morning sickness" can occur at any time of the day; it does not have to be in the morning only! It lasts for a few days or weeks and it is best **not** to schedule dentistry during this period of discomfort.

Urinary frequency

Urinary frequency exists throughout the pregnancy and the patient may need to excuse herself during dental treatment.

Fatigue

The patient complains of fatigue in the first and third trimester more commonly. It is better to schedule shorter appointments to prevent further exhaustion.

Pregnancy Tests

Tests confirming pregnancy are:

1. **Urine Pregnancy Test:** This test detects the monoclonal antibodies in the urine and it becomes positive 2 weeks after conception, which is just around the time of the missed menstrual period.
2. **The Serum Pregnancy Test:** This test detects β-HCG; the test becomes positive 9 days after conception.

PREGNANCY-ASSOCIATED CHANGES

Pregnancy-associated changes experienced by the mother are generalized and knowing what areas are affected will help you better manage your patient. The changes that occur are dietary, cardiovascular, gastrointestinal, and oral cavity changes.

Dietary Changes

The daily caloric, protein, and folic acid requirements increase, and lack of folic acid can lead to spina bifida in the fetus. The patient gains about 25–35 lb throughout the pregnancy.

Cardiovascular Changes

Several cardiovascular changes occur as the pregnancy advances, as described in the following sections.

Pulse

The pulse rate increases by 10–15 beats/min during pregnancy. Having knowledge of the baseline pulse rate **prior** to pregnancy always helps to calculate the actual change in pulse rate for the patient.

It is always advisable to **decrease** the amount of **epinephrine** in the local anesthetic or to avoid epinephrine in a patient visibly affected with tachycardia.

Cardiac Output

The cardiac output increases by 40% in the first trimester and this causes increased vascularity in all areas of the body, including the gum tissue.

Cardiac output changes cause blood pressure changes in the mother. It is always important to monitor the blood pressure throughout the pregnancy.

A diagnosis of hypertension is made when the current BP shows changes compared to the prepregnancy BP or the BP prior to 20 weeks of pregnancy.

An increase in the systolic BP by 30 mmHg and/or the diastolic BP by 15 mmHg spells hypertension. Any BP reading >140/90 mmHg, if previous readings are unknown, also indicates hypertension.

It is important to remember that the blood pressure usually decreases in the second trimester because of vasodilatation. You need to stop all dental treatment and refer the patient to the obstetrician immediately **if the second trimester BP shows no change or an increase** when compared to the first trimester BP readings. The obstetrician needs to evaluate and treat this patient for pregnancy-associated hypertension before you can continue with dentistry.

Supine Hypotension

Supine hypotension usually occurs in the third trimester due to compression of the inferior vena cava by the gravid uterus.

Supine hypotension must be prevented in the dental chair because it can cause the patient to pass out. When she passes out, the uterine blood flow gets affected and this causes the baby's heart rate to decrease.

The best preventive treatment for supine hypotension is to turn the patient, preferably to the left side, to displace the uterus away from the inferior vena cava. The patient can also be placed in a sitting position with the knees flexed.

Gastrointestinal Changes

The gums can become hyperemic and bleed during pregnancy. It is advisable to stress good daily oral hygiene and schedule hygiene appointments at shorter intervals. The gastric emptying is delayed and this accounts for the increased risk of aspiration during general anesthesia, which is contraindicated in the dental setting.

Oral Cavity Changes

Pregnancy-related oral cavity changes seen are pregnancy gingivitis, pregnancy tumor, and periodontal disease.

Pregnancy Gingivitis

There is an increased incidence of inflammation, erythema, edema, and hypertrophy of the gums with pregnancy gingivitis.

Pregnancy-associated hormonal changes cause a shift in the bacterial flora and increased bacterial growth at the gumline. The gums swell, bleed easily, and become sensitive.

The process begins around the second month of pregnancy and peaks in the middle of the third trimester. Pregnancy gingivitis, however, usually disappears postpartum.

The dentist may need to implement scaling and root planing to correct or improve the gingivitis and prevent plaque growth.

Pregnancy gingivitis can cause premature birth and low birth weight. The bacteria from the pregnancy gingivitis–associated plaque enter the bloodstream and stimulate the patient's immune system to produce prostaglandins. Prostaglandins in turn can trigger uterine contraction leading to early labor, premature birth, and a small-sized baby. Thus, meticulous oral hygiene can prevent and minimize the symptoms experienced by the patient and prevent premature birth.

Pregnancy Tumor

The pregnancy tumor or "pyogenic granuloma" is a pedunculated outgrowth from the palatal surface of the gingiva and is usually found between the teeth. It is an inflammatory immune system response to an irritant and in this case it is the plaque that acts as an irritant. Pregnancy tumors occur in 3–5% of all pregnancies but they disappear after birth.

The pregnancy tumor appears as a soft, gray tissue mass with a red border. Surgical excision after birth is the treatment of choice, but it can recur.

Periodontal Disease

Increased incidence of periodontal disease during pregnancy is associated with adverse pregnancy outcomes: preterm birth, low birth weight, miscarriage, or preeclampsia because of increased inflammation and infection in the mother's oral cavity. This causes interference with placental and fetal development triggering uterine contractions leading to prematurity, as discussed above. Emphasis on good daily oral health and appropriate dental treatment can prevent these negative outcomes.

TERATOGENIC DRUGS AND FDA DRUG CATEGORIES

Teratogenic Drugs Facts

Teratogens are drugs or factors that can cause permanent alteration in the formation or anchoring of the fetus. Organogenesis occurs during **weeks 3–10,** and it is best to **avoid** dental drugs and routine dentistry during these weeks.

The baby is completely formed at 35 weeks, and prior to this point the fetus is vulnerable to changes by adverse teratogenic drugs or factors.

Some of the **category B opioid** pain medications that are safe during pregnancy **become category C/D** toward the time of delivery and should not be used **closer to term**. These specific drugs are discussed later in this section.

To have a better understanding of what medications to use and what to avoid in the pregnant patient, one has to have a good understanding of the FDA drug categories and specific drug facts. Drugs that are category A or B are safe drugs to use during pregnancy.

FDA Drug Categories

The following are FDA drug categories:

Category A: Drugs in this category demonstrate no fetal risk and the safety of these drugs have been documented by controlled studies.

Category B: Animal studies have shown no risk with the drugs in this category, but there are no well-documented human studies to demonstrate safety of these drugs.

Category C: Animal studies have shown adverse effects; no controlled studies have been done in women and there are no studies available in animals or women to show safety with these drugs.

Category D: Drugs in this class have evidence of human risks, but benefits sometimes may outweigh the risks when the drug is needed.

Category X: There is definite demonstration of risks, and the risks far outweigh the benefits. These drugs should not be given to pregnant mothers.

DRUGS ABSOLUTELY AND RELATIVELY CONTRAINDICATED DURING PREGNANCY

Drugs Absolutely Contraindicated During Pregnancy

The following are drugs that are absolutely contraindicated:

- **Accutane:** Accutane is associated with severe congenital abnormalities.
- **Amiodarone:** Amiodarone is an antiarrythmia drug.
- **Angiotensin-converting enzyme (ACE) inhibitors**
- **Ciprofloxacin (Cipro):** Cipro affects fetal kidneys and it should be avoided completely during pregnancy.
- **Live attenuated vaccines:** Included are Varicella and MMR.
- **Methotrexate:** Methotrexate is associated with a high rate of miscarriage.
- **Oral hypoglycemic drugs:** These drugs can cause hypoglycemia in the fetus.
- **Prostaglandins:** These drugs promote miscarriage.
- **Radioactive iodine:** Radiation exposure occurs.
- **Sumatriptan Succinate (Imitrex):** It is an antimigraine drug, vasoconstrictor in action, and it can cause growth restriction.
- **Tetracyclines:** These affect teeth and bone growth.
- **Warfarin (Coumadin):** Heparin is used instead if blood-thinning is required.

Drugs Relatively Contraindicated During Pregnancy

Aspirin and NSAIDS are contraindicated, particularly in the first trimester during the weeks of organogenesis because of the risk of miscarriage.

Aspirin and NSAIDS can promote placental bleeding. Avoid aspirin use for dental pain control in *all* dental patients because of the permanent dysfunction affect by aspirin on the platelets, which can potentiate bleeding.

Occasionally, you might need to prescribe NSAIDS for 2–3 days for moderate to severe dental inflammation, but do so only after consulting with the patient's obstetrician.

RADIATION AND PREGNANCY

The following are important facts to know about radiation:

- The unsafe radiation dose is >10 rads, but newer studies now indicate an unsafe level to be >5 rads.
- Estimated fetal exposure during dental series radiographs with lead shield is 0.00001 rad.
- Daily background radiation is 0.0004 rad.
- Chest x-ray exposure radiation dose is 0.008 rad.

Fetal Risks with Radiation Exposure

The following are fetal risks with radiation exposure:

1. **Embryonic death resulting in miscarriage:** This occurs if there is too much radiation exposure in the first trimester and especially in the first week of pregnancy.
2. **Congenital abnormalities:** Congenital abnormalities occur mostly during weeks 3–10 of the pregnancy, when organogenesis occurs.
3. **Intrauterine growth:** Intrauterine growth restriction occurs after the first trimester.
4. **Leukemia:** There is a slightly increased risk of childhood leukemia with fetal radiation exposure.

Antepartum Dental Radiography and Low Birth Weight Infant

Maternal exposure >0.4 mGy antepartum can be associated with low birth weight.

The full mouth x-ray radiation dose is 1.6 mGy and periapical x-ray radiation dose is 0.08 mGy.

GENERAL ANESTHESIA AND PREGNANCY

The general anesthetic can affect the fetus if it crosses over through the placental circulation. General anesthesia should not be given near the time of delivery because it will impair the infant's breathing. General anesthesia will also prolong the gastrointestinal transition time in the mother and thus increase the risk of aspiration.

Chronic N_2O exposure can be hazardous. This is more so for women working in the office than the pregnant patient herself. Women chronically exposed to N_2O have an increased rate of spontaneous abortions or give birth to infants with congenital abnormalities. Chronic N_2O exposure also accounts for the reduced rate of fertility among such women.

SUGGESTED PRINCIPLES OF PREGNANT PATIENT CARE DURING DENTISTRY

Follow these guidelines:

1. Always have the patient sign a case note in the dental record giving consent to dentistry before you start the dental treatment.
2. Dental treatment can be conducted throughout pregnancy with the exception of the following periods:
    a. Organogenesis or fetal organ formation occurs in weeks 3–10, and the highest risk to the fetus is during these weeks. Consequently, all potentially harmful drugs should be avoided during the organogenesis weeks; this is also true for drugs used for dentistry.

b. Avoid treatment during the weeks of morning sickness in the first trimester for obvious reasons.

3. The safest and most comfortable time for dentistry during pregnancy is the last 2–3 weeks of the first trimester, the entire second trimester, and the first half of the third trimester.

4. Give the patient a left lateral position during dental treatment in the latter half of the third trimester. Dentistry is not contraindicated in the latter half of the third trimester, but it may just be uncomfortable for the patient. The lateral position displaces the gravid uterus and prevents putting pressure on the inferior vena cava.

5. Provide dental treatment only if the patient is comfortable going through it.

6. Do not use O_2+N_2O, because N_2O has teratogenic effects.

7. Restrict the taking of excessive radiographs during pregnancy, and take only those that are needed. If absolutely needed, a full-mouth radiographic survey can be done as long as you protect the patient with a full body and thyroid lead shield. The full mouth survey radiation dose is 1.6 mGy.

8. All essential dental treatment can continue during pregnancy. This includes routine extractions, periodontal treatment, restorations, continuation of orthodontic treatment, and placement of removable and fixed prosthodontics and crowns.

9. In general during dentistry, use a minimum amount of epinephrine and minimum number of carpules of the local anesthetic.

Dentistry and Semesters Approach

Follow these guidelines:

1. **During the First Trimester:** Evaluate the dentition and perform ongoing and maintenance dentistry.

2. **During the Second Trimester:** Perform any routine or major procedures necessary because this is the best time to treat the pregnant patient.

3. **During the Third Trimester:** Continue established maintenance programs and perform only major required procedures.

Suggested Anesthetics, Analgesics, Antibiotics (AAAs) Guidelines During Pregnancy (Table 49.1)

Safe Local Anesthetics

The following are safe category B local anesthetics used during pregnancy:

1. 2% lidocaine (Xylocaine) with 1:100,000 epinephrine
2. 4% prilocaine HCL with 1:200,000 epinephrine (Citanest Forte)
3. 4% prilocaine HCL without epinephrine (Citanest Plain)
   a. It is best to use local anesthetics with less or no epinephrine, particularly in the presence of an increased pulse rate during the pregnancy.
   b. With any one of the anesthetics, use a maximum of 2 carpules only.
   c. Avoid epinephrine completely when treating a mild to moderate hypertensive pregnant patient. Use 4% prilocaine HCL without epinephrine (Citanest Plain) after obtaining a clearance for dentistry from the patient's obstetrician.

Unsafe Local Anesthetics

The following are category C local anesthetics contraindicated during pregnancy:

Table 49.1. Suggested safe anesthetics, analgesics, and antibiotics during pregnancy

Safe Medications	Precautions/Remarks
LOCAL ANESTHETICS	
1. 2% Lidocaine (Xylocaine), 1:100,000 epinephrine 2. 4% Prilocaine HCL with 1:200,000 epinephrine (Citanest Forte) 3. 4% Prilocaine HCL without epinephrine (Citanest Plain)	It is best to use local anesthetics with less or no epinephrine in the presence of tachycardia. Use a maximum of 2 carpules. Avoid epinephrine in presence of mild to moderate hypertension. Use 4% Prilocaine HCL without epinephrine (Citanest Plain) after obtaining a **clearance** for dentistry from the patient's obstetrician.
ANALGESICS	
1. Acetaminophen (Tylenol) 2. Codeine + Tylenol 3. Hydrocodone + Tylenol (Vicodin) 4. Oxycodone + Tylenol (Percocet)	Percocet and Vicodin are category B drugs that are safe when used **short-term** and in **smaller doses.** Avoid Vicodin and Percocet just prior (2–4 weeks) to delivery to prevent breathing problems in the newborn. Avoid aspirin and NSAIDS.
ANTIBIOTICS	
Use standard dose of 1. All Penicillins 2. All Cephalosporins 3. Erythromycin (not used now) 4. Azithromycin (Zithromax) 5. Clindamycin (Cleocin)	Use Pen VK to treat acute oral infections (symptomatic for less than 3 days). Use Clindamycin with Penicillin or if the infection has been symptomatic for more than 3 days. Avoid Clarithromycin (Biaxin) and Tetracyclines.

1. 0.5% bupivacaine (Marcaine)
2. 4% septocaine (Articaine) with 1:100,000 or 1:200,000 epinephrine
3. 2% mepivacaine (Carbocaine) with 1:20,000 levonordefrin (NeoCobefrin)
4. 3% mepivacaine HCL (Carbocaine)

Safe Analgesics During Pregnancy

The following are safe analgesics:

1. Acetaminophen (Tylenol)
2. Codeine + Tylenol
3. Hydrocodone + Tylenol (Vicodin)
4. Oxycodone + Tylenol (Percocet)

Percocet and Vicodin are category B drugs that are safe when used short-term and in smaller doses.

Unsafe Analgesics

Analgesics contraindicated during pregnancy are

1. Aspirin
2. NSAIDS
3. Long-term or high-dose Percocet or Vicodin at term

Long-term or high-dose Percocet or Vicodin at Term are category B drugs, but when they are used for a prolonged period at term or in high doses they can become category D drugs causing breathing difficulty and even death in the newborn.

To be conservative, avoid opioid analgesics Vicodin and Percocet just prior to delivery (2–4 weeks prior) to prevent breathing problems in the newborn.

Safe Antibiotics During Pregnancy

The following are safe antibiotics:

1. All penicillins
2. All cephalosporins
3. Erythromycin (not used any more in dentistry)
4. Azithromycin (Zithromax)
5. Clindamycin (Cleocin)

Category C/D Antibiotics Contraindicated During Pregnancy

The following are contraindicated:

1. Clarithromycin (Biaxin)
2. Tetracycline HCL
3. Doxycycline (Vibramycin)

Potentially Toxic Antibiotics to Avoid During Pregnancy

The following are potentially toxic antibiotics to avoid during pregnancy:

1. **Sulfa antimicrobials:** They cause hyperbilirubinemia and kernicterus.
2. **Tetracyclines:** Tetracyclines are associated with discoloration of teeth and they affect growing bones.
3. **Nitrofurantoin:** It can cause hemolytic anemia in an infant with G6PD deficiency.

LACTATION/BREAST-FEEDING

The following sections itemize the anesthetics, analgesics, and antibiotics to use in the lactating patient **after** breast-feeding.

Safe Local Anesthetics During Lactation (Table 49.2)

The following local anesthetics are safe during lactation:

1. 2% lidocaine with 1:100,000 epinephrine (Xylocaine)
2. 0.5% bupivacaine with 1:200,000 epinephrine (Marcaine)
3. 4% septocaine with 1:100,000 or 1:200,000 epinephrine (Articaine)
4. 4% prilocaine HCL with 1:200,000 epinephrine or without epinephrine (Citanest Forte/Citanest Plain)
5. 2% mepivacaine (Carbocaine) with 1:20,000 levonordefrin
6. 3% mepivacaine (Carbocaine)

In a hypertensive lactating patient with Stage I hypertension use a local anesthetic with 1:200,000 epinephrine, and avoid epinephrine in the local anesthetic in the Stage II hypertension patient.

Table 49.2. Suggested anesthetics, analgesics, and antibiotics guidelines during lactation

Safe Medications	Precautions/Remarks
LOCAL ANESTHETICS	
1. 2% Lidocaine, 1:100,000 epinephrine (Xylocaine)	Inject the local anesthetic **after** the baby has been fed.
2. 0.5% Bupivacaine with 1:200,000 epinephrine (Marcaine)	For Stage I hypertensive lactating patient: Use a local anesthetic with 1:200,000 epinephrine.
3. 4% Septocaine with 1:100,000 or 1:200,000 epinephrine (Articaine)	Avoid epinephrine in the Stage II hypertension patient.
4. 4% Prilocaine HCL with 1:200,000 epinephrine or without epinephrine (Citanest Forte/Citanest Plain)	Defer routine dental treatment in a Stage III hypertensive lactating patient.
5. 3% Mepivacaine (Carbocaine)	
6. 2% Mepivacaine (Carbocaine) with 1:20,000 Levonordefrin (NeoCobefrin)	
ANALGESICS	
1. Acetaminophen (Tylenol)	The patient should take the pain medication **after** breast feeding and keep a **2 h** interval with the next feed.
2. Codeine + Tylenol (Tylenol #1–3)	
3. Hydrocodone + Tylenol (Vicodin)	
4. Oxycodone + Tylenol (Percocet)	Opioids pass through the breast milk. Use lower doses and prescribe opioids only when absolutely needed.
ANTIBIOTICS	
1. All Penicillins	The patient should take the antibiotic **after** breast feeding and keep a **2 h** interval with the next feed.
2. All Cephalosporins	
3. All Macrolides	
4. Clindamycin	Minimize antibiotic use because of the risk of altering the baby's intestinal flora and promoting the growth of resistant pathogens.

Safe Analgesics During Lactation (Table 49.2)

The following analgesics are safe during lactation:

1. Acetaminophen (Tylenol)
2. Codeine + Tylenol (Tylenol #1–3)
3. Hydrocodone + Tylenol (Vicodin)
4. Oxycodone + Tylenol (Percocet)

Opioids pass through the breast milk, accordingly use lower doses and prescribe opioids only when absolutely needed.

Safe Antibiotics During Lactation (Table 49.2)

The following antibiotics are safe during lactation:

1. All penicillins
2. All cephalosporins
3. All macrolides
4. Clindamycin

Unsafe Antibiotics During Lactation

The following antibiotic is unsafe during lactation: tetracycline HCL and doxycycline (Vibramycin).

ORAL AND SYSTEMIC CONTRACEPTIVES

To better understand how oral contraceptives are affected with dental treatment, it is important to review the mechanism of oral contraceptive action and the effect of oral antibiotics on oral contraceptive potency.

Oral Contraception Activation Mechanism

Oral contraceptives are absorbed into the bloodstream on ingestion and delivered to the liver. They are inactivated in the liver and delivered back to the gut where the intestinal bacteria reactivate the birth control pill, rendering it effective. If bacteria in the gut are insufficient to reactivate the pill, it remains inactive and is excreted without providing adequate contraceptive effect.

Oral Antibiotics and Oral Contraceptive Interaction

Oral contraceptives are rendered less effective when taken with **oral** antibiotics. You must warn your patient to use added external contraception when taking the oral contraceptives.

Systemic contraceptives etonogestrel implant (Implanon) or levonorgestrel implant (Norplant) are not affected with oral antibiotic use.

Contraceptive Facts and Suggested Precautions During Dentistry

Follow these precautions:

1. Always determine whether your patient is using oral or systemic contraceptives. As discussed above, concurrent use of oral antibiotics with oral contraceptives (OCs), decreases the potency of the OC. Ampicillin and tetracycline are the most implicated antibiotics, but in general, all antibiotics affect oral contraceptive potency.

   Always explain this adverse DDI causing decreased potency of OCs to the patient and note in the record that you have informed the patient. Let the patient know that she will have to take **extra** barrier precautions till the **end** of the **next** cycle to prevent pregnancy.

   As discussed above, parentally or systemically administered contraceptives' potency is not affected by OCs.
2. Levonorgestrel (Norplant) is an implanted systemic contraceptive that is effective for 5 years. Norplant production was stopped by the manufacturer in 2000 because the drug was not completely effective.
3. Etonogestrel (Implanon) is a new systemic contraceptive that just got FDA approval. Implanon is inserted under the skin of the upper arm and there is a continuous release of a low dose of etonogestral into the bloodstream. Implanon provides contraceptive protection for 3 years.
4. Implanon and Norplant are not affected by oral antibiotics; **however,** Norplant and Implanon contain progestin, which can predispose the patient to gingival bleeding during dentistry.

XVII

Rheumatology: Diseases of the Joints, Bones, and Muscles

Classic Rheumatic Diseases: Assessment of Disease States and Associated Dental Management Guidelines

RHEUMATOLOGY OVERVIEW, FACTS, AND DISEASE CLASSIFICATION

Rheumatic diseases are chronic conditions that cause significant morbidity and affect the patient's quality of life. The patient is often on immunosuppressants to control the underlying inflammation and improve the long-term outcome with the disease.

It is important to remember that immunosuppressants **decrease** inflammation but **increase** the incidence of infections. This increased incidence of infections, coupled with the poor oral hygiene and increased dental decay found in this population, stresses the importance of regular dental intervention for these patients.

Arthritis affecting the hands can also make it difficult for the patient to keep up with the routines of daily oral care. Extractions are often needed when the decay is extensive because the patient has neglected going to the dentist. Thus, the patient must incorporate regular dental visits as an important part of the multidisciplinary care to stay dentally healthy.

Classification of Joints, Bones, and Muscle Diseases

Rheumatology diseases are classified as the following:

A. **The classic "rheumatic diseases" that commonly affect the joints:** systemic lupus erythematosus (SLE), scleroderma, Sjögren's syndrome, Reiter's syndrome, Behçet's syndrome, temporal or giant cell arteritis, rheumatoid arthritis (RA), osteoarthritis, ankylosing spondilitis, diffuse idiopathic skeletal hyperostosis (DISH), or Forestier disease and gout
B. **Diseases affecting the bones:** Paget's disease
C. **Diseases affecting the muscles:** Malignant hyperthermia, polymyositis, Parkinson's disease, myasthenia gravis, and multiple sclerosis.

SYSTEMIC LUPUS ERYTHEMATOSUS (SLE)

Systemic Lupus Erythematosus (SLE) Overview

Systemic lupus erythematosus (SLE) is a chronic autoimmune condition associated with a hyperactive immune system that attacks normal tissue and the exact cause for this adverse action is unknown. Systemic lupus is a multisystem disease that can affect the skin, joints, blood, lungs, kidneys, heart, brain, and the nervous system.

SLE typically affects women in the child-bearing age and it is postulated that perhaps estrogen plays a role with this disease state. Antibody production is important for the diagnosis of SLE.

The 11 Criteria Associated with SLE

To make a diagnosis of SLE the patient must have at least 4 of the following 11 criteria present:

1. **Anemia:** Lupus-associated CBC will show leukopenia, lymphopenia, and thrombocytopenia.
2. **Arthritis:** SLE-associated arthritis affects the major and minor joints.
3. **Discoid rash:** Discoid lupus or cutaneous lupus affects the skin causing a discoid rash. The discoid lupus patient experiences increased photosensitivity.
4. **Increased photosensitivity:** The least amount of sun exposure causes blistering and sunburn with lupus.
5. **Neurological disorder:** SLE can be associated with seizures and/or psychosis.
6. **Oral ulcers:** Lupus-associated ulcers are rather nonspecific, shallow, and painless. Nasal ulcerations also can often coexist.
7. **Renal disease:** Lupus-associated renal disease is demonstrated by an elevated serum creatinine and BUN levels.
8. **Serositis:** SLE causes inflammation of the pericardial and pleural linings.
9. **The malar or the butterfly rash:** This lupus-associated rash occurs on the face, spanning over the nose and the cheeks but not going downward below the nasolabial fold.
10. **Positive ANA test:** The antinuclear antibody (ANA) test is a screening test for lupus. Active lupus is associated with high levels of antinuclear antibodies. The majority of patients with SLE have a positive ANA test at some point during their disease. The ANA test is not specific, however, for lupus. It can be positive in healthy people and in patients suffering from other connective tissue disorders.
11. **Other blood tests:** Other blood tests that can assist with the diagnosis of lupus are the LE test, the anti-ds DNA test, the anti-Sm test, the anti-Ro test, and the anti-La test.

The LE (lupus erythematosus) cell test is positive in only 50% of patients with SLE. In some cases the patient may be tested for specific ANA subtypes. Anti–double-stranded DNA (anti-ds DNA) is usually found only in SLE patients. Anti-Sm antibodies are also usually found only with SLE. When the ANA is negative and there is a strong suspicion for lupus, the anti-Ro and anti-La antibodies, when detected, can identify a rare form of lupus called *Ro lupus*.

Lupus Symptoms and Signs

No two patients with lupus will have similar symptoms. Symptoms will vary according to the organ systems affected. Additionally, these patients can have alopecia and may present with oral candidiasis due to the underlying xerostomia experienced by a majority of these patients.

Overwhelming infection and kidney failure are two of the common causes of death in people with lupus.

Lupus Treatment

The treatment is aimed at decreasing inflammation with NSAIDS, corticosteroids, and cytotoxic drugs.

Drug Precautions with Lupus

Patients with lupus are **often** allergic to multiple agents. Always go through the allergy history very carefully.

Drug history may show that the patient has responded adversely to sulpha antimicrobials and penicillin in the past. All drugs causing even a minimal form of allergy should be avoided.

SCLERODERMA

Scleroderma is an autoimmune condition associated with excessive fibrosis or scar tissue formation involving organs and the skin of the face and distal extremities. Scleroderma causes thickness and firmness of the affected areas. Vascular reactivity causing Raynaud's phenomenon is quite significant with scleroderma.

Auto-antibodies are useful in the diagnosis of the disease.

Forms of Scleroderma

There are two forms of the disease: diffuse scleroderma and limited scleroderma.

Diffuse Scleroderma

Diffuse scleroderma is the more severe form of scleroderma, which begins with thickening of the skin of the trunk and extremities. This rapidly progresses to fibrosis and involvement of vital organs. Heart, lungs, esophagus, and kidneys can be affected. Renal insufficiency occurs in >10% of patients. 40% of the patients have antiscleroderma-70 antibodies.

Limited Scleroderma/Limited Form (CREST)

This is the more benign form of scleroderma and it affects mainly the skin of the face and the digits. This form progresses slowly. CREST represents the clinical pattern associated with this form and it stands for calcinosis, Raynaud's phenomenon, esophageal involvement, slerodactyly, and telangiactasias.

There is less cardiac and pulmonary involvement with this form of scleroderma. 80% of the patients exhibit anticentromeric antibodies.

Scleroderma Clinical Features

The scleroderma patient can present with the following:

1. **Microstomia:** Microstomia is a classic oral manifestation of scleroderma.
2. **Retracted skin of the face and hands:** The skin on the face is retracted, the lips are pursed, and the skin is tightly bound around the digits. This can cause a "mouse face" appearance in the late stages.
3. **Swollen hands:** Swollen hands are caused by diffuse edema.
4. **Raynaud's Phenomenon:** Raynaud's Phenomenon causes the patient to experience white painful fingers and toes.

5. **Arthritis:** Scleroderma-associated arthritis affects the major and the minor joints.
6. **Dysphagia or regurgitation:** Smooth muscle dysfunction involving the lower two-thirds of the esophagus occurs causing dysphagia or regurgitation. The patient can swallow but cannot get the food down.
7. **Pulmonary fibrosis:** Pulmonary fibrosis is progressive and is associated with significant breathing difficulty as the condition worsens.
8. **Myocardial fibrosis:** Myocardial fibrosis causes arrhythmia, which indicates poor prognosis.
9. **Kidney disease:** Renal involvement also indicates poor prognosis.

Scleroderma Diagnosis

The diagnosis of scleroderma is based on the presence of the clinical features of the disease and specific blood tests. Most scleroderma patients are antinuclear antibody (ANA)–positive.

The CREST or the limited form is exclusively positive for the anticentromere antibody. The Anti-Scl 70 antibody (anti–topo-isomerase I antibody) is positive in most cases of the diffuse form of scleroderma.

Scleroderma Treatment

Treatment is directed toward the organs affected. Special emphasis is placed on monitoring and control of the blood pressure (BP) to slow the progression of the associated kidney disease.

SJÖGREN'S SYNDROME

Sjögren's syndrome is an autoimmune condition where autoimmune cells destroy the salivary and tear glands causing decreased saliva and tear production.

Sjögren's syndrome also causes dryness of the skin, nose, and other mucus membranes. Sjögren's syndrome may affect the kidneys, blood vessels, lungs, liver, pancreas, and brain.

The dentist must pay close attention to any abnormal lymph gland swelling in the head and neck region of a Sjögren's syndrome patient because this may be a sign of lymphoma.

Sjögren's Syndrome Classification

Sjögren's syndrome is classified as follows:

1. Primary Sjögren's syndrome
2. Secondary Sjögren's syndrome

The secondary form is typically associated with other autoimmune conditions such as rheumatoid arthritis, SLE, or scleroderma.

Sjögren's Syndrome Clinical Features

All forms are associated with ocular and oral dryness and salivary gland enlargement.

Sjögren's Syndrome Diagnosis

The SSA and SSB antibodies are frequently positive in the primary form of Sjögren's syndrome. The ANA can also be positive.

Sjögren's Syndrome Treatment

Treatment is usually symptomatic. Saliva and tear substitutes provide relief for dryness of the mouth and eyes, respectively. The patient may be on NSAIDS for symptomatic relief of musculoskeletal symptoms. Corticosteroids or immunosuppressive drugs may be prescribed to the severely symptomatic patient.

REITER'S SYNDROME

Reiter's syndrome or reactive arthritis is an autoimmune condition that affects white males, most commonly, age 20–40. It occurs in response to a genitourinary or gastrointestinal infection. It is an HLA-B27-linked inflammatory arthritis that damages the cartilage of the joints, and this triggers subacute or chronic inflammatory disease. The inflammatory response triggers a triad of symptoms: arthritis, uveitis, and urethritis.

Reiter's Syndrome Characteristic Features

The characteristic features associated with Reiter's syndrome are conjunctivitis, nonspecific urethritis, arthritis affecting mostly the joints of the lower extremities (feet and heels), and painless shallow oral and genital ulcers.

Reiter's Syndrome Treatment

Treatment consists of providing adequate antibiotics to treat the precipitating infection, NSAIDS, and corticosteroids.

BEHÇET'S SYNDROME

Behçet's syndrome or Behçet's disease is associated with inflammation of the blood vessels. Behçet's syndrome affects patients in their 20s and 30s.

The disease is chronic and recurrent with asymptomatic periods in between, but the flare-ups are unpredictable. It is prevalent in North Africa, Turkey, the Middle East, Korea, and Japan.

Behçet's Syndrome Clinical Features

Behçet's syndrome is characterized by the following:

1. Features include painful deep oral ulcers involving the mucous membrane of lips, gingiva, cheeks, and tongue; painful genital ulcers; and anterior or posterior uveitis that can lead to blindness.
2. **Pathergy:** This is a hyperirritable reaction to needle puncture such that blistering occurs at the puncture site.
3. **Arthritis:** Pain and swelling of the joints is quite significant.
4. Thrombophlebitis
5. Meningitis
6. Thrombosis
7. Neurological symptoms: Neurological symptoms are rare.

Behçet's Syndrome Treatment

Treatment is symptomatic and focuses on pain relief and prevention of serious problems.

TEMPORAL OR GIANT CELL ARTERITIS

Temporal or giant cell arteritis is a vasculitis that affects medium and large blood vessels, particularly in the head. It is called *temporal arteritis* because the temporal artery is frequently affected. The alternate name, giant cell arteritis reflects the cells seen on biopsy of the affected blood vessel.

It is not a permanent disease because it completely disappears in 1–2 years. The disease affects the elderly, and women are more affected than men are. It is rare before age 50 and is most common around age 70.

Temporal or Giant Cell Arteritis Classic Features

The patient typically complains of temporal headache and this is associated with a tender, thickened, and nodular temporal artery.

Temporal arteritis, however, may also affect other vessels such as the opthalmic, facial, or lingual arteries.

Ophthalmic and posterior ciliary arteries, when involved, can lead to blindness.

Facial artery involvement is rare, but when it occurs it is associated with painful jaw swelling or claudication. Lingual artery involvement is rare and, when affected, it causes color change, paresthesias, and necrosis of the tongue. Oral pain may be prominent at the level of the gums.

Temporal or Giant Cell Arteritis Diagnostic Test

Temporal or giant cell arteritis characteristically shows immediate elevation of the ESR, with values rising at the rate of 100 mm/hr. Definitive diagnosis is established only with tissue biopsy of the affected vessel.

Temporal or Giant Cell Arteritis Treatment

Treatment consists of high-dose corticosteroids, which rapidly correct the symptoms and prevent blindness. Steroids should be given immediately even before the return of biopsy results, if the suspicion is high. The corticosteroids are continued if the biopsy results are positive and discontinued with negative results. Once started, however, the steroids are gradually decreased over months.

RHEUMATOID ARTHRITIS (RA)

Rheumatoid arthritis affects women more than men, and at age 30 or greater.

Rheumatoid Arthritis (RA) Clinical Features

The patient experiences symmetrical inflammation of the distal joints: digits, wrists, feet, and knees. The pain in the joints the is worst on waking up. The knuckles and the proximal interphalangeal joints of the hands and feet are affected. The cervical spine is involved in severe cases, but involvement of the spine is rare. Lumber spine is always spared. The patient complains of prolonged morning stiffness, malaise, and sometimes low-grade fever.

Rheumatoid Arthritis (RA)–Associated Cervical Spine Involvement

RA-associated cervical spine changes are prominent at the uncovertebral joints and bursae. The synovial bursae surrounding the dens are often affected, causing lysis and disruption of the transverse ligament of atlas and atlantoaxial subluxation. This can lead to impingement of the spinal cord.

Cervical spine involvement is associated with the **Lehrmitte's sign**: The patient experiences flashes of pain in all four extremities.

Rheumatoid Arthritis (RA)–Associated Cervical Spine Involvement Diagnosis

RA-associated cervical spine involvement is diagnosed with review of the cervical spine films taken with the neck in forward flexion. Diagnosis is confirmed by identifying an increased distance between the dens and the anterior arch of atlas.

Rheumatoid Arthritis (RA)–Associated Cervical Spine Involvement Treatment

Treatment consists of prompt surgical stabilization and consists of wiring of the C-1 and C-2 posterior arches.

Rheumatoid Arthritis (RA)–Associated Cricoaritenoid Arthritis

This is a frequent manifestation of RA. The patient experiences pain, dysphagia, fullness or tension in the throat, hoarseness, and stridor.

Rheumatoid Arthritis (RA) Blood Tests

CBC often shows thrombocytopenia and anemia in patients with RA.

Rheumatoid Arthritis (RA) Treatment

Treatment is symptomatic and focuses on pain relief: NSAIDS, corticosteroids, and chemotherapeutic drugs.

OSTEOARTHRITIS

Osteoarthritis Facts

Osteoarthritis is differentiated from RA in that osteoarthritis is associated with pain on rotation, negligible morning stiffness, and bony enlargements, especially affecting the hands. The pain of osteoarthritis is most pronounced at the end of the day.

Joint involvement is unilateral and the major joints or distal interphalyngeal joints of the hands are affected. The patient does not experience any systemic, symptoms and there are no associated changes seen on the CBC. Treatment is symptomatic with NSAIDS or steroids.

ANKYLOSING SPONDILITIS

Young men are more affected than women and the majority of these patients are HLA-B28 positive.

Ankylosing spondilitis is associated with inflammation of vertebral attachment or outermost fibers of intervertebral discs. This results in ossification and spinal fusion.

Ankylosing Spondilitis Clinical Features

The patient experiences lack of motion and brittle cervical spine due to lack of muscle pulling. The patient finds it difficult to turn and complains of a stiff back and prolonged morning stiffness lasting more than 30 min.

Ankylosing Spondilitis Diagnosis

Classic "bamboo spine" is seen on radiographs.

Ankylosing Spondilitis and General Anesthesia

These patients present significant risk during general anesthesia because minor forces can fracture the neck precipitating quadric-paresis.

DIFFUSE IDIOPATHIC SKELETAL HYPEROSTOSIS (DISH) OR FORESTIER DISEASE

DISH Facts

DISH is characterized by the fusion of four vertebrae that are welded together by heavily ossified anterior longitudinal ligaments. This condition is limited to the dorsal spine area, and the cervical spine is often involved. Massive flame-shaped anterior osteophytes (bone spurs) can produce dysphagia. Compression of the cord is rare.

GOUT

Gout Facts

Gout is an inherited disorder associated with an abnormality in the body's ability to process uric acid. Thus, there is an overload of uric acid in the body, recurring attacks of joint inflammation, and gouty arthritis.

Chronic gout is associated with kidney stones, decreased renal function, and progressive renal failure.

Gouty arthritis is precipitated by deposits of uric acid crystals in the synovial fluid and the synovial lining. Intense joint inflammation occurs as white blood cells engulf the uric acid crystals and release lysosomal enzymes associated with inflammation, causing pain, heat, and redness of the joint tissues.

Gout is more common in males. The numbers do, however, go up in females after menopause.

Diseases often associated with gout are hypertension, obesity, leukemia, and lymphomas.

Gout Symptoms and Signs

Gout attacks are very sudden in onset. The pain escalates rapidly as the joint gets inflamed. It is characteristic for only a single joint to be affected. The big toe, knees, ankle, small joints of the hands, etc., can be affected.

Gout Clinical Features

During an attack, the joint swells and the skin over the joint becomes red, hot, and extremely painful.

Chronic deposition of uric acid crystals causes tophi (tiny nodules/outgrowths), and these can be found at the outer rim of the pinna on examination of the head and neck.

Gout Diagnosis

Diagnosis of gout is established with the following:

1. **Medical history** The medical history will show the classic disease presentation and joint involvement history of sudden onset and single joint involvement.
2. **Blood test: A** blood test will show increased uric acid levels.
3. **Arthrocentesis:** Finding uric acid crystals in the fluid aspirate from the joint confirms the diagnosis.

Gout Treatment

Treatment consists of the following:

1. **Weight reduction:** Weight loss along with decreased alcohol consumption helps control the disease state.
2. **Dietary changes:** Diet should be low in animal proteins and purine-containing food items.
3. **Water consumption:** The water intake should be increased to dilute the urine and decrease the formation of renal stones. Literature shows that dehydration increases the incidence of gout attacks.

Gout Medications: Acute and Maintenance Drugs

Acute Gout Medications

Treatment is provided with medications that treat acute gout and maintenance drugs that keep the patient symptom free between attacks. The following are classic acute gout medications:

1. **NSAIDS:** NSAIDS are given till symptoms abate. NSAIDS are contraindicated in the presence of kidney disease.
2. **Corticosteroids:** Steroids are given short-term to decrease the inflammation and are a useful alternative to NSAIDS in patients with associated kidney disease.
3. **Colchicine:** As stated earlier, during an acute gout attack intense joint inflammation occurs as white blood cells engulf the uric acid crystals and release lysosomal enzymes associated with inflammation, causing pain, heat, and redness of the joint tissues. Colchicine helps suppress inflammation associated with the acute attack by decreasing WBC motility and phagocytosis in the joint. It also inhibits lactic acid production, and this in turn slows down the deposition of urate crystals in the joints. Colchicine is very effective in the management of an acute attack and it is given every few hours till the symptoms resolve.

Gout Maintenance Drugs

The following are drugs used to prevent gout:

1. **Allopurinol (Zyloprim):** Allopurinol is a maintenance drug that causes decreased uric acid production.
2. **Probenecid (Benemid) and sulfinpyrazone (Anturane):** These are maintenance drugs and are uricosuric agents that increase the clearance of uric acid and thus prevent gout.

ANTIRHEUMATIC MEDICATIONS

Rheumatic disease management drugs are not just used for the classic rheumatic diseases, but they are also used for diseases affecting the bones and muscles. They can be classified into three basic classes of drugs:

1. **Biologic response modifiers (BRMs)**
2. **NSAIDS**
3. **Older Drugs:** corticosteroids (see Chapter 40, "Adrenal Gland Cortex and Medulla Disease States: Assessment, Analysis, and Associated Dental Management Guidelines")

BIOLOGIC RESPONSE MODIFIERS (BRMS)

The BRMs stimulate or restore the ability of the immune system to fight arthritis, rheumatic diseases, and infections. BRMs interfere with inflammatory activity by binding to and inactivating TNF-alpha, thus ultimately decreasing joint damage.

BRM Classification

BRMs can be classified into:

1. Tumor Necrosing Factor (TNF) Blockers
2. The Biologic Disease-Modifying Antirheumatic drugs (DMARDs)

Common Tumor-Necrosing Factor (TNF) Blockers

TNF blockers are often first-line drugs and the common drugs in this category are

1. D2E7/Adalimumab (Humira)
2. Etanercept (Enbrel)
3. Infliximab (Remicade)

TNF Blockers Side Effects

The side effects associated with TNF blockers are leukopenia and risk of serious infection such as MTB and lymphoma.

DMARDs (Disease-Modifying Antirheumatic Drugs)

DMARDs are often prescribed early on in the treatment of rheumatic diseases, in addition to NSAIDS.

Common DMARDs

The common DMARDs prescribed are azathioprine (Imuran), chlorambucil (Leukeran), cyclophosphamide (Cytoxan), hydroxychloroquine (Plaquenil), injectable gold (Myochrysine), leflunomide (Arava), methotrexate (Rheumatrex, Trexall), minocycline (Minocin), mycophenolate (CellCept), penicillamine (Cuprimine, Depen), ridaura/oral gold (Auranofin), gold injections (they cause metallic taste and stomatitis), cyclosporine (Sandimmune), and sulfasalazine (Azulfidine).

Methotrexate Facts

Methotrexate blocks purine synthesis and inhibits the activity of the immune system, thus reducing inflammation. As a cytotoxic drug it may slow the rapid growth of cells in the synovial membrane that lines the joints. Methotrexate is a potent drug, and a low dosage level of it is used for arthritis. Only 1/100 the amount used for cancer chemotherapy is used, thus decreasing its toxic side effects.

Methotrexate is the most commonly used drug for rheumatic diseases.

Methotrexate Side Effects

Common side effects associated with methotrexate are nausea, severe forms of anemia, lung disease, liver damage that is irreversible, and sores on the skin and inside the mouth. Folic acid use can decrease the side effects during treatment.

Alcohol should be **avoided** with methotrexate. TNF blockers become the first line of therapy if the patient cannot avoid alcohol.

NSAIDS

NSAIDS Classification

NSAIDS interfere with the inflammatory process. They are classified into the following:

1. Acetylated salicylates: aspirin
2. Nonacetylated salicylates
3. Traditional NSAIDS
4. COX-2 selective inhibitors: celecoxib (Celebrex), etoricoxib (Baxtra)

Acetylated Salicylate: Aspirin

Aspirin permanently affects platelets and often these patients are on large doses of aspirin. Consult with the M.D. when major surgery is planned; it may take 7–10 days to reverse the effects of high doses of aspirin if the go-ahead is given to stop the aspirin.

Nonacetyl Salicylates

Common nonacetyl salicylates are the following:

1. Choline salicylate (Arthropan)
2. Magnesium salicylate (Magan/Mobidin)
3. Nonprescription magnesium salicylate (Arthritab or Bayer Select or Doan's Pills)

Nonacetylated Salicylates Facts

These drugs are not used as much now. Choline and magnesium salicylate **do not** affect platelets and **do not** affect the bleeding time (BT). Nonacetylated salicylates **do not** need to be stopped prior to any kind of dental surgery.

Traditional NSAIDS

The traditional NSAIDS include diclofenac potassium (Cataflam), diclofenac/misoprostol (Arthrotec) (the first NSAID protective against ulcers), diclofenac sodium (Voltaren), diflunisal (Dolobid), etodolac (Lodine), fenoprofen (Nalfon), flurbiprofen (Ansaid), ibuprofen (Motrin, Advil), indomethacin (Indocin), ketoprofen (Orudis, Oruvail), meclofenamate sodium (Meclomen), mefanamic acid (Ponstel), meloxicam (Mobic), nabumetone (Relafen), naproxen (Naprosyn, Aleve), oxaprozin (Daypro), piroxicam (Feldene), sulindac (Clinoril), and tolmetin sodium (Tolectin).

NSAIDS Facts

NSAIDS affect platelet adhesivenes, resulting in prolonged bleeding. Ibuprofen has reversible inhibitory effect that lasts only hours.

All NSAIDS, with the exception of aspirin and nonacetylated salicylates, should be stopped for at least 24 hr prior to major surgery, after consulting with the patient's M.D.

Cyclo-oxygenase (COX)-2 Inhibitors

The only COX-2 inhibitor prescribed today is celecoxib (Celebrex). Valdecoxib (Baxtra) and Vioxx were recently withdrawn.

COX-2 Inhibitors Facts

COX-2 inhibitors are associated with some extent of increased cardiovascular complications and potentially life-threatening gastrointestinal bleeding.

Baxtra was withdrawn because it had increased cardiovascular events. Vioxx was associated with deaths from sudden cardiac arrythmias. Thus, Baxtra and Vioxx were withdrawn because the risks with both the drugs far outweighed the benefits.

Celebrex also was temporarily withdrawn, but because the benefits outweighed the risks, Celebrex was reintroduced with specific warning labels about its side effects.

COX-2 inhibitors act by inhibition of prostaglandin synthesis via inhibition of cyclooxygenase-2 (COX-2). COX-2 inhibitors do not affect COX-1.

COX-2 inhibitors are metabolized in the liver by the CYP 450 enzyme and are excreted through the kidneys.

The COX-2 inhibitors are primarily used to treat pain associated with osteoarthritis and rheumatoid arthritis. These drugs do not cause GI ulcers, nor do they affect platelet aggregation, so they do not need to be stopped prior to major surgery.

50% dose reduction of COX-2 inhibitors is recommended in patients with hepatitis, and they are contraindicated in patients with cirrhosis or any form of kidney disease.

COX-2 Inhibitors and DDIs

Do not prescribe the following drugs to patients on COX-2 inhibitors:

- Fluconazole (Diflucan)
- Tetracycline HCL
- Doxycycline (Vibramycin)
- Clarithromycin (Biaxin)

SUGGESTED DENTAL GUIDELINES FOR RHEUMATIC DISEASES

These guidelines in general are applicable for diseases of the joints, bones, or muscles:

1. Always determine the type of rheumatic disease affecting your patient and know the extent of the disease.
2. Determine what organ systems are affected because this will help guide you in the request of laboratory tests to determine the patient's current medical and vital organ status.
3. At the minimum, request the CBC, serum creatinine, and LFTs. Review the CBC and determine whether the patient has anemia, thrombocytopenia, or increased monocyte count.
4. Incorporate the anemia and thrombocytopenia suggested anesthetics, analgesics, and antibiotics (AAA) guidelines if either or both changes are seen on the CBC.

5. Increased monocyte count is associated with flare-ups, and routine dental treatment must be deferred for 4–6 weeks till the acute state resolves.

6. Always calculate the absolute neutrophil count (ANC) count and follow the ANC guidelines when the immunity is affected (not uncommon with these diseases).

7. Follow the kidney and liver AAA suggested guidelines if the serum creatinine and LFTs are affected.

8. Discuss with the patient whether the spine is affected and what is the patient's mobility status as far as the TMJ, cervical, and lumbar spine areas are concerned. Provide TMD care if the TMJ is affected.

9. Patients with limited cervical spine mobility should be asked to move their neck themselves when you need a change of position. Do not rotate the neck yourself because this could negatively affect the patient and cause nerve pains in the upper extremities.

10. A patient with lumbar spine involvement may not be able to stay in the chair for too long and may need help to get out of the chair. Have the patient bring in a lumbar pillow if the patient uses one.

11. A patient with moderate to severe arthritis-associated hand deformities may need to use an electric toothbrush or have a bulky taped wrapping around the toothbrush handle for a better grip. The toothbrush can also be taped in place after inserting it through small cuts into the top and bottom of a tennis ball.

12. Know and analyze each medication the patient is on for the management of the underlying rheumatic disease.

13. Always confirm whether the patient is currently on corticosteroids or has been on steroids for 2 weeks or longer, in the past 2 years. If the response is positive, you will have to follow "the rule of two's" for major surgery, after consulting with the patient's physician.

14. Patients on bisphosphonates must be educated about maintaining a healthy dental status and have more frequent hygiene recalls to prevent any adverse side effects from the drug. All infections must be aggressively treated with antibiotics and pain medications, in the presence of bisphosphonates.

15. Patients experiencing xerostomia should be treated with saliva substitutes. Optimal oral hygiene should be maintained and any oral candidiasis that develops should be immediately treated as outlined in Chapter 48, "Therapeutic Management of Oral Lesions in the Immune-Competent and the Immune-Compromised Patient in the Dental Setting."

16. As discussed earlier, there are several antirheumatic medications and the specifics of each should be noted and implemented appropriately during patient care. Of particular importance are the TNF-blockers, which usually need to be stopped 2 weeks prior to dentistry, if the WBC count is low. This temporary cessation will help increase the WBC count and promote healing.

DISEASES OF THE BONES: PAGET'S DISEASE

Paget's is a bone disease that is more common in people over 40, and men are more frequently affected than women. The exact etiology is not known, but it does seem to run in families. The bones affected are the skull, extremities, pelvis, and spine. The disease could be limited to one or two bones or it could be widespread, affecting several bones.

Paget's Disease Pathophysiology

Paget's disease is associated with a disruption of bone remodeling. In the initial stages of the disease bone breakdown is more rapid than bone remodeling. With time, however, bone remodeling is rapid but the new bone formed is soft and weak. This leads to bone pain, bone deformity, and fractures.

Paget's Disease Symptoms and Signs

Symptoms and signs associated with Paget's depends on the extensiveness of the disease. Some patients can be asymptomatic; others are quite bothered by their symptoms.

Common Symptoms

The following are common symptoms:

1. **Bone pains:** The pains may be constant and deep and are more aggravating at night.
2. **Joint pains:** Joint pains are due to the loss of cartilage and the progressive osteoarthritis that follows.
3. **Nerve pains:** Enlargement of the bones causes compression of the nerves in close proximity to the spine. This causes severe radiating pains, tingling, numbness, and weakness along the distribution of the nerves affected.
4. **Neurological symptoms:** Headaches, vision problems, facial weakness, and hearing loss are the neurological symptoms experienced.
5. **Other symptoms:** Fractures, increased head size, loss of teeth, and bowlegs are some of the symptoms that are classically associated with the disease as it progresses with time.

Paget's Disease Diagnosis

Paget's disease diagnosis is established with the following:

1. **Blood tests:** The alkaline phosphatase levels are markedly increased, indicating rapid bone turnover.
2. **Radiographs:** Radiographic survey of the affected bone can show enlargement, resorption, and deformities.
3. **Bone scans:** Bone scans can detect changes in bones due to Paget's disease, much earlier than standard radiographs. Another advantage is that a bone scan is able to detect all bones affected with the disease.

Paget's Disease Complications

The disease progresses slowly. Osteoarthritis, cardiac failure, and osteosarcoma, however, are some of the complications that are associated with Paget's disease.

Paget's Disease Treatment

A slowly progressing disease process may not need much care, but a progressive disease may need some or all of the treatments listed in the following sections.

Surgery

Surgical intervention may be needed to correct bone deformity or relieve osteoarthritis-associated joint problems with joint prostheses. Patients with a joint prosthesis will have to be *premedicated for life*, according to the AHA guidelines, for all invasive dentistry because Paget's is a chronic systemic disease that affects bones.

Medical Management

The following medications are used to manage Paget's disease–associated symptoms: NSAIDS, bisphosphonates, and calcitonin.

NSAIDS

NSAIDS are given to control arthritis-associated pain. Refer to the previous section, "Classic Rheumatic Diseases" for a detailed discussion on NSAIDS.

Bisphosphonates

Bisphosphonates help decrease the bone activity and are the **main** class of drugs used in the management of Paget's disease. Refer to Chapter 41, "Parathyroid Dysfunction Disease States: Assessment, Analysis, and Associated Dental Management Guidelines," for a detailed discussion on bisphosphonates.

Calcitonin

Calcitonin is given to patients who have Paget's and associated renal disease when bisphosphonates are contraindicated. Thus, it serves as an **alternate** drug. Calcitonin (Miacalcin) regulates calcium and bone metabolism. Refer to Chapter 41, "Parathyroid Dysfunction Disease States: Assessment, Analysis, and Associated Dental Management Guidelines," for a detailed discussion on calcitonin.

Paget's Disease Alert: Paget's disease is associated with increased vascularity in the affected areas. Any one of these two medications, when given for some time prior to surgery, will help reduce the number of blood vessels in the area and associated bleeding with surgery.

SUGGESTED DENTAL GUIDELINES FOR PAGET'S DISEASE

Follow these guidelines:

1. Prior to treatment, obtain the CBC with platelets and WBC differential, serum creatinine, and LFTs. Calculate the ANC and implement the ANC guidelines when the WBC count is decreased. Assess the status of the liver and kidney and implement appropriate guidelines when either or both organs are compromised.
2. In the early osteolytic stage, bone resorption predominates and there may be much bleeding because of greatly increased vascularity seen in the affected tissue during this stage.
3. In the later sclerotic stage, the affected bones become enlarged and dense, and because of poor blood supply to the bones, surgery in this stage can predispose to suppurative osteomyelitis. Antibiotic coverage **prior** to surgery will prevent infection and promote the healing process.
4. The maxilla is more affected than the mandible, but jaw involvement is less in general with Paget's disease.
5. Dentures frequently have to be replaced in patients with Paget's disease because the alveolar bone resorption continues over time and proper fitting of the dentures becomes an issue.

6. Patients with a joint prosthesis need to be premedicated prior to all invasive procedures. Amoxicillin does not have as good a bone penetration when compared to all the other antibiotics on the AHA list. It is better to use cephalosporins, clindamycin, azithromycin, or clarithromycin instead.
7. Occasionally, steroids may also be prescribed, and you have to consider "the rule of twos" prior to major surgery.
8. Patients on bisphosphonates must be educated about maintaining a healthy dental status and have more frequent hygiene recalls to prevent any adverse side effects from the drug. All infections must be aggressively treated with antibiotics and pain medications in the presence of bisphosphonates.

DISEASES AFFECTING MUSCLES: MALIGNANT HYPERTHERMIA (MH)

Malignant hyperthermia (MH) is an autosomal dominant disorder that causes severe muscle contractions on exposure to specific general anesthetics and a sudden sharp rise in body temperature. Once a patient is diagnosed with MH, all family members are considered to have MH.

Malignant Hyperthermia (MH) Pathophysiology

The basic defect is an inability of the skeletal muscles to regulate calcium. **Reuptake** of calcium is necessary for the **termination** of skeletal muscle **contraction,** and with MH there is a **reduction in the reuptake** of calcium by the sarcoplasmic reticulum. The skeletal muscle contraction is thus sustained, causing a rapid rise in body temperature. With the associated hypermetabolic crisis there is a constant demand for oxygen by the skeletal muscles. Initially, the body tries to compensate but eventually the patient experiences a circulatory collapse.

Malignant Hyperthermia (MH) Causative Factors

Malignant hyperthermia patients become symptomatic **within 1 hr** when exposed to the following:

1. Succinylcholine: a depolarizing muscle relaxant.
2. Specific volatile anesthetics: halothane, desflurane, enflurane, isoflurane, and sevoflurane.

Malignant Hyperthermia (MH) Diagnostic Tests

The two muscle biopsy-associated tests that aid in MH diagnosis are:

1. The In Vitro Contracture Test (IVCT)
2. The Caffeine-Halothane Contracture Test

Malignant Hyperthermia (MH) Symptoms and Signs

MH is characterized by a rapid rise in body temperature with associated skeletal muscle rigidity, lockjaw, tachycardia, cardiac arrythmias, hypotension, hypoxemia (low oxygen in the blood), hypercarbia (increased carbon dioxide in the blood), respiratory and metabolic acidosis, and skeletal muscle breakdown in the blood.

Malignant Hyperthermia (MH) Treatment

Treatment must be immediate and consists of the following:

1. Call for help immediately.
2. Hyperventilate the patient with 100% oxygen.
3. Cool down the patient with cold blankets.
4. Give **cold** intravenous (IV) fluids 15 cc/kg.
5. Inject IV Dantrolene immediately.

Dantrolene

Dantrolene is a muscle relaxant that works directly on the ryanodine receptor and prevents the release of calcium. Listed are the bolus, follow-up, and maintenance doses of Dantrolene:

1. **Dantrolene Bolus Dose:** Give Dantrolene 2.5 mg/kg IV stat.
2. **Dantrolene Follow-Up Dose:** Give Dantrolene 2 mg/kg every 5 min, till the patient is stable.
3. **Dantrolene Maintenance Dose:** The patient is maintained at Dantrolene, 1–2 mg/kg/h.

Malignant Hyperthermia (MH) and Suggested Safe Drugs During Dentistry

1. **Anxiety-relieving medications:** lorazepam (Ativan), diazepam (Valium), triazolam (Halcion), and midazolam (Versed)
2. **Barbiturates/intravenous anesthetics:** diazepam (Valium), methohexital (Brevital), midazolam (Versed)
3. **Inhaled nonvolatile general anesthetics:** nitrous oxide
4. **Local anesthetics:** bupivicaine (Marcaine), lidocaine (Xylocaine), mepivicaine (Carbocaine), prilocaine (Citanest), Septocaine (Articaine)
5. **Narcotics (opioids):** codeine (Methyl Morphine), fentanyl (Sublimaze), hydromorphone (Dilaudid), meperidine (Demerol), methadone (Dolophine), morphine, naloxone (Narcan), and oxycodone (Percocet)
6. **Antibiotics: All** antibiotics used in the dental setting are safe with MH.
7. **Analgesics/antipyretics:** All analgesics-antipyretics used in the dental setting are safe with MH.

DISEASES AFFECTING MUSCLES: POLYMYOSITIS AND DERMATOMYOSITIS

Polymyositis

Polymyositis is an inflammatory myopathy that is considered to be an autoimmune disease. The exact etiology is not clear. It is thought to occur secondary to a viral or bacterial infection.

It is more common in the black compared to the white population, and women are more frequently affected than men. Patients are usually in their 40s or 50s at the onset of the disease.

Polymyositis Symptoms and Signs

The symptoms of polymyositis are gradual in onset. The patient usually experiences weakness in the hip and shoulder muscles, making it difficult for the patient to get in and out of bed or a chair. Mild joint pains, muscle tenderness, fatigue, generalized malaise, and difficulty swallowing are also experienced.

Dermatomyositis Symptoms and Signs

Dermatomyositis is associated with specific skin lesions, commonly a butterfly rash, **and** all the symptoms and signs associated with polymyositis. Etiology for dermatomyositis is the same as the etiology for polymyositis.

Dermatomyositis usually affects patients in their 50s and 60s and females are more frequently affected than males. Other collagen vascular disorders can also be associated with dermatomyositis.

Polymyositis and Dermatomyositis Diagnosis

Diagnosis of both disease states is made with the following:

1. **Medical History:** The classic presentation is often very suggestive of either of the two diseases.
2. **Muscle Biopsy:** Muscle biopsy may reveal muscle changes suggestive of the disease.
3. **Electromyography:** Different muscles are tested with electromyography to reveal the underlying disease state.
4. **Blood Tests:** Blood tests show increased levels of creatinine kinase and aldolase, indicating muscle damage.

Polymyositis and Dermatomyositis Complications

Polymyositis and Dermatomyositis are often associated with other connective tissue disorders. These patients can also have associated heart disease, cardiac arrythmias, heart failure, and interstitial lung disease with fibrosis.

Polymyositis and Dermatomyositis Management

Medical management frequently involves medications, along with physical therapy. Physical therapy is provided to tone and loosen the muscles and joints. The following are the drugs most often prescribed:

1. **Corticosteroids and Bisphosphonates:** Steroids are given long-term and bisphosphonates are often prescribed along with the steroids to counteract the steroid-associated osteoporosis.
2. **Immunosuppressants:** Azathioprine (Imuran) or methotrexate (Rheumatrex) are prescribed as alternates if steroids are ineffective or not well tolerated by the patient.

Polymyositis and Dermatomyositis Suggested Dental Alerts

The following are dental alerts:

1. Follow the suggested guidelines outlined for the earlier section "Classic Rheumatic Diseases."
2. Take into consideration the associated anemia, collagen-vascular abnormalities, and corticosteroid or immunosuppressant therapy.
3. These patients benefit when given shorter appointments because this prevents undue exhaustion.

DISEASES AFFECTING MUSCLES: PARKINSON'S DISEASE (PD)

Parkinson's disease is a motor system disorder, caused by loss of dopamine-producing brain cells in the basal ganglia. This thus results in localized deficiency of dopamine.

Parkinson's disease is also called *paralysis agitans* and it usually affects patients in their 50s.

Some patients progress slowly with the disease while others progress quite rapidly. It is not uncommon for these patients to experience infrequent blinking, drooling due to poor swallowing, emotional and sleep disturbances, and with bowel and bladder control problems.

Parkinson's Disease Presentation

Parkinson's disease primarily presents in one of four ways:

1. **Tremors:** The patient experiences trembling in the hands, arms, legs, jaw, and face when Parkinson's presents as tremors. Hands and arm tremors cause a pin-rolling movement pattern and the tremors are worst at rest.
2. **Rigidity:** There is stiffness of the limbs and trunk when Parkinson's presents with rigidity. The patient's arms are flexed and held to the sides. Cogwheel rigidity is seen during movement of the limbs, and a stooping posture occurs because of rigidity.
3. **Bradykinesia:** There is slowness of movement in this form of Parkinson's presentation and slowness in initiation and execution of movements, and the patient often shuffles when walking.
4. **Postural instability:** Another form of presentation is when the patient experiences impairment of balance and coordination.

Parkinson's Disease Diagnosis

Diagnosis is made by the following:

1. Evaluation of the medical history
2. Thorough neurological examination

   Parkinson's Disease Management: Parkinson's disease is managed with the following:

1. **Dopamine precursors:** Levodopa or levodopa combined with carbidopa is the first choice medication. Carbidopa slows the conversion of levodopa to dopamine until it reaches the brain. Nerve cells convert levodopa to dopamine. Bradykinesia and rigidity respond best to levodopa.
2. **Anticholinergics:** Trihexyphenidyl HCL (Artane) and benzotropine mesylate (Cogentin) are the drugs from this category used for the management of Parkinson's disease.
3. **Dopamine antagonists—bromocriptine (Parlodel), pramipexole (Mirapex), and ropinirole (Requip):** These drugs simulate the action of dopamine in the brain and may help control the tremor and rigidity.
4. **Catechol-O-Methyl-Transferase (COMT) inhibitors:** Entacapone (Comtan) and tolcapone (Tasmar) are the COMT drugs used in the management of Parkinson's disease.

5. **Neurotransmitter inhibitor:** Amantadine, an antiviral drug, also appears to decrease Parkinson's symptoms.
6. **Rasagiline with levodopa:** This combination is usually the treatment for advanced PD or it can be used as a single-drug treatment for early PD.
7. **Deep brain stimulation (DBS):** Electrodes implanted into the brain are connected to a small electrical device that is externally programmed.

DBS helps decrease tremors, slowness of movements, gait problems, and the need for medications.

Parkinson's Disease Suggested Dental Guidelines

The following are dental guidelines:

1. Follow the suggested dental guidelines outlined for "Classic Rheumatic Diseases."
2. Additionally, a Parkinson's patient with mild tremors may need to be strapped in the chair with a Velcro belt so the head can be stable during treatment.
3. Patients experiencing significant tremors will need to be sedated for dentistry. Low-dose sedation should be used to minimize the additive sedation with anti–Parkinson's disease drugs.
4. Minimize the amount of epinephrine use in the patient on COMT inhibitors and use local anesthetics with 1:200,000 epinephrine or without epinephrine, maximum 2 carpules.
5. Avoid clarithromycin, tetracycline, doxycycline, and azole antifungals with the dopamine antagonist drugs.

DISEASES AFFECTING MUSCLES: MYASTHENIA GRAVIS

Myasthenia gravis is a condition associated with muscle weakness due to poor response of the muscle receptor to the neurotransmitter acetylcholine. Autoantibodies to the acetylcholine receptor protein are often found in many cases.

The weakness and fatigue of affected muscles is gradual or insidious in onset. The weakness may be localized or more generalized, when several muscles are affected. It is often unmasked and/or exacerbated by certain stress factors such as infection, pregnancy, or menstrual periods. Muscle weakness becomes more pronounced as the day progresses.

Myasthenia gravis can occur at all ages, but it is most common in young females who have the HLA-DR3 gene. Myasthenia gravis can occasionally be associated with other conditions such as SLE, RA, thyrotoxicosis, or thymoma. Myasthenia gravis affects men more commonly in their 60s when present with thymoma.

Myasthenia Gravis Symptoms and Signs

Symptoms experienced are associated with the muscles involved: involvement of the ocular muscles results in ptosis and vision problems; involvement of the muscles of mastication and pharyngeal muscles causes the patient to complain of difficulty chewing and swallowing. A very lax jaw can be found on physical examination. Respiratory muscles involvement causes breathing impairment, and involvement of the muscles in the extremities causes weakness in the limbs. There is difficulty supporting the neck when the neck muscles are affected. The gag reflex can be absent or poor, and the ability to cough may be compromised in the Myasthenia gravis patient, causing an increased risk of aspiration.

Myasthenia Gravis Diagnostic Tests

The following are tests to diagnose myasthenia gravis:

1. **Endrophonium (Tensilon) injection test:** The diagnosis of myasthenia gravis is confirmed by demonstration of improved patient response to IV Endrophonium, a short-acting anticholinesterase.
2. **Acetylcholine receptor antibody test:** Blood tests showing elevated levels of circulating acetylcholine receptor antibodies confirms the diagnosis of myasthenia gravis.

Myasthenia Gravis Treatment

Myasthenia gravis treatment considerations are the following:

1. **Anticholinesterases, neostigmine, and pyridostigmine:** Anticholinesterases increase the amount of available acetylcholine (ACh) at the myoneural junction by inhibiting the degradation of ACh.
2. **Neostigmine (Prostigmin)** and **pyridostigmine (Mestinon):** These drugs are used alone or in combination and provide symptomatic relief by enhancing neuromuscular transmission, but they do not affect the course of the disease.
3. **Corticosteroids or cyclosporine (Sandimmune) or azathioprine (Imuran):** Occasionally, the treatment is supplemented with corticosteroids or cyclosporine or azathioprine to suppress the abnormal antibody production and provide symptomatic relief.
4. **Surgery:** Surgical removal of a myasthenia-associated thymoma causing significant symptoms can result in disease remission, postsurgery.

Myasthenia Gravis Suggested Dental Guidelines

Follow these guidelines:

1. Always confirm the extent of disease affecting the entire body and particularly the head and neck region.
2. Check for the gag reflex plus the ability to cough and confirm that both are adequate before you begin treatment.
3. Anticholinesterases increase salivation, and you may often have to provide active suction during dental treatment.
4. Morning appointments are recommended because the weakness is least in the morning and worsens as the day progresses.
5. Follow "the rule of twos" if the patient is currently on steroids or has been on steroids for 2 weeks or longer within the past 2 years.
6. Any form of infection, emotional stress, or certain medications can worsen the status of the disease. Explain the procedure for the day to help relax the patient and decrease any anxiety.
7. Avoid all types of muscle relaxants.
8. Use a minimal dose of local anesthesia, limit it to 2 carpules only, and avoid lidocaine.

9. Avoid macrolides, tetracycline, aminoglycosides, and fluoquinolones diazepam (Valium), lorazepam (Ativan), and general anesthesia because these drugs can aggravate myasthenia gravis symptoms.

DISEASES AFFECTING MUSCLES: MULTIPLE SCLEROSIS (MS)

Multiple sclerosis, a central nervous system disease is considered to be an autoimmune condition that causes progressive antibody-mediated damage of the nerve fibers in the brain and spinal cord. Antibodies are directed against the myelin-producing cells causing inflammation of the myelin sheaths. Multifocal plaques of demyelination occur in the CNS causing patchy areas of sclerosis with resultant motor and sensory dysfunction. The demyelination causes decreased nerve conduction velocity, a differential rate of impulse transmission, partial conduction blocking, or complete failure of impulse transmission.

The exact cause of MS is not known, but viruses (Epstein-Barr virus most often) have often been implicated as either triggering the onset of the disease or triggering an exacerbation of the disease. Pregnancy is also known to worsen the disease. The disease can be progressive and debilitating; however, spontaneous remission is known to occur in some patients.

Multiple Sclerosis (MS) Types

The disease can present in one of four ways:

1. **Relapsing-remitting:** Most patients give a history of frequent flare-ups that last weeks, followed by phases of remission.
2. **Primary progressive:** A few patients especially those that experience initial symptoms after age 40, can have progressively deteriorating symptoms as a primary form of presentation.
3. **Secondary progressive:** A small number of the relapsing-remitting patients can ultimately go on to develop progressively deteriorating symptoms, and this form of the disease is the secondary progressive form of MS.
4. **Progressive relapsing:** This is a variant of primary progressive MS. The patient experiences periodic flare-ups causing worsening of existing, or the occurrence of new, symptoms.

Multiple Sclerosis Age of Onset

MS primarily affects patients between the ages of 20 and 40. Females are more affected than males.

Multiple Sclerosis Symptoms and Signs

The wide range of symptoms experienced depend on the neurological areas affected and the severity of the disease. Excessive fatigue, vision problems, and problems with gait are the common initial symptoms experienced.

The specific symptoms that may be experienced however are blurring of vision; colored halos; impaired vision; unilateral blindness; paresthesias and "pins and needles" sensations in the extremities; tremors and dizziness; hearing loss; speech problems; progressive muscle weakness affecting the limbs; impaired coordination and balance; impaired walking; partial or complete paralysis; impairment of the bowel and bladder function; depression; and difficulty with concentration, memory and judgment.

Multiple Sclerosis Diagnosis

The diagnosis of MS can be established with the following:

1. **Medical history:** There are no specific tests that can diagnose MS, but a thorough medical history can unearth the motor and sensory deficits, neuromuscular symptoms affecting the extremities, vision problems, and problems with gait or coordination.
2. **Magnetic resonance imaging (MRI):** MRI will help detect areas of sclerosis or evidence of plaques in the brain.
3. **Spinal tap:** A spinal tap is done only when the diagnosis is questionable. The CSF will show elevated levels of proteins and mononuclear WBCs.

Multiple Sclerosis Treatment

There is no known effective treatment that can eradicate the disease. There are, however, two basic forms of MS therapy:

1. Drugs used to slow the progression of MS
2. Treatment modalities for symptoms associated with MS

Drugs Used to Slow the Progression of Multiple Sclerosis

The following are drugs are used to slow the progression:

1. **Beta interferon:** Beta interferon preparations decrease exacerbations or severity of symptoms and slow the progression of MS. They help fight viral infections and enhance the immune system. FDA-approved beta interferons available for the management of MS are
    a. Interferon beta-1a injection (Avonex or Rebif)
    b. Interferon beta-1b injection (Betaseron)
2. **Copolymer 1/Glatiramer acetate (Copaxone):** Copolymer I (Copaxone) injection, a synthetic form of basic myelin protein, decreases the relapse rate by one-third. This drug prevents the immune system from attacking myelin.
3. **Mitoxantrone injections (Novantrone):** Mitoxantrone (Novantrone), an immunosuppressive drug, is used short-term (2–3 years) for the treatment of advanced progressive MS.

Treatment Modalities for Symptoms Associated with Multiple Sclerosis

Treatment modalities for MS are

1. **Steroids:** Steroids, when given, are used to reduce the severity and duration of attacks. Occasionally, a patient experiencing troublesome optic symptoms can benefit from a short course of IV methylprednisolone (Solu-Medrol) followed by oral steroids.
2. **Muscle relaxants:** Beclofen (Lioresal) and tizanidine (Zanaflex) muscle relaxants are dispensed for the treatment of muscle stiffness, muscle spasms, and increased muscle tone. Be aware that these drugs can cause **drowsiness and xerostomia.**
3. **Anticonvulsants:** The patient may be on carbamazepine (Tegretol) or phenytoin sodium (Dilantin) for the treatment of trigeminal neuralgia or neuropathy. Refer to Chapter 43, "Classic Seizures Petit Mal and Grand Mal Epilepsy: Assessment,

Analysis, and Associated Dental Management Guidelines," for suggested dental guidelines.

4. **Antidepressant medications:** Tricyclic antidepressants are often prescribed to overcome the associated depression.

5. **Physical therapy and exercise:** Physical therapy and exercise is provided to help maintain muscle function and mobility.

SUGGESTED DENTAL ASPECTS AND GUIDELINES FOR MULTIPLE SCLEROSIS

Follow these guidelines:

1. Patients with severe MS will need shorter appointments because they are unable to keep their mouth open for a longer duration.

2. It is best to treat these patients during morning appointments because fatigue experienced is more pronounced in the afternoon.

3. These patients may need assistance with transfer from the wheelchair to the dental chair.

4. Evaluate the CBC, serum creatinine, and LFTs prior to the start of dental treatment.

5. The patient can experience abnormal facial pain or intraoral pain and discomfort that may be localized or generalized. The patient must be thoroughly evaluated to determine the cause and be referred to the medical side for further evaluation. Incomplete assessment could lead to unnecessary extractions or endodontic treatment.

6. MS can trigger the development of trigeminal neuralgia that is often **bilateral**. It causes paroxysmal pain that simulates electrical shocks, and it can be brought on by chewing or stroking of the cheek. The pain when it occurs is severe and recurring.

7. The trigeminal sensory neuropathy-associated parasthesia is progressive and the maxillary and mandibular divisions of the trigeminal nerve are frequently affected.

8. Significant facial anesthesia can also occur in the severe cases of MS.

9. Numbness of the lower lip and chin with or without pain can occur if the mental nerve is involved.

10. A significant number of patients may be affected with facial palsy, which occurs later in the disease.

11. Severe respiratory problems can occur when the respiratory muscles are affected. The gag reflex may be lacking or impaired. These patients can also suffer from vertigo, which can worsen in the lying-down position. For all these reasons the patient should be treated in a semi-sitting position. The rubber dam should be used only if the patient can adequately breathe through the nose.

12. There is a higher incidence of caries in patients with MS because there is significant xerostomia.

13. It is not uncommon to find stomatitis, ulcerations, gingivitis, herpes infection, candidiasis, and parotid gland enlargement in addition to the xerostomia.

14. Dentistry for severe cases may have to be done under general anesthesia in a hospitalized setting.

15. Interferon and many of the immunosuppressant drugs can cause changes in the CBC affecting the WBCs (neutropenia and/or lymphopenia), hemoglobin, hematocrit, and platelets. Always evaluate the CBC prior to dentistry and stringently implement the ANC guidelines when indicated. All infections should be aggressively treated because infections can worsen the status of the disease. Also adequately compensate for thrombocytopenia, when present.
16. Interferon beta-1a (Avonex/Rebif) causes leukopenia, anemia, thrombocytopenia, and alteration of the LFTs. All hepatotoxic drugs must be avoided with Avonex/Rebif.
17. Interferon beta-1b (Betaseron) causes significant lymphopenia and neutropenia.
18. Copolymer-1/Glatiramer acetate (Capoxone) can cause enlargement of the parotid glands and severe stomatitis.
19. Mitoxantrone (Novantrone) can cause changes in the LFTs plus significant pancytopenia, stomatitis, and mucositis.
20. Evaluate the oral cavity for candida infection in patients on steroids.
21. Follow "the rule of twos" during major dentistry if the patient is currently on steroids or has been on steroids for 2 weeks or longer within the past 2 years. Always provide antibiotic coverage for 5 days, following major dentistry to prevent any postop infection.
22. Steroids mask the symptoms and signs of infection; be extra vigilant. Carefully examine and treat any infection found in the oral cavity.

Multiple Sclerosis and Anesthetics

Follow these guidelines:

1. Limit the anesthetic to a maximum of 2 carpules per visit.
2. Avoid articaine (Septocaine) and prilocaine (Citanest) because both these local anesthetics are known to cause parasthesias.
3. Avoid epinephrine-containing local anesthetics in the presence of tricyclic antidepressants.

Multiple Sclerosis and Analgesics

Follow these guidelines:

1. Avoid aspirin and NSAIDS because these drugs can promote gastric ulceration.
2. Meperidine (Demerol) and propoxyphene (Darvon) should be avoided because the MS drugs affect the LFTs.
3. Follow the liver dosing guidelines when prescribing acetaminophen, acetaminophen + codeine (Tylenol #3), oxycodone + acetaminophen (Percocet), or hydrocodone + acetaminophen (Vicodin) in the presence of abnormal liver enzymes.
4. Use regular-strength acetaminophen (Tylenol) in the presence of antiseizure medications.

Multiple Sclerosis and Antibiotics

No specific antibiotic contraindication exists; however, avoid antibiotics metabolized and cleared by the liver if the LFTs are affected.

XVIII

Oncology: Head and Neck Cancers, Leukemias, Lymphomas, and Multiple Myeloma

51

Head and Neck Cancers and Associated Dental Management Guidelines

ONCOLOGY OVERVIEW

Cancers of the mouth, salivary glands, sinuses, nose, throat, and lymph nodes in the neck are designated *head and neck cancers*.

The dentist plays a very important role in the detection of head and neck cancers because of oral cancer screening as a routine part of patient examination and because of the frequency with which a patient visits a dentist compared to a physician.

Difficulty swallowing, hoarseness, lesions in the oral cavity, and lymph node enlargements in the neck are frequently how head and neck cancers present.

Cancer care is multifaceted and multidisciplinary; this chapter discusses cancer terminology; cancer staging; cancer treatment principles and goals, cancer treatment options and treatment response definitions. This will enable the reader to understand and participate in the cancer patient's care as and when needed.

HEAD AND NECK CANCER DETECTION AND THE DENTIST

The dentist might be the first provider to track and follow through with a patient experiencing difficulty swallowing. The dentist can also identify hoarseness that is of concern and request further evaluation; the dentist can identify suspicious oral lesions because of their color, shape, or size and refer the patient for biopsy.

The dentist can focus on lesions associated with poor healing and triage the patient to the medical side for further assessment. The dentist can find lymph node enlargements that do not fit the picture of infection-associated enlargements, but rather have cancer-associated features. Thus, the dentist is often the first provider to refer the patient to the medical side for further evaluation.

A dentist can also aid in the diagnosis of leukemias and lymphomas by detecting the following:

1. Enlargement of the lymph nodes in the head and neck region associated with sudden onset of systemic symptoms.
2. Oral findings that frequently accompany lymphomas and leukemias due to associated acute deficiency of RBCs and platelets.
3. Oral findings due to lack of normal functioning WBCs, RBCs, and platelets.

NEOPLASMS OF THE ORAL CAVITY

To understand cancer growth one has to understand tumor biology. One malignant cell creates 10^9 cells. These cancer cells grow faster than normal cells and have unstable DNA that cannot be repaired.

Head and neck cancers account for 6% of all cancers, and of these 30% of the cancers occur in the oral cavity.

Males are more often affected than females. The patients are usually in their 40s to 50s.

The most common tumor of the oral cavity is a squamous cell carcinoma in the upper aerodigestive tract.

NEOPLASMS OF THE NASAL CAVITY

Neoplasms of the nasal cavity are rare. There are two types:

1. **Juvenile Nasopharyngeal Angiofibroma:** Juvenile nasopharyngeal angiofibroma can sometimes affect adolescent males. It is often benign and the patient frequently experiences recurrent epitaxis.
2. **Nasopharyngeal Carcinoma:** Nasopharyngeal carcinoma can be due to exposure to hardwood or heavy chemicals, particularly metals. Nasopharyngeal carcinoma is frequently seen in males from the Canton Province of China.

HEAD AND NECK CANCER SYMPTOMS AND SIGNS

Symptoms and signs frequently experienced are localized pain; odynophagia (pain on swallowing); dysphagia (difficulty swallowing); hoarseness; dyspnea (shortness of breath); coughing up blood; and referred pain to the ear from the upper digestive tract, especially in patients with alcohol and tobacco use.

LYMPH NODES OF THE HEAD AND NECK

A dentist needs to know about cancers of the head and neck region *and* the associated lymphatic drainage so the two can be correlated to assist in the diagnosis, treatment, and follow-up of benign or malignant tumors.

The lymph nodes surrounding the base of the skull and the cervical chains of lymph nodes are *the* nodes of great importance for head and neck tumors. A dentist should have a clear understanding of what specific areas each set of nodes drains. Thus, when a lesion is detected on physical examination, the appropriate lymph nodes should be palpated to determine the extent of involvement.

Lymph Nodes Surrounding the Base of the Skull

These nodes include the following:

- The preauricular or superficial parotid node
- The postauricular nodes
- The occipital nodes
- The deep parotid nodes
- The retropharyngeal nodes
- The submandibular nodes

- The submental nodes
- The tonsilar/jugulodigastric node
- The juguloomohyoid node
- The para- and pretracheal nodes

The Cervical Chain of Lymph Nodes

These nodes include the following:

- The superficial cervical chains
- The deep cervical chains

The Superficial Cervical Chains

The superficial cervical chains receive drainage from the preauricular, postauricular, and occipital nodes. The superficial cervical chains, in turn, drain into the deep cervical chains.

The Deep Cervical Chains

The deep cervical nodes receive drainage from the salivary glands, thyroid gland, tongue, tonsils, nose, pharynx, and larynx (Table 51.1).

On the left side the deep cervical chain drains into the thoracic duct. On the right side the deep cervical chain drains into the right lymphatic duct, or the internal jugular, subclavian, or brachiocephalic veins.

GENERAL CANCER RISK FACTORS AND PREVENTION

The general risk factors for cancer are **smoking, alcohol, and miscellaneous other causes.**

Smoking as a Cancer Factor

Smoking accounts for 170,000 deaths/year. 30% of all cancers are due to tobacco and 80% of all lung cancers are due to smoking.

Examples of Tobacco-Related Cancers

Tobacco-associated cancers are lung, mouth/pharynx; esophageal cancers; pancreatic cancer; uterus/cervix/kidney/bladder cancers; oral cancer because of chewing tobacco; and lung, oral, larynx, and esophageal cancers due to cigar smoking.

Alcohol as a Cancer Factor

Alcohol accounts for 19,000 deaths/year and alcohol is an important etiological factor for many cancers, especially cancers of the head and neck.

Oral cancer risk is highest in patients using both alcohol and tobacco, compared with those using just one or the other.

Miscellaneous Risk Factors

Other risk factors for head and neck cancers are obesity, viruses, ultraviolet light, and immune conditions.

Table 51.1. Head and neck lymph nodes identifying tissues drained and specifying direct or indirect drainage into the deep cervical chains

Lymph Nodes	Areas Drained	Drainage
Preauricular or Superficial Parotid Nodes	Drain the external ear canal, front of auricle, and adjacent scalp.	**Indirect drainage** from superficial cervical to deep cervical nodes.
Postauricular Nodes	Drain the external ear canal, back of auricle, and adjacent scalp.	**Indirect drainage** from superficial cervical to deep cervical nodes.
Occipital Nodes	Drain the posterior part of scalp and adjacent region of the neck.	**Indirect drainage** from superficial cervical to deep cervical nodes.
Deep Parotid Nodes	Drain the anterior half of the scalp, infratemporal region, orbit, lateral eyelids, maxillary molar teeth, external ear canal, and parotid gland.	**Direct drainage** deep parotid nodes directly drain into the deep cervical nodes.
Retropharyngeal Nodes	Drain the upper part of the pharynx and adjoining structures.	**Direct drainage:** These nodes drain directly into the deep cervical nodes.
Submandibular Nodes	Drain anterior nasal cavities, tongue, teeth, gums, submandibular and sublingual glands, and all of the face except the lateral eyelids and medial lower lip and chin.	**Direct drainage:** These nodes drain directly into the deep cervical nodes.
Submental Nodes	Drain the tip of the tongue, floor of the mouth, lower lip, and chin.	**Direct drainage:** These nodes drain directly into the deep cervical nodes.
Tonsillar/Jugulodigastric Nodes	Drain the tonsils and lateral part of the tongue.	**Direct drainage:** These nodes drain directly into the deep cervical nodes.
Jugulo-omohyoid Nodes	Drain the tongue via the submental and submandibular nodes.	**Direct drainage:** These nodes drain directly into the deep cervical nodes.
Para and Pretracheal Nodes	Drain the trachea and thyroid gland.	**Direct drainage:** These nodes drain into the tracheobronchial nodes in the mediastinum.

CANCER PREVENTION

The risk of cancer can be lowered with smoking cessation, screening tests, sunscreen use, diet modification, and healthy lifestyle.

SCREENING TESTS FOR CANCER DETECTION AT SPECIFIC BODY SITES

A dentist has to be very familiar with oral cancer screening, and as a health care provider the responsibility extends to knowing other forms of cancer screenings too. Your patient may provide information about having had specific tests or may question you about other screening methods or tests. The following are tests for cancer screening in all parts of the body:

1. **Breast:** Screening is done by self exam and mammogram.
2. **Testicular:** Screening is done by self exam.
3. **Cervix:** Screening is done by Pap smear.
4. **Colon:** Screening is done by colonoscopy and fecal occult blood test.
5. **Skin:** Screening is done by dermatological examination.
6. **Oral:** Screening is done by oral examination.
7. **Prostate:** Screening is done by digital rectal examination.
8. **Lungs:** There is no good screen as yet for lung cancer.

CANCER MANAGEMENT

Cancer management is multitiered and consists of the following:

1. Cancer diagnostic aids
2. Cancer staging
3. Cancer treatment

CANCER DIAGNOSTIC AIDS

To confirm cancer pathology, tissue samples can be obtained using any of the following options; biopsy of suspect tissue, bone marrow aspiration, blood sample, assessment of cell surface markers, and cytogenics or DNA analysis.

CANCER STAGING

Tumor staging can be done using the Broder's classification and/or the TNM staging system.

Broder's Classification

Tumor grading using the Broder's classification (Tumor Grade [G]) is as follows:

G1:   Tumor that is well-differentiated
G2:   Tumor that is moderately well-differentiated
G3:   Tumor that is poorly differentiated
G4:   Tumor that is undifferentiated

The TNM Staging System

The TNM staging system is a clinical staging system that helps estimate the extent of disease *prior* to treatment. The staging process helps determine the treatment choice, the predictive treatment response, and survival. The tumor and nodes are assessed by inspection and palpation when possible. The status of the tumor must be confirmed histopathologically before treatment options are explored. Additional tests that help with the staging process are biopsy, x-ray, CT scan, MRI, nuclear study, or surgery.

Magnetic resonance imaging (MRI) is a better option compared to CT scans for detection and localization of head and neck tumors. MRIs are also better than CT scans in distinguishing lymph nodes from blood vessels in the assessment of head and neck cancers. In the event of a relapse, restaging of the cancer is done to determine appropriate additional treatment that will be required.

American Joint Committee on Cancer (AJCC) TNM Classification

TNM Staging is done using the listed definitions for tumor, lymph nodes, and metastasis:

1. **Tumor Definitions:**
   - Primary tumor (T) represents the extent of the primary tumor
   - TX: Primary tumor cannot be assessed
   - T0 (T zero): No evidence of primary tumor
   - TIS: Carcinoma in situ
   - T1: Tumor ≤2 cm in its greatest dimension
   - T2: Tumor >2 cm but ≤4 cm in its greatest dimension
   - T3: Tumor >4 cm in its greatest dimension
   - T4: Invasive tumor
2. **Regional Lymph Nodes (N) Definitions:**
   - N represents the degree of lymph node involvement
   - NX: Regional lymph nodes cannot be assessed
   - N0 (N zero): No regional lymph node metastasis present
   - N1: Metastasis present in a single ipsilateral (same side) lymph node, ≤3 cm in its greatest dimension
   - N2a: Metastasis in a single ipsilateral (same side) lymph node >3 cm but ≤6 cm in dimension
   - N2b: Metastasis in multiple ipsilateral lymph nodes, ≤6 cm in greatest dimension
   - N2c: Metastasis in bilateral or contralateral (on the opposite side) lymph nodes, ≤6 cm in greatest dimension
   - N3: Metastasis in a lymph node >6 cm in greatest dimension.
3. **Distant Metastasis (M) Definitions:**
   - M represents the presence of metastasis
   - MX: Distant metastasis cannot be assessed
   - M0 (M zero): No distant metastasis present
   - M1: Distant metastasis present

The TNM Stages

The TNM Stages are:

Stage 1: Primary tumor
Stage 2: Large primary tumor with or without lymph node involvement
Stage 3: Primary tumor plus lymph node involvement
Stage 4: Indicates metastasis

American Joint Committee on Cancer (AJCC) Stage Groupings

The stage groupings indicate the TNM definitions associated with each of the TNM stages:

Stage 0:   TIS, N0, M0
Stage I: T1, N0, M0

Stage II: T2, N0, M0
Stage III: T3, N0, M0; T1, N1, M0; T2, N1, M0 **or** T3, N1, M0
Stage IVA: T4a, N0, M0; T4a, N1, M0; T1, N2, M0; T2, N2, M0; T3, N2, M0 **or** T4a, N2, M0
Stage IVB: Any T, N3, M0 or T4b, any N, M0
Stage IVC: Any T, any N, M1

The Eastern Cooperative Oncology Group Scale

The Eastern cooperative oncology scale helps decide which patients can receive treatment. It does so by classifying the patient's level of activity with the associated cancer. According to the scale, it is appropriate to treat only stage 2 or better because the patient loses one level during treatment. The following are the stages according to the Eastern cooperative oncology scale:

Stage 0:   This scale represents working full time.
Stage 1:   This scale represents working part time.
Stage 2:   This scale represents a patient disabled with cancer therapy and spending <50% time in bed or a chair.
Stage 3:   This scale represents a patient who spends >50% time in bed or a chair.
Stage 4:   This scale represents a bedridden patient.

CANCER TREATMENT

Cancer treatment entails establishment of the following:

1. Cancer treatment options and goals
2. Principles of treatment
3. Treatment response definitions
4. Head and neck cancer treatment options

Cancer Treatment Options and Goals

Cancer treatment options and their respective goals are

1. **Curative:** This option completely gets rid of the cancer.
2. **Adjuvant:** This option prevents relapse once the cancer is removed.
3. **Palliative:** With this option, although the cancer cannot be gotten rid of, disease progression is prevented.
4. **Supportive care:** Supportive care is needed for cancer treatment–associated side effects, such as nausea, anorexia, weight loss, etc.
5. **Hospice:** When the cancer cannot be controlled, hospice care treats the pain and suffering to make the end stage comfortable for the patient.

Cancer Treatment Principles

Cancer treatment options depend on the invasiveness of the cancer; the options offered are

1. **Localized cancer:** The treatment option for localized cancer is surgery and/or radiation.
2. **Systemic Cancer:** The options for systemic cancer are chemotherapy, radiation, hormonal therapy, or immunotherapy.

Cancer Treatment Response Definitions

The dentist plays a very important role in managing and maintaining the oral health status of the cancer patient, during chemotherapy and/or radiotherapy.

The treating oncologist can sometimes forward the patient's records to the dental provider to assist with the care. Familiarity with the treatment response definitions often used by the treating oncologists is thus helpful in evaluating the records and assessing the patient's status. Common treatment response definitions used are

1. **CR:** Complete remission
2. **PR:** Partial remission
3. **SD:** Stable disease and one that is not progressing
4. **DP:** Disease progression
5. **Relapse:** Disease occurrence after complete remission (CR)
6. **Refractory:** Disease never in complete remission (CR)

Head and Neck Cancer Treatment Options

The treatment options for cancer care are

1. Surgery
2. Radiation therapy
3. Chemotherapy
4. Chemotherapy plus radiation

Stage I and Stage II cancers are highly curable by surgery or radiation therapy. Stage III or Stage IV cancer patients are candidates for treatment by a combination of surgery and radiation therapy. They should also be considered for a combination of chemotherapy with surgery and/or radiation therapy to improve local control and to decrease the frequency of distant metastases.

HEAD AND NECK CANCER TREATMENT

Surgery

Advantages of Surgical Therapy

Surgical therapy is curative and ideal for early-stage cancer with limited involvement.

Risks of Surgical Therapy

Risks are limited to what can be removed, the microscopic disease status, and the operating room risks. Surgery is not a useful choice in widespread disease.

Radiation Therapy

Advantages of Radiation Therapy

Radiation works differently in different cancers but is a good choice for tumors that cannot be removed. The mechanism of action of radiotherapy is different than that for chemotherapy. The response is fast and with minimal side effects.

Risks of Radiotherapy

Radiotherapy damages the surrounding normal tissues and it is useless in widespread cancers.

Radiation Therapy Options

A dentist should be familiar with all forms of radiation therapy to the head and neck region and **know the amount** of radiation the patient has received during cancer care. Radiation options available are:

1. **External-Beam Radiation Therapy:** This is the treatment option for large tumors. The area radiated includes the tumor and regional lymph nodes even if they are not clinically involved.
2. **Interstitial Implantation Radiation Therapy:** Interstitial implantation alone is a treatment option for small superficial cancers.
3. **Both External-Beam and Interstitial Implantation Radiation Therapy:** This form of combined radiation is needed for large primary tumors and/or bulky nodal metastases.

Chemotherapy

Knowledge of the following chemotherapy-associated topics is important for patient care:

1. Chemotherapy schedules
2. Chemotherapy vascular access
3. Chemotherapy choices

Chemotherapy Schedules

For provision of dental care during chemotherapy, it is always important to know the patient's chemotherapy schedule and the terms used to describe the schedules. Some of the terms used are:

1. **Chemotherapy cycle:** A chemotherapy cycle represents one treatment. Usually the treatment consists of multiple cycles.
2. **Chemotherapy frequency:** Frequency defines the rate at which chemotherapy is given. The frequency can be monthly, weekly, or continuous.

Chemotherapy Vascular Access

Multiple (four in all) vascular accesses are established **prior** to the start of chemotherapy. The reason multiple accesses are established is that if one line gets infected, it has to be removed and another line gets inserted. To create a new access during chemotherapy is not possible because of tissue scarring. Two jugulars and two subclavial vascular lines are needed for blood draws.

Presence of a vascular access requires that you premedicate the patient prior to dental treatment.

Chemotherapy Choices

Chemotherapeutic choices are determined by identifying the cycle specificity and the phase specificity:

1. **Cycle nonspecific choice:** Corticosteroid is the cycle nonspecific choice drug.
2. **Cycle-specific, phase-nonspecific:** Alkylating agents are the cycle-specific, phase-nonspecific choices.
3. **Cycle-specific, phase-specific:** Antimetabolites are the cycle- and phase-specific choices.

BONE MARROW TRANSPLANT (BMT)

Bone marrow transplant is another option available for cancer care. High-dose chemotherapy, usually 10 times the normal dose is needed for BMT. Stem cells used are taken from the patient or from a donor.

In donor cells BMT, one can get a host-graft in which the donor cells see the cancer cells as bad and attack it.

Posttransplant immunosuppression is always needed to prevent rejection.

Bone Marrow Transplant Complications

Significant complications associated with bone marrow transplantation are: xerostomia, mucositis, and infections: fungal, viral, or bacterial infections and graft versus host disease.

Graft versus host disease is an adverse reaction wherein donor cells attack the healthy cells of the host. The right thing to happen with BMT is for donor cells to see tumor cells as bad and attack them. This is the graft versus tumor attack.

IMPORTANT HEAD AND NECK CANCER FACTS

Most head and neck cancers are of the squamous cell variety. Patient factors and local expertise influence the choice of treatment. When the tumor invades the vasculature, the prognosis is bad. Leukoplakia as a descriptive term indicates a white patch that does not rub off. Early cancers of the buccal mucosa are equally curable by radiation therapy or by adequate excision. The treatment options for lip and oral cavity cancer may be surgery alone; radiation therapy alone; or a combination of surgery, radiation, and chemotherapy.

Larger cancers require composite resection with reconstruction of the defect by pedicle flaps. Moderate excisions of tongue, even hemiglossectomy, often results in little speech disability. With extensive tongue resection there can be problems with aspiration, difficulty swallowing, and speech difficulties.

Patients who **smoke** while on radiation therapy have **lower** response and survival rates, and patients should be counseled to stop smoking before starting radiation therapy. Additionally, poor oral hygiene and tobacco or alcohol use during radiation can accelerate the onset of ORN.

Be aware that patients with head and neck cancers have an **increased incidence** of developing a **second** primary tumor of the upper aerodigestive tract.

Surgery for parotid tumor can lead to **facial paralysis** because the facial nerve goes through the gland.

Dental status evaluation should be performed **prior** to radiation or chemotherapy. Prosthodontic rehabilitation posttreatment is implemented for better quality of life.

Head and Neck Cancer Therapy Localized and Systemic Complications

Localized and systemic complications associated with head and neck cancer therapy are mucositis, xerostomia, xerostomia-associated rampant caries and periodontal disease, infection (viral, fungal, and bacterial), pain, nausea and vomiting, malnutrition, deformity, trismus, microvascular injury, osteoradionecrosis, bone marrow suppression, and death.

HEAD AND NECK CANCERS AND DENTISTRY

Dentistry in a patient with a current or past history of head and neck cancer has to be a well-thought-out, planned process. Several aspects associated with the cancer care have to be evaluated **prior** to implementation of dentistry.

Head and neck radiation therapy causes short- and long-term side effects. Short-term side effects associated with radiation therapy are

1. Mucositis and mucosal infections
2. Altered salivary gland function

Mucositis usually begins by the **third week** of radiation and it presents as an inflammation or ulceration of the oral mucosa. Patients suffering from mucositis often benefit from using a mouthwash prepared as follows: Mix 2 tsp salt and 2 tsp baking soda in 8 oz cold water. The patient should gargle and expectorate the mixture.

Altered salivary gland function causes xerostomia, and xerostomia in turn leads to oral candidiasis. It is absolutely necessary to avoid alcohol-based mouth rinses at this time because further drying of the oral mucosa can occur.

The long-term side effects of radiation occur because of progressive vascular and cellular changes in the bones and soft tissue. There is slow remodeling of the bone and soft tissue, and this leads to necrosis and an increased rate of infection. Salivary gland damage and increased fibrosis also occurs.

The hallmark features of long-term radiation-associated side effects are hypoxic, hypovascular, and hypocellular tissues, the classic "3H's." These side effects **worsen with time**, and this fact **must always** be factored in and appropriately addressed during patient care.

Provide an antibiotic coverage starting 1 hr prior to dentistry and prescribe penicillin VK or clindamycin for 5 days postop to promote the healing process and prevent the occurrence of any infection.

OSTEORADIONECROSIS (ORN)

Osteoradionecrosis is a serious consequence of radiation to the head and neck region. **Lifelong** risk exists with high doses of radiation, and invasive surgical procedures such as extractions and periodontal surgery should be avoided with high doses of radiation.

Necrosis is **more pronounced** and the healing is **more depressed** as the postradiation time interval increases. The bone becomes susceptible to infection and the ability to repair is compromised.

The mandible is most commonly affected because the bone density is high and the vascularization is poor. Patients receiving radiation for tumors anatomically related to the mandible develop necrosis five times more frequently than patients with tumors at other sites.

ORN is more common in the anterior part of the mandible due to limited vascular supply. Osteoradionecrosis of the maxilla is rare.

Radiation by implants is more often associated with osteoradionecrosis compared to radiation from an external source. Consultation with the radiologist **prior** to dentistry is therefore a must to determine the duration and type of radiation planned or given. The radiologist will inform you whether radioactive implant or external beam radiotherapy is planned or was used. The consult will also provide the location and size of the treatment fields plus the total radiation dose.

When the radiation dose has been <6,500 rads, extractions, when required postradiation, should be done **1 year after** radiation, using antibiotic coverage. Usually penicillin or clindamycin can be given for 5 days to promote the healing process.

A radiation dose >6,500 rads/65 Gy is associated with an increased incidence of osteoradionecrosis. If a patient has to have extractions after having undergone radiation to the head and neck region using doses **>6,500** rads, hyperbaric O_2 therapy is strongly suggested.

The patient has to have hyperbaric O_2 dives or treatment cycles during the preop and postop time period. 100% O_2 is provided at 2–2.5 atmospheres of pressure for 90 min per dive, to prevent osteoradionecrosis. The patient needs up to 20 dives prior to surgery and 10 dives after surgery for a good outcome.

Hyperbaric O_2 treatment stimulates tissue angiogenesis in the hypovascular irradiated tissue. Intermittent high O_2 tissue levels stimulate fibroblasts to secrete a collagen matrix, which capillaries follow during angiogenesis, and this leads to more fibroblastic activity. The cost for each dive is $500–700.

It should be clear that to prevent problems postradiation, nonrestorable teeth should be extracted at least **2 weeks prior** to radiation so healing can occur.

CHEMOTHERAPY-ASSOCIATED LOCALIZED AND SYSTEMIC SIDE EFFECTS

Chemotherapy-associated side effects are discussed in the following sections.

Myelosuppression

Myelosuppression occurs for 10–14 days following chemotherapy, when there is a *drop* in the blood counts. As discussed earlier, this pattern of myelosuppression also occurs with radiotherapy. Low WBC increases the potential for infection; low RBC causes anemia and low platelets are associated with easy bruising and bleeding. Thus, dental intervention is not recommended during the first 2 weeks following chemotherapy/radiotherapy.

Fever and Oral Infections

Fever may have an oral origin in chemotherapy patients. Immunosuppressed patients usually have less swelling, pain and fever, so it makes it harder to detect an infection. Always be vigilant and treat all infections aggressively and completely.

As mentioned earlier, conventional symptoms and signs associated with infections are usually absent because of decreased immunity during chemotherapy. Oral flora is different compared to the normal patient and anaerobic organisms abound. Broad-spectrum systemic antibiotics are usually administered. Generally Carbenicillin, a semi-synthetic penicillin is used. Carbenicillin, 1–2 tablets q6h for 5–7 days or aminoglycosides Gentamycin or Tobramycin are prescribed.

Graft Versus Host Disease

Graft versuss host disease is seen more if the patient has periodontal disease and it can last for years in severe cases.

Organ Damage

Chemotherapeutic agent toxicity can sometimes adversely affect the liver and the kidneys.

Neurotoxicity

Neurotoxicity can cause the patient to experience persistent deep aching and burning pain. A certain class of drugs, vancomycins and alkaloids, are more commonly associated with these side effects. Benzodiazepines are usually prescribed, when possible, to control the discomfort.

Integument Involvement

Integument involvement results in mucositis, diarrhea, nausea, vomiting, and alopecia. Mucositis when present should be treated with lidocaine + Benadryl + Maalox rinse. An antifungal rinse should also be given to prevent superinfection.

Toothache

The patient can experience dental discomfort that **mimics** a toothache. It is important therefore to evaluate and treat the patient's dental needs **before** starting chemotherapy.

SUGGESTED DENTAL GUIDELINES OF THE CHEMOTHERAPY- AND/OR RADIOTHERAPY-TREATED HEAD AND NECK CANCER PATIENT

Follow these guidelines:

1. The dentist must intervene in the chemotherapy/radiotherapy schedule with minimal disruption and work as a team.
2. The dentist must consult with the oncologist and do so frequently when needed.
3. Chemotherapy is given in cycles as discussed earlier and one cycle equals one treatment. The treatment can be continuous, weekly, or monthly. Determine the patient's chemotherapy schedule and plan the dental treatment during weeks 3 and 4.
4. The majority of cancer patients receiving chemotherapeutic agents have an **Infusaport or a Hickmann Venous** access for administration of the drugs. Use **SBE prophylaxis** when providing dental treatment in these patients.
5. All head and neck radiation patients **and** 75% of the blood and bone marrow transplant patients are patients at risk for oral complications. 40% of chemotherapy patients have a higher rate of myelosuppression.
6. Bone marrow transplant (BMT) patients have an increased incidence of host versus graft disease if periodontal disease is present. Transplant patients must have dental assessment and care **before** transplant.
7. Always determine the platelet count, absolute neutrophil count (ANC), and PT/INR prior to dentistry in these patients. Calculate the ANC and follow the ANC guidelines if the WBC count is ≤3,500 cells/mm^3. Counts are highest prior to the next cycle so obtain blood tests **within 24 hr** of providing treatment.

You can treat a patient with an ANC as low as 500 cells/mm³ in the outpatient dental setting, with adequate antibiotic use. Patients with an ANC <500 cells/mm³ need to be hospitalized. You can treat a patient with platelets as low as 50 K.

8. The WBC count can decrease with radiation/chemotherapy, and the count is lowest during the first 2 weeks after treatment. The counts begin to rise during the 3rd to 4th week posttreatment period. Any emergent dental work, when needed, should therefore be done in weeks 3–4, posttreatment.

9. Educate the patient about the importance of hygiene and good home care. Treat all sources of oral infection **prior** to chemotherapy, radiotherapy, or bone marrow transplant. It is critical to treat periodontal disease early and conservatively. To minimize complications, do not introduce new practices.

10. Before chemotherapy or radiation therapy, do caries control, control all lesions, complete all dental needs, and provide fluoride trays.

11. **Fluoride care:** Prescription-strength fluoride toothpastes and varnish are better than rinses during chemotherapy or radiotherapy, but there is low patient compliance with these products. Fewer root caries occur with fluoride use. Fluoride increases mineralization and this decreases associated mucositis.

12. Dental extractions in the field of radiation should be done **prior** to radiation if the teeth are nonrestorable, need excessive restoration, or need periodontal or endodontic treatment. Also remove orthodontic bands when present.

13. Treat pericoronitis or deep periodontal pockets immediately. Do scaling and root planing and prescribe metronidazole (Flagyl) treatment for 5 days.

14. For deep pockets, dental minocycline (Arestin) is placed in the pockets and repeated weekly until the condition resolves.

15. Prescribe the nonalcoholic (alcohol prevents mucositis from healing) chlorhexidine rinse bid to degerm the oral cavity and schedule frequent recalls. Also have the patient use a nonalcoholic mouth rinse prior to treatment.

16. **Trismus:** Fibrosis around the muscles of mastication can cause trismus. The patient must be advised to open and close the mouth frequently during the entire radiation period.

17. **Sedation:** The patient should be provided with sedation for dental procedures.

18. **Analgesics:** The following pain management options should be used when needed: codeine alone or in combination with Tylenol can be given q4–6 h. Additionally, morphine, meperidine (Demerol), or a fentanyl patch may also be used.

19. **Vomiting during chemotherapy:** Advise the patient to rinse with the following mixture: Add 1/4 tsp baking soda and 1/8 tsp salt to 1 cup warm water and rinse several times a day. Each mixture use should be followed by rinsing with plain water.

CHEMOTHERAPY- OR RADIOTHERAPY-ASSOCIATED ORAL LESIONS OR SIDE EFFECTS AND SUGGESTED MANAGEMENT GUIDELINES (TABLE 51.2)

Mucositis

Mucositis Overview

Mucositis is associated with white ropy thickening of the mucosa and formation of a pseudomembrane. When this membrane sloughs off, large areas of raw underlying tissue get exposed, causing extreme pain that needs IV morphine for control. Burned tissue from radiation appears red, and tissue turnover occurs every 5 days.

Table 51.2. Summary of chemotherapy- or radiotherapy-associated oral lesions or side effects and suggested management guidelines

Oral Side effects	Prescriptions
Mild Mucositis	**Alkaline saline:** Use 2% sodium bicarbonate in Normal Saline as mouth rinse q4h. **Hydrogen Peroxide (Peroxyl) rinse:** In the presence of dried mucus, rinse with 1.5% H_2O_2 in mint base. Use Peroxyl **first** and then alkaline saline rinse. **Mouthwash mixture for Mucositis:** Swish with 5 cc of a mouthwash mixture consisting of 4 oz Diphenhydramine (Benadryl) elixir + 1 oz Nystatin + 1500 mg Tetracycline + 60 mg Hydrocortisone + 7 oz Water. Add 10 cc **Nystatin (Nilstat)** PO tid if thrush is present and avoid spicy foods.
Moderate Mucositis: The patient has ulcers but can eat.	**Hydrogen Peroxide (Peroxyl) rinse:** Use Hydrogen Peroxide (Peroxyl) rinse diluted 1:1 followed with copious amounts of alkaline saline rinses for general care. **Phenol (Ulcerease):** Swish and hold 5–10 cc topical Phenol mouth rinse (Ulcerease) for 30 sec PRN to alleviate ulcer pain. Follow with mouthwash mixture for mucositis, as specified under mild mucositis.
Severe Mucositis: The patient has severe ulcerations and is not able to eat.	Treatment is the same as with moderate mucositis, plus: **Mylanta-Lidocaine-Benadryl Paste:** A paste consisting of 3 parts Mylanta, 2% viscous Lidocaine and 1 part Diphenhydramine (Benadryl) can be applied over the ulcers. **Consider IV nutrition** supplementation if unable to eat.
Xerostomia Treatment Please see Chapter 48, "Therapeutic Management of Oral Lesions in the Immune-Competent and the Immune-Compromised Patient in the Dental Setting," for more complete prescription details.	**Give sialogogues** 1 h prior to radiotherapy to spare some of the salivary glands. **Xylitol:** Xylitol is a natural sugar substitute that increases saliva flow and does not promote caries. Xylitol actually decreases caries. Use Xylitol following meals after rinsing, 3–5 times/day and use it in place of chewing gum or candy. **Mouth guards and sonic toothbrush:** Recommend mouth guards and sonic toothbrush use because they increase saliva flow. **Chlorhexidine (Peridex) rinse:** Rinse and expectorate with nonalcoholic, 0.12% Chlorhexidine (Peridex) gargles bid. This helps tremendously and degerms the oral cavity. **Lubricants:** Saliva flow can also be increased with lubricants like vitamin E or borage seed oil to decrease discomfort. **Gene therapy:** Gene therapy–associated insertion of Aquoporin-1 helps increase saliva flow and overcome xerostomia.
Herpes Simplex/Herpes Zoster Please see Chapter 48 for more complete prescription details.	Provide prophylactic treatment with antiviral medications **Valacyclovir (Valtrex) or Acyclovir (Zovirax)** to prevent complication during treatment.

Table 51.2. *Continued*

Oral Side effects	Prescriptions
Oral/Esophageal Candidiasis Please see Chapter 48 for more complete prescription details.	**Topical antifungal therapy:** **Clotrimazole cream:** Clotrimazole cream is good for angular cheilitis. **Nystatin oral suspension:** Nystatin rinse is preferred because the mouth is dry during cancer treatment. **Clotrimazole troche:** Clotrimazole troche is **not** the first drug of choice because it does not dissolve well in a dry mouth. **Systemic antifungal therapy:** 1. **Fluconazole:** Consider Fluconazole if the patient is unable to keep up with home care. It should not be the first choice because Fluconazole can affect the liver and the patient can develop resistance to the drug. 2. **Itraconazole (Sporanox):** 20 mL of Sporanox liquid or 200 mg bid, Sporanox capsules. 3. **Amphotericin B IV:** If all else fails, use IV Amphotericin B.
Trismus	Teach stretching exercises and provide mechanical devices like Therabite or stacked popsicle sticks.
Vomiting with Chemotherapy	Add 1/4 tsp of baking soda and 1/8 tsp salt to 1 cup of warm water and rinse several times a day. Then rinse with plain water, each time.

There can be DNA injury from chemotherapy or radiation. This leads to clonogenic cell death associated with destruction of the tissues, which then become an open window for infection.

Ragged restorations and sharp teeth can cut the mucosa. Oral bleeding because of low platelets can occur due to chemotherapy or bone marrow transplant.

Mild Mucositis

The patient has erythematous areas of burn or white plaques that can be treated with the following: **Mild mucositis prescriptions:**

1. **Alkaline saline rinse:** Use 2% sodium bicarbonate in Normal Saline (NS) as mouth rinse q4h.
2. **Hydrogen peroxide (Peroxyl) rinse:** With the presence of dried mucus, rinse with 1.5% H_2O_2 hydrogen peroxide (Peroxyl) in mint base **first** and then use the alkaline saline rinse.
3. **Prepared mouthwash for mucositis:** Swish with 5 cc of a mouthwash mixture consisting of the following: Mix 4 oz diphenhydramine (Benadryl) elixir **plus** 1 oz nystatin **plus** 1500 mg Tetracycline **plus** 60 mg Hydrocortisone **plus** 7 oz water. Add 10 cc nystatin (Nilstat) liquid, PO tid if thrush is present and avoid spicy foods.

Moderate Mucositis

With moderate mucositis the patient has ulcers but can eat.
Moderate mucositis prescriptions:

1. **Hydrogen peroxide (Peroxyl) rinse:** Use hydrogen peroxide (Peroxyl) diluted 1:1 followed with copious amounts of alkaline saline rinses for general care, as with mild mucositis.
2. **Phenol (Ulcerease) mouth rinse:** Have the patient swish and hold 5–10 cc of topical phenol mouth rinse (Ulcerease) for 30 sec PRN to alleviate pain from ulcers.
3. **Prepared mouthwash for mucositis:** Follow with use of prepared mouthwash mixture specified under mild mucositis.

Severe Mucositis

The patient with severe mucositis has severe ulcerations and is not able to eat.
  Severe mucositis prescriptions:

1. Treatment for severe mucositis is the same as for moderate mucositis.
2. **Mylanta-Lidocaine-Benadryl paste:** The paste is applied over the ulcers to numb the pain and it is prepared by mixing the following: Mix 3 parts Mylanta **plus** 2% viscous lidocaine **plus** 1 part diphenhydramine (Benadryl).
3. **IV nutrition:** Consider IV nutrition supplementation in cases where the patient is unable to eat because of the severe mucositis.

Xerostomia

Saliva and Xerostomia Facts

Saliva is medically necessary for optimal health of the oral cavity. Severe abrasion and attrition of tissues can occur with xerostomia. Patients can have toothbrush abrasion and caries at the same time because of xerostomia.

  Provide treatment with fluoride, lubrication, or sialogogue to prevent adverse effects associated with xerostomia. Fluoride acts as a catalyst for remineralization.

Consequences of Reduced Saliva

Reduced saliva flow can be associated with the following:

1. There is increased incidence of infection, either candidiasis or periodontal disease or both.
2. Loss of remineralization is responsible for the very high incidence of caries among these patients compared with the normal population.
3. Decreased lubrication causes difficulty speaking and trouble swallowing.
4. Xerostomia creates an acidic environment.
5. There is poor stability of dentures.
6. Poor salivation is also associated with mucositis, ulcerations, halitosis, altered taste, and sleeping problems.

Xerostomia Prevention During Radiotherapy

Prevention includes the following:

1. Use of computer-assisted 3-D confocal radiation (IMRT) during radiotherapy helps reduce destruction of the salivary glands as it varies the shape and intensity of radiation.
2. Give sialogogues **1 hr prior** to radiotherapy to spare some of the salivary glands from destruction. Once the glands are destroyed they cannot regenerate.

Xerostomia Prescriptions

Chemotherapy- or radiotherapy-associated xerostomia can be corrected with the following:

1. **Xylitol:** Xylitol is a natural sugar substitute that increases saliva flow and does not promote caries. Xylitol actually decreases caries. Use Xylitol following meals after rinsing, 3–5 times/day, and use it in place of chewing gum or candy.
2. **Mouth guards and sonic toothbrush:** Recommend mouth guards and sonic toothbrush use because they increase saliva flow.
3. **Chlorhexidine (Peridex) rinse:** Rinse and expectorate with nonalcoholic, 0.12% chlorhexidine (Peridex) gargles bid. This helps tremendously and degerms the oral cavity.
4. **Lubricants:** Saliva flow can also be increased with lubricants such as vitamin E or borage seed oil to decrease discomfort.
5. **Gene Therapy:** Gene therapy–associated insertion of Aquoporin-1 helps increase saliva flow and overcome xerostomia.

Infections

Herpes Simplex/Herpes Zoster

The virus can be reactivated during radiation and shows up in unusual places. It is best to provide prophylactic treatment with antiviral medications, valacyclovir (Valtrex) or acyclovir (Zovirax), to prevent complication in the midst of treatment.

Candidiasis

Candidiasis has many presentations, and if caught early it is easier to treat. In the neutropenic patient, systemic spread of candidiasis can lead to death.

Topical Antifungal Therapy

Use the following for topical antifungal therapy:

1. **Clotrimazole cream:** Clotrimazole cream is good for angular cheilitis.
2. **Nystatin oral suspension:** Nystatin rinse is **preferred** because the mouth is dry during cancer treatment.
3. **Clotrimazole troche:** Clotrimazole troche is **not** the first drug of choice because it does not dissolve well in a dry mouth.

Systemic Antifungal Therapy

Use the following for systemic therapy:

1. **Fluconazole:** Fluconazole is an option to consider if the patient is unable to keep up with home care. It should not be the first choice, because Fluconazole can affect the liver and the patient can develop resistance to the drug.
2. **Itraconazole (Sporanox):** 20 mL of Sporanox liquid or 200 mg Sporanex capsules is dispensed bid.
3. **Amphotericin B IV:** If all fails, the patient is put on IV Amphotericin B.

With all three preparations, continue treatment for at least 2 weeks until the condition is eradicated. The infection is very hard to treat and comes back easily when the patient does not have proper saliva.

If the saliva is low, infections can get precipitated in the salivary ducts causing stones and blockage. The patient is treated with doxycycline when this occurs.

Trismus

Trismus Definition

Trismus is restricted opening of the mouth, and it often is secondary to surgery.

Fibrosis due to radiation treatment has an effect on the muscles of mastication and it occurs 6–12 months after radiation.

Trismus causes problems with chewing, and it is difficult to do dentistry in the presence of trismus.

Trismus Treatment

Treatment consists of teaching stretching exercises and providing mechanical devices such as Therabite or stacked Popsicle sticks.

LEUKEMIA

Leukemia or liquid cancer of the blood and bone marrow can present as, acute lymphoblastic/lymphocytic leukemia, chronic lymphocytic leukemia, acute myelocytic leukemia, or chronic myelocytic leukemia.

Acute Leukemias Overview

The acute forms of leukemia are associated with rapid accumulation of dysfunctional, immature cells in the blood and the bone marrow and an associated reduction in the number of normal, functioning, mature white blood cells.

In addition to the inadequate number of normal white blood cells, there is often an associated reduction in the number of red blood cell and platelet production. Thus, increased susceptibility to infection, anemia, and platelet deficiency–associated bleeding; bruising; and petechiae are often seen in patients suffering from the acute forms of leukemia.

Chronic Leukemias Overview

The chronic forms of leukemia progress slowly and consequently the bone marrow is able to produce more mature functional cell lines. The patient is less symptomatic and it is not uncommon for the leukemia to be accidentally detected on routine examination.

Leukemia Prevalence

Leukemia affects males more than females and patients of African descent are more likely to be affected, compared to those of European descent.

Acute Lymphoblastic Leukemia (ALL) is the most common form of leukemia affecting children ages 0–19 years, and ALL is now considered a curable cancer in the majority of patients affected by the disease.

Acute myelogenous leukemia (AML) and chronic lymphocytic leukemia (CLL) are the most common forms of leukemia affecting adults. Chronic myelogenous leukemia (CML) affects people above age 60.

AML, CML, and CLL are most common in the 7th, 8th, and 9th decades of life. Leukemias thus occur more commonly in the elderly, after age 60.

Leukemia Symptoms and Signs

Symptoms and signs associated with acute leukemia reflect the lack of normal levels of WBCs, RBCs, and platelets. The patient experiences anemia-associated fatigue, pallor and decreased ability to perform routine chores; platelet deficiency–associated mucosal bleeding, petechiae, easy bruising, easy bleeding, plus increased susceptibility to infection and poor wound healing due to the decreased number of mature, normal, functioning WBCs.

Chronic leukemia in many patients is often asymptomatic and is an accidental discovery during routine medical examination.

Leukemia Diagnosis

Leukemia diagnosis is made by pathological examination of the peripheral smear and the bone marrow aspirate.

Leukemia Treatment Terminology

A dental provider helps manage the oral side effects caused from leukemia and also helps maintain ongoing oral health for optimal outcome. It thus becomes important to clearly understand leukemia remission and leukemia relapse, as discussed in the following sections.

Leukemia Remission

With remission, treatment causes complete recovery of the blood and bone marrow to normal and the patient becomes fully functional. Palliative and supportive dental intervention is done during the acute stage, and subsequently the patient is kept on 4–6 months maintenance recall to access ongoing status.

Leukemia Relapse

Relapse is a return of the leukemia and abnormal cells are seen again in the circulation and the bone marrow. Palliative and supportive dental intervention is done during the acute and relapse stages, and maintenance is provided if recovery occurs subsequently after the relapse.

Leukemia Treatment

When there is **complete remission for 5 years** after treatment, the acute forms of leukemia are said to be cured. The 5-year survival rate has improved for all forms of leukemia.

Treatment Protocols

Discussed in the next sections are treatment protocols for the following:

1. Acute Lymphoblastic Leukemia (ALL)
2. Acute Myeloid Leukemia (AML)

ACUTE LYMPHOBLASTIC LEUKEMIA (ALL) TREATMENT PROTOCOL

Treatment options offered for ALL depend on the patient's age and the health status at the time of diagnosis.

The treatment protocol for ALL is a **3-step** process:

1. Induction chemotherapy
2. Consolidation chemotherapy
3. Maintenance chemotherapy

ALL Induction Chemotherapy

Induction chemotherapy is usually done with daunorubicin, vincristine, prednisone, asparaginase, and occasionally cyclophosphamide (Cytoxan).

Neupogen, red cell and/or platelet transfusion are often used as adjunct supports to compensate for the associated lack of functioning WBCs, RBCs, and platelets.

ALL Consolidation Chemotherapy

The consolidation chemotherapy follows the induction chemotherapy. The patient is given multiple cycles of intensive chemotherapy for a period of 6–9 months.

ALL Maintenance Chemotherapy

The third step of ALL care is the maintenance chemotherapy that is done with oral chemotherapeutic drugs for a period of 18–24 months.

ACUTE MYELOID LEUKEMIA (AML) TREATMENT PROTOCOL

Treatment of AML consists of the following:

1. Remission induction
2. Consolidation

AML Remission Induction Therapy

Intensive chemotherapy is provided over 1 week, to induce remission with two chemotherapy drugs, Cytarabine (ara-C) and daunorubicin/idarubicin (Daunomycin, Idamycin). Occasionally a third drug, 6-Thioguanine, may be added.

AML Consolidation Therapy

Consolidation therapy follows remission induction therapy. It is provided by using multiple cycles of the drug Cytarabine (ara-C). This form of therapy is used to destroy any remaining leukemia cells and prevent relapse.

Leukemia and Suggested Dental Guidelines

Follow the same guidelines as those discussed under head and neck cancers.

HODGKIN'S LYMPHOMA

Hodgkin's Lymphoma Overview

Hodgkin's and non-Hodgkin's lymphomas are common cancers of the lymphatic system; Hodgkin's lymphoma is less common in occurrence than non-Hodgkin's lymphoma. Early diagnosis and excellent treatment options available are responsible for the significantly lower death rates today with Hodgkin's lymphoma. Hodgkin's lymphoma is now considered a highly treatable disease.

Hodgkin's Lymphoma Pathophysiology

B cell dysfunction results in accumulation of abnormal B cells. The abnormal B cells also called *Reed-Sternberg cells*, are responsible for the occurrence of the malignancy.

Hodgkin's Lymphoma Risk Factors

Risk factors associated with Hodgkin's lymphoma are:

1. **Sex:** Males are more affected than females.
2. **Age:** Patients age 15–40 years and beyond 55 are more prone to develop the malignancy.
3. **Immune status:** Reduced immunity from HIV/AIDS, chemotherapy, radiotherapy, or organ transplant increases the susceptibility to Hodgkin's lymphoma.
4. **Family history:** Family history of Hodgkin's lymphoma increases the risk for Hodgkin's in another member of the family.
5. **Infection:** Past history of infectious mononucleosis can predispose to the development of Hodgkin's lymphoma.

Hodgkin's Lymphoma Symptoms and Signs

The patient usually presents with tiredness, weakness, fatigue, night sweats, anorexia, weight loss, and flulike symptoms.

These symptoms are associated with an **organized**, progressive, **painless** enlargement of the lymph glands in the visible areas of the body, such as the neck, axilla, or groin. Lymph glands in the nonvisible areas, such as the thoracic cavity and the abdomen, can also be affected.

Hodgkin's Lymphoma Diagnosis

Diagnosis is confirmed with demonstration of the Reed-Sternberg cells on examination of a lymph node biopsy specimen.

Complete blood count (CBC), bone marrow biopsy, computerized tomography (CT) scan, radiographs, magnetic resonance imaging (MRI), and positron emission tomography (PET) scans are additional tools that can assist with the diagnosis of Hodgkin's lymphoma.

Hodgkin's Lymphoma Staging

The extent of tissue involvement or spread of Hodgkin's lymphoma defines the disease stage. The I-IV staging helps with determination of treatment options available for the patient. Stage I and Stage II have the best 10-year survival rates.

Hodgkin's Lymphoma Stage I: Only one set of lymph nodes are involved with this stage.

Hodgkin's Lymphoma Stage II: Two sets of lymph nodes in one given area, either above or below the diaphragm, are affected during this stage.

Hodgkin's Lymphoma Stage III: Lymph nodes above and below the diaphragm are affected with total sparing of all organ involvement.

Hodgkin's Lymphoma Stage IV: This stage has all the findings of Stage III plus involvement of the liver and/or the bone marrow.

Hodgkin's Lymphoma Treatment

Treatment options include

1. **Radiation therapy:** Radiation therapy alone is reserved for Stage I Hodgkin's lymphoma. More commonly, however, radiation in combination with chemotherapy is used to completely eradicate the cancer.
2. **Combined chemotheraphy:** Combined chemotherapy is the best option for progressive disease and the preferred treatment of choice is Mechlorethamine, Oncovin, Procarbazine, and prednisone (MOPP).
3. **Bone marrow transplant (BMT):** BMT is an option used for recurrent cases of Hodgkin's lymphoma.

Hodgkin's Lymphoma and Suggested Dental Guidelines

The suggested dental guidelines for Hodgkin's lymphoma are the same as those discussed collectively for head and neck cancers.

NON-HODGKIN'S LYMPHOMA (NHL)

NHl Pathophysiology

NHL can be a B or T cell-associated cancer and more than 30 different types of non-Hodgkin's lymphomas have been identified.

NHLs can be aggressive or of the slow-growing type. NHL has a greater tendency to go toward extranodal sites compared to Hodgkin's lymphoma. Thus, the treatment options and outcomes of care depend on the aggressive or nonaggressive nature of the cancer.

Aggressive NHLs occur more commonly in the HIV/AIDS patients, and Burkitt's lymphoma is an example of a B cell lymphoma.

Non-Hodgkin's Lymphoma Etiology

Non-Hodgkin's lymphoma can occur at any age, but it is more common in individuals above age 60.

Infectious mononucleosis, H. pylori infection, malaria, and decreased immunity from HIV/AIDS or organ transplant are all risk factors increasing the incidence of non-Hodgkin's lymphoma.

Non-Hodgkin's Lymphoma Symptoms and Signs

Symptoms and signs associated with NHL are the same as with Hodgkin's lymphoma.

Non-Hodgkin's Lymphoma Diagnosis

The diagnostic criteria (x-rays, scans and biopsy) are also the same as with Hodgkin's lymphoma.

Non-Hodgkin's Lymphoma Staging

NHL staging is also the same as with Hodgkin's lymphoma.

Non-Hodgkin's Lymphoma Treatment

There are two NHL Treatment options available:

1. Treatment as outlined for Hodgkin's lymphoma
2. Newer forms of NHL treatment

Treatment as Outlined for Hodgkin's Lymphoma

As with Hodgkin's lymphoma, radiation therapy is the option for early, slow-growing/low-grade tumors. Combination chemotherapy is the option for high-grade, aggressive tumors, and bone marrow transplant is the option for recurrent cancers. Radiation and combination chemotherapy, when instituted immediately, can also improve the survival rate in affected patients with early-detected aggressive NHLs. Early-detected low-grade, nonaggressive Stage I and II tumors have the best 10-year survival rates.

Newer Forms of NHL Treatment

The newer forms of NHL treatment are:

1. **Biological treatment:** Rituximab (Rituxan), a type of monoclonal antibody, is used in combination with chemotherapy.
2. **Radioimmunotherapy:** Radioimmunotherapy with ibritumomab (Zevalin) and tositumomab (Bexxar) is used for aggressive and recurrent NHLs.

NHL and Suggested Dental Guidelines

The suggested dental guidelines for NHL are the same as those discussed collectively under head and neck cancers.

MULTIPLE MYELOMA (MM)

Multiple Myeloma is a form of cancer that is associated with a proliferation of malignant plasma cells resulting in an overabundance of monoclonal paraprotein. The exact cause for MM is not known, but genetic predisposition, viruses, chemicals, and exposure to radiation have been implicated as precipitating factors.

To better understand MM, it is important first to discuss the **normal** bone and immunoglobulin production cycles, the **normal** immunoglobulins, and the pathophysiology associated with MM.

Normal Bone Cell Activity

Osteoclasts normally function with bone-forming cells or osteoblasts to rebuild areas of bone that are wearing out. This process is called *bone remodeling*, and healthy bone is continuously being remodeled.

During the normal bone-remodeling process, osteoclasts are attracted to the area of fatigued bone. There they remove the worn out bone by breaking it down and creating a cavity in the bone.

Osteoblasts get attracted to the cavity in the bone. They fill in the cavity with a matrix or framework and eventually new bone forms.

Normally, the activity of the osteoclasts and osteoblasts is well balanced. The osteoclasts clear out the fatigued bones and the osteoblasts begin the rebuilding of new bones immediately.

In patients with multiple myeloma, bone resorption by the osteoclasts is **increased and exceeds** bone reformation. Calcium lost from the bones appears in increasing amounts in the patient's serum and urine. This increase in bone resorption can result in pain, bone fractures, spinal cord compression, and hypercalcemia.

Normal Immunoglobulin Production Cycle

Stem cells from the bone marrow develop into B and T lymphocytes. B cells go on to mature in the lymph nodes and then travel throughout the body. When foreign substances or antigens enter the body, B cells develop into plasma cells that produce immunoglobulins or antibodies that help fight infection and disease. Plasma cells therefore develop from B cells, and it is the **plasma cells** that **produce the antibodies** that help fight infections or diseases.

Immunoglobulins

Every infection or disease triggers its own specific antibody production. With time, the plasma cells produce many different immunoglobulins in the body.

Antibodies or immunoglobulins are made up of two long protein chains called *heavy chains* and two shorter chains called *light chains*. Immunoglobulin light chains are labeled as kappa (κ) or lambda (λ).

Immunoglobulin Types

The five major classes of antibodies or immunoglobulins made by the plasma cells are gamma (IgG), alpha (IgA), mu (IgM), epsilon (IgE), and delta (IgD). IgG is normally present in the largest amounts in blood, followed by IgA and IgM. IgD and IgE are present in very small amounts in the blood.

Malignant Plasma Cells Formation Cycle and Associated Pathophysiology

Multiple genetic abnormalities transform a normal B cell into a malignant plasma cell that continues to divide unchecked, generating more malignant plasma or myeloma cells. The myeloma cells collect in the bone marrow via the blood and cause permanent damage to healthy tissue.

Myeloma plasma cells target the stromal cells of the bone marrow and this triggers an unchecked growth of the myeloma cells.

The myeloma and stromal cells produce cytokines that stimulate the growth of myeloma cells and inhibit natural cell death or apoptosis, causing excess production of MM cells that ultimately cause bone destruction.

Myeloma cells also produce growth factor that promotes angiogenesis or new blood vessels. These new blood vessels provide the nutrition that promotes tumor growth.

Mature myeloma cells often produce substances that decrease the body's normal immune response and, with the defense being down, the cells grow unchecked.

The myeloma cells affect all the large bones of the body, forming multiple small lesions.

Myeloma cells produce an abnormal immunoglobulin protein called *monoclonal* or *M protein*, and these M proteins show up as a spike during electrophoresis.

In addition to the abnormal plasma cells that overwhelm the bone marrow, MM is also associated with an overproduction of Bence Jones proteins that are free monoclonal κ and λ light chains.

The malignant cells lack normal function and cause excess production of immunoglobulins of a single type and reduced numbers of normal immunoglobulins. The abnormal antibody production leads to impaired humoral immunity and an increased incidence of infection. The overproduction of these antibodies may also lead to hyperviscosity, amyloidosis, and renal failure.

The malignant plasma cells additionally cause leukopenia, anemia, and thrombocytopenia.

Multiple Myeloma Prevalence

Multiple myeloma is the second most common blood cancer after non-Hodgkin's lymphoma and it occurs more frequently in men than women.

It occurs most commonly around age 60 and beyond, but some cases do occur in patients under age 40. The median age of occurrence is 68 years for men and 70 years for women.

It is more prevalent in African-Americans and Native Pacific Islanders compared to Asians. Myeloma is one of the leading causes of cancer deaths among African Americans.

Multiple Myeloma Clinical Features

Multiple myeloma can be asymptomatic or insidious in onset. It may be discovered accidentally during routine blood testing because symptoms are uncommon in the early stages of myeloma. When symptoms are present, however, they are often vague and simulate those caused by many other conditions.

Multiple Myeloma–Associated Symptoms and Signs

Amyloid Deposits

Amyloidosis is a rare complication that occurs in patients with light chain myeloma because the light chains can combine with other serum proteins to produce amyloid.

Macroglossia is a common finding in patients with amyloidosis. Bilateral swelling of the shoulder joints secondary to amyloid deposition can cause the shoulder pad sign. The swelling is hard and rubbery.

The amyloid protein may be deposited in the nerves, kidneys, liver, and heart, disrupting the organ's normal functions. Amyloid can also stick to the walls of blood vessels, causing them to lose their elasticity; the patient is then unable to maintain the blood pressure.

Amyloidosis can thus produce neuropathies; low blood pressure; and kidney, heart, or liver failure.

Alert: **Avoid Extra Strength Tylenol, aspirin, NSAIDS, meperidine, and propoxyphene in the presence of kidney disease.**

Anemia and Ecchymosis

Excess production of abnormal plasma cells causes decreased production of normal RBCs, WBCs, and platelets. Patients can present with pallor, ecchymoses, or purpura resulting from thrombocytopenia.

A complete blood count (CBC) will confirm the presence of anemia, thrombocytopenia, or leucopenia.

Fatigue

Anemia causes tiredness, weakness, fatigue, and pallor. Anemia, when present, is treated with erythropoietin and/or transfusions.

Infection

Impaired production of normal immunoglobulins results in an increased susceptibility to viral and bacterial infections. Aggressive treatment is provided with antivirals, antibiotics, and IV immunoglobulin therapy.

Clotting Factor Deficiency–Associated Bleeding

In some patients the monoclonal protein can rarely absorb the clotting factors and cause bleeding.

Blood Hyperviscosity

High protein concentration in the blood causes the blood to become very thick and sticky. This can cause the patient to experience shortness of breath, confusion, and chest pain.

Bone Pain

MM patients experience pain in the ribs or lower back due to tiny fractures of bones weakened with plasma cell infiltration.

Physical therapy, surgical correction of fractures, radiation, and bisphosphonates are treatment options for patients experiencing bone pains.

Osteoporosis

Diffuse osteoporosis involves the pelvis, spine, ribs, and skull.

Hypercalcemia

Excessive bone breakdown causes elevated calcium levels in the blood. The patient can experience tiredness, weakness, fatigue, anorexia, confusion, nausea, vomiting, constipation, increased thirst, and excessive urination.

Hypercalcemia is usually treated with steroids, furosemide, (Lasix), and bisphosphonates.

Renal Damage

The MM patient can experience kidney disease, renal failure or hypercalcemia-associated renal symptoms.

Additionally, the Bence Jones proteins deposit in the kidney causes kidney damage and consequent renal failure.

Cryoglobulinemia

Cryoglobulinemia occurs when the abnormal protein comes out of the solution as particles on exposure to cold temperatures. These particles can block small blood vessels and cause pain, tingling, and numbness in the fingers and toes in cold weather.

Neurological Deficits

Neurologic findings may include sensory changes due to spinal cord compression, weakness, or carpal tunnel syndrome. Nerve impingement associated with collapsing bones is not uncommon with this disease.

Plasmacytomas

Plasmocytomas are soft tissue masses of plasma cells and they are a common finding in myeloma patient.

Skin Lesions

Wax papules or nodules may occur on the back, ears, or lips and the papules are painful.

Multiple Myeloma Types

Overview

The most common types of myeloma are the IgG and IgA types. IgG myeloma accounts for about 60–70% of all cases of myeloma, and IgA accounts for about 20% of cases. A few cases of IgD and IgE myeloma have also been reported.

Multiple Myeloma Classification

The three types of multiple myeloma are:

1. **The M protein myeloma:** This is the classic or the most common type of myeloma that is associated with a high level of M protein in the blood.
2. **Light chain or Bence Jones myeloma**: A small percentage of patients have only the light chain portion of the immunoglobulin called the *Bence Jones proteins*. Bence Jones proteins in these patients are detected by immunoelectrophoresis of the urine.
3. **Nonsecretory myeloma:** This is a rare form of myeloma that affects an extremely small percentage of myeloma patients. The plasma cells in this form **do not** produce M protein or light chains.

Multiple Myeloma Diagnosis

Diagnosis is made with medical evaluation/assessment and bone studies.

Medical Evaluation/Assessment

The presence of anemia and a high serum protein can alert the physician to further evaluate the patient. A diagnosis of multiple myeloma is difficult to make on the basis of any single laboratory test result. Currently, the diagnosis requires one major *and* one minor criterion *or* three minor criteria.

Multiple Myeloma–Associated Major Criteria

The findings classified as major criteria are:

1. A biopsy confirming plasmacytoma
2. A bone marrow aspiration showing 30% plasma cells
3. Elevated monoclonal immunoglobulin levels in the blood or urine

Multiple Myeloma–Associated Minor Criteria

The findings classified as minor criteria are:

1. A bone marrow sample showing 10–30% plasma cells.
2. Minor monoclonal immunoglobulin levels in blood or urine.
3. Imaging studies showing holes in bones due to tumor growth.
4. Normal antibody levels that are abnormally low in the blood.
5. Detection of serum levels of beta-2 microglobulin (β2-M) that reflect the tumor mass and are a standard measure of tumor burden.
6. Detection of C-reactive protein that is a surrogate marker for IL-6, a growth factor for myeloma cells.
7. Quantitive immunoglobulins (QIGs): QIGs measure the levels of different types of antibodies—IgG, IgA, IgM.
8. Serum protein or urine protein electrophoresis (EP): serum/urine protein EP measures the levels of various proteins in the blood or urine, respectively.
9. Immunoelectrophoresis (IEP): IEP also detects the presence of abnormal antibody M protein. IEP helps track the progression of myeloma disease and response to treatment. M protein appears as a spike on electrophoresis.
10. 24-hr urine protein: 24-hr urine protein determination helps stage the patient's status and assess the progression of the disease and the patient's response to treatment.
11. The FREELITE™ Test: A new serum-based assay, FREELITE, helps detect and quantify free light chains.

Bone Studies

The following tests performed on the bone help with the diagnosis of MM:

1. X-rays of affected bone
2. Total body bone survey
3. Magnetic resonance imaging (MRI)
4. Computerized axial tomography
5. Bone marrow biopsy taken from the hip

Multiple Myeloma Treatment

Multiple Myeloma Treatment Overview

The patient can be asymptomatic, minimally symptomatic, or significantly symptomatic with MM. Chemotherapy is the ultimate treatment for MM, and chemotherapy has its own significant side effects. Determination of how debilitating the MM symptoms are for the patient is therefore one way to decide when to begin chemotherapy.

In the initial stages some patients decide to get bisphosphonates for the associated osteoporosis; others prefer supportive care for symptoms and complications.

In all these cases, postponing therapy may help avoid the risk of complications associated with chemotherapy and may also delay development of resistance to chemotherapy.

Multiple Myeloma Treatment Classification

For decisions on treatment, MM patients are classified into one of three myeloma categories:

1. The Monoclonal Gammopathy of Undetermined Significance (MGUS) Category
2. The Asymptomatic Category
3. The Symptomatic Category

The Monoclonal Gammopathy of Undetermined Significance (MGUS) Category

The MGUS category is a common finding among patients suspected of having MM. Patients in this category demonstrate the presence of a monoclonal protein but **no cause** for the increased protein can be identified. There are **no symptoms** and other criteria for myeloma diagnosis are absent.

MGUS occurs in about 1% of the general population and in about 3% of normal individuals over 70 years of age.

MGUS by itself is harmless, but after many years approximately 16% of patients with MGUS progress toward a malignant plasma cell disorder.

The Asymptomatic Multiple Myeloma Category

Patients with asymptomatic multiple myeloma have a monoclonal protein and slightly increased numbers of plasma cells in the bone marrow.

They may have mild anemia and/or a few bone lesions, but they do not exhibit the renal failure and frequent infections that characterize active multiple myeloma.

In these patients the myeloma is static and may not progress for months or years.

Symptomatic Multiple Myeloma (MM)

Patients who present with symptoms typically have a monoclonal protein and increased numbers of plasma cells in the bone marrow. They also have anemia, kidney failure, and hypercalcemia or bone lesions. Patients with symptomatic myeloma require immediate treatment.

Multiple Myeloma Treatment Options

Although patients benefit from treatment, currently there is no cure. The currently available therapies for multiple myeloma are

1. **Chemotherapy:** When therapy is indicated, the patient typically receives chemotherapy. Chemotherapeutic agents are used to reduce the disease burden. Trimethoprim-sulfamethoxazole is commonly used as prophylaxis for P. carinii pneumonia during chemotherapy. The chemotherapy choices offered are:
    a. Melphalan and prednisone (M and P): This is the most commonly used regimen.

    b. Vincristine, bischloroethylnitrosourea, melphalan, cyclophosphamide, and prednisone.

    c. Vincristine, doxorubicin [Adriamycin], and dexamethasone [VAD].

    d. Vincristine, bischloroethylnitrosourea, doxorubicin, and prednisone

2. **Radiotherapy**

3. **Stem cell transplantation**

4. **Thalidomide (Thalomid):** Thalidomide is now often used as first-line therapy either as a single agent or in combination with steroids.

5. **Bisphosphonates:** Zoledronic acid (Zometa) is a very potent bisphosphonate and is commonly used in MM patients.

6. **Erythropoietin:** Erythropoietin corrects the anemia resulting from either myeloma alone or from chemotherapy and has been shown to improve the patient's quality of life.

Multiple Myeloma Suggested Dental Guidelines

Follow these guidelines:

1. Thoroughly assess the patient and note the significant medical history and physical examination findings already discussed.

2. Communicate with the patient's physician to understand the extent of the disease.

3. Evaluate the CBC with differential and platelet counts, PT/INR, serum creatinine, and LFTs, and note vital organ status.

4. Specifically determine the patient's cardiac status by communication with the patient's physician.

5. Incorporate the suggested anemia, thrombocytopenia, ANC, serum creatinine, PT/INR, and LFT guidelines when the tests indicate abnormality. In the presence of neutropenia the patient may need premedication, per ANC guidelines.

6. Always have the patient use a nonalcoholic mouth rinse prior to every dental visit to degerm the oral cavity.

7. Follow stringent asepsis guidelines and treat all infections aggressively.

8. Always check whether the patient has a portacatheter or IV line for chemotherapy. Premedication prophylaxis should be provided when present.

9. Check whether the patient is on bisphosphonates and for how long. Review and follow the bisphosphonates suggested guidelines outlined in Chapter 41, "Parathyroid Dysfunction Disease States: Assessment, Analysis, and Associated Dental Management Guidelines."

10. Significant osteoporosis can cause jaw pains and frequent denture adjustments.

11. Significant neuropathies can shorten chair time or may require adaptation of proper positioning in the chair.

12. **Anesthetics:** The local anesthetic use will be dictated by the extent of anemia or kidney, liver, cardiac diseases, when present.

13. **Analgesics:** Avoid extra strength Tylenol aspirin, NSAIDS, meperidine, and propoxyphene because of the anemia, kidney disease, and/or associated liver disease.

14. **Antibiotics:** The antibiotic use will be dictated by the extent of anemia, kidney disease, or liver disease, when present, and by the PCP prophylaxis, when used. When the patient is on PCP prophylaxis, determine whether the antibiotic used is a cidal or a static antibiotic. The antibiotic you prescribe should preferably match the PCP antibiotic type (cidal with cidal, static with static). Maintain an interval of 6 hr when the two antibiotics are different.

XIX

Psychiatry

Psychiatric Conditions: Assessment of Disease States and Associated Dental Management Guidelines

ANXIETY DISORDERS

Anxiety is a normal healthy reaction to stress and it helps a patient deal with stressful situations. When anxiety becomes excessive or irrational it becomes a disabling disorder. Intensity of symptoms experienced is directly related to the patient's ability to cope.

Anxiety Disorder Classification

The five major types of anxiety disorders are:

1. Generalized anxiety disorder
2. Obsessive-compulsive disorder (OCD)
3. Panic disorder
4. Posttraumatic stress disorder (PTSD)
5. Social phobia or social anxiety disorder

Generalized Anxiety Disorder (GAD)

GAD is associated with excessive, unrealistic anxiety that lasts 6 months or more. These patients also experience trembling, muscle aches, insomnia, bowel movement upsets, dizziness, and irritability.

Obsessive-Compulsive Disorder (OCD)

The OCD patient is plagued by obsessions due to increased anxiety or fears. The obsessions lead the patient to perform a ritual to relieve the anxiety caused by the obsession.

Panic Disorder

Patients with panic disorders go through a phase of extreme anxiety when faced with a specific situation, e.g., fear of heights or closed spaces. They experience severe palpitations, chest discomfort, sweating, trembling, tingling sensations, feeling of choking, fear of dying, and fear of losing control.

Posttraumatic Stress Disorder (PTSD)

PTSD can follow an exposure to a traumatic event, such as an assault of any kind, unexpected death of a family member/spouse, or experiencing a natural disaster.

The patient relives the traumatic event by experiencing flashbacks and nightmares. The patient avoids places related to the trauma and becomes emotionally detached from others. The patient also experiences difficulty sleeping, irritability, and poor concentration. Internal or external stimuli can trigger an attack of PTSD. Drug and alcohol abuse is a **common** occurrence with PTSD.

Social Anxiety Disorder (SAD)

SAD is associated with extreme anxiety about being judged by others or having extreme anxiety about behaving in a way that might cause embarrassment or ridicule. The patient experiences blushing, palpitations, and sweating. Good history-taking will show that the patient starts to avoid situations that will cause SAD.

Treatment of Anxiety Disorders

Anxiety disorders are treated with the following:

1. Psychosocial therapies
2. Medications
3. Both psychosocial therapies and medications

Anxiety Medications

Combination therapies are often utilized in the management of anxiety. Drugs used to treat anxiety disorders are:

1. Benzodiazepines
2. Beta blockers
3. Monoamine oxidase inhibitors (MAOIs): an antidepressant with antianxiety effects
4. Selective serotonin reuptake inhibitors (SSRIs): antidepressants with antianxiety effects
5. Tricyclic antidepressants: antidepressants with antianxiety effects

Anxiety Disorders and Alcohol Abuse

Patients with anxiety and alcohol abuse could present with the following complications:

1. These patients often have poor treatment compliance.
2. They have an increased risk of relapse into alcohol abuse following detoxification.
3. They can have severe drug interactions between prescription medication and alcohol.
4. Patients with social anxiety disorder (SAD), posttraumatic stress disorder (PTSD), generalized anxiety disorder (GAD), and panic disorder often abuse alcohol.
5. Substance abuse or alcohol abuse is treated with group or individual therapy utilizing the 12-step programs used by Alcoholics Anonymous.
6. SSRIs are often prescribed in conjunction with therapy to assist with the recovery process. Common SSRIs prescribed are fluoxetine (Prozac), sertraline (Zoloft), flu-

voxamine (Luvox), paroxetine (Paxil), citalopram (Celexa), and escitalopram (Lexapro).

7. Benzodiazepines should be avoided in these patients as they can increase the risk of abuse, tolerance, and physical dependence.

Anxiety Disorders and Suggested Dental Alerts

The following are dental alerts for anxiety disorders:

1. The anxious individual will tend to be very alert, quite hyperactive, and fidgety in the dental environment. It is best to address the anxiety with the patient before you begin treating the patient.
2. Always establish good communication and trust with these patients. Show genuine concern and offer stress management.
3. $O_2 + N_2O$ or benzodiazepines can be used to control the anxiety with the following precautions: Use benzodiazepines for stress management **only** if the patient is **not** on any medications to control the anxiety or the patient is already on benzodiazepines to control the anxiety. Use $O_2 + N_2O$ for patients on antidepressant medications.
4. An occasional physician may allow the use of low-dose benzodiazepines in conjunction with the patient's antianxiety or antidepressant medications. You are advised, therefore, to always check with the patient's M.D.
5. Benzodiazepine use is contraindicated in the pregnant patient, the elderly patient, the obese patient, the alcoholic patient, the patient on centrally acting drugs, and the patient on H_2 blockers for GERD or peptic ulceration or gastritis. When benzodiazepines have to be used in the presence of H_2 blockers, keep an interval of **2 hr** between both the medications.
6. **Anesthetics:** Avoid epinephrine in the local anesthetic and epinephrine cords in the presence of TCAs and MAO-Is. Epinephrine is not contraindicated with the SSRIs.
7. Patients suffering from anxiety often experience aphthous ulcerations, ulcerative gingivitis, TMJ problems, lichen planus, geographic tongue, and myofacial pain. These conditions should also be additionally addressed in the dental setting.
8. Xerostomia is a genuine concern in patients taking all kinds of antipsychiatric medications. Follow the suggested xerostomia management guidelines in Chapter 48, "Therapeutic Management of Oral Lesions in the Immune-Competent and the Immune-Compromised Patient in the Dental Setting."
9. Antipsychiatric medications cause postural hypotension. Assist the patient out of the chair to prevent a fall or collapse.

Anesthetics, analgesics, and stress management summary: Avoid sedatives, epinephrine (except with SSRIs), narcotic analgesics, sedating antihistamines, and epinephrine cords with antipsychiatric medications.

MOOD DISORDERS: DEPRESSION

Depression is a condition where a patient feels sad, hopeless, and/or disinterested in life in general. Depression is an illness that affects the way a person thinks, feels, behaves, and functions.

When these feelings last for more than 2 weeks and when the feelings interfere with daily living, it is called a *major depressive episode.*

Major Depressive Episode Symptoms

Symptoms experienced are persistent sadness, hopelessness, pessimism, worthlessness, decreased energy, fatigue, difficulty concentrating and making decisions, insomnia, early-morning awakening or oversleeping, decreased appetite and/or weight loss, overeating and weight gain, thoughts of death or suicide, suicide attempts, restlessness, and irritability.

The patient experiences persistent physical symptoms such as headaches, digestive disorders, and pain for which no other cause can be determined. The patient does not respond to treatment for any of these symptoms.

Depression Disorder Classification

The three main types of depressive disorders can occur with any of the major anxiety disorders:

1.   Major depression
2.   Dysthymia/chronic depression
3.   Bipolar disorder

Major Depression

Major depression is diagnosed when the patient is symptomatic for a 2-week period.

Major depressive episodes may occur once or twice in a lifetime, or may recur frequently throughout life. They may occur spontaneously and some patients may attempt suicide.

Dysthymia/Chronic Depression

Dysthymia is a less severe and more chronic form of depression. The patient mainly experiences decreased energy, poor appetite or overeating, insomnia or oversleeping, and extreme pessimism.

Bipolar Disorder/Manic-Depressive Psychosis

Bipolar disorder formerly called *manic-depression* is characterized by shifting mood cycles. The mood cycles associated with bipolar disorder are:

1.   Severe highs or mania
2.   Mild highs or hypomania
3.   Severe lows or depression

Manic Phase

The disorder here can manifest itself as a "manic state" during which there is an excessive, endless enthusiasm for interacting.

During the manic phase a patient experiences abnormal or excessive elation, a decreased need for sleep, grandiose ideas, increased racing thoughts, markedly increased energy, poor judgment, and inappropriate social behavior.

Hypomania Phase

The disorder here may manifest itself as a "mixed state": Initially the individual shows a tremendous mood upswing and this is followed by an episode of depression.

Depressive Phase

A third way in which this disorder can manifest itself is a "depressed state" during which there are multiple episodes of depression with at least one manic episode. During the depressive phase, the patient experiences the symptoms of major depression.

Mood swings from manic to depressive are often gradual, but they can occasionally occur abruptly. Management of the depressed state is the same with depression.

Depression Treatment Options

Depression is treated with the following:

1. Cognitive-behavioral therapy
2. Medications

Antidepressant Medications

The following medications have antianxiety and antidepressants effects: tricyclic anti-depressants (TCAs), mono amine oxidase inhibitors (MAO-I), selective serotonin reuptake inhibitors (SSRIs), lithium, or phenothiazines.

Tricyclic Antidepressants (TCAs) or Heterocyclic Antidepressants (HCAs)

Drugs included in this class are amytriptyline (Elavil), imipramine (Tofranil/Norpramine), nortriptyline (Aventyl), and doxepin (Sinequan).

MAO Inhibitors

Drugs included in this class are phenelzine (Nardil), isocarboxazid (Marplan), and tranylcypromine (Parnate).

Selective Serotonin Reuptake Inhibitors (SSRIs)

Drugs included in this class are paroxetin (Paxil), fluoxetin (Prozac), sertraline (Zoloft), and citalopram (Celexa).

Lithium or Phenothiazines

These drugs are used for the treatment of the manic state. Patients unable to take lithium are given the phenothiazines.

Lithium takes 7–12 days to become effective.

The more common side effects associated with lithium are tremors, anxiety, and memory impairment. The less common side effects associated with lithium are skin rash, impairment of the renal function, excessive loss of potassium, xerostomia, and stomatitis.

Phenothiazines can cause bone marrow depression resulting in thrombocytopenia and leucopenia.

Treatment for Bipolar or Manic-Depressive Psychosis

Bipolar or manic-depressive psychosis is treated with lithium carbonate (Lithane or Lithobid or Lithonate or Eskalith), carbemazepine (Tegretol), and valproic acid (Depakote).

DEPRESSION AND SUGGESTED DENTAL ALERTS

The following are dental alerts for depression:

1. Poor personal and oral hygiene, decreased salivary flow, increased dental caries, increased periodontal disease and facial pain syndromes are common in patients suffering from depression.
2. Patients suffering from anxiety or depression often experience aphthous ulcerations, ulcerative gingivitis, TMJ problems, lichen planus, geographic tongue, and myofacial pain. These conditions must also be addressed in the dental setting.
3. Always show empathy toward the patient and try to clearly understand the patient's problems.
4. Injury to the oral cavity may occur during mania. Overbrushing can cause abrasion of the teeth and overflossing can injure gingival tissue in bipolar patients.
5. Antidepressants have anticholinergic side effects and this can precipitate xerostomia. MAO-Is and TCAs induce significant xerostomia. Patients on antidepressants should therefore use fluoride rinses on a regular basis.

    Xerostomia is actually a genuine concern in patients taking all kinds of antipsychiatric medications. Follow the suggested xerostomia management guidelines in Chapter 48, "Therapeutic Management of Oral Lesions in the Immune-Competent and the Immune-Compromised Patient in the Dental Setting."
6. **Anesthetics with MAO-Is:** MAO inhibitors interact with epinephrine. Vasoconstrictors in the local anesthetics are contraindicated with MAO-Is, due to the possibility of hypertensive episodes.
7. **Sedatives and narcotic analgesics with MAO-Is:** Sedatives and narcotic analgesics are strictly contraindicated in patients on MAO-Is.
8. **Anesthetics with TCAs:** Tricyclic antidepressants enhance the effect of catecholamines. Avoid vasoconstrictors in the local anesthetics with TCAs.

    In conclusion, avoid epinephrine in the local anesthetic and epinephrine cords in the presence of TCAs and MAO-Is. No epinephrine contraindications with the SSRIs.
9. **Sedatives and narcotic snalgesics with TCAs:** Sedatives and narcotic analgesics should also be avoided with tricyclics.
10. Antipsychiatric medications cause postural hypotension. Assist the patient out of the chair to avoid collapse.

   In conclusion, avoid sedatives, epinephrine (except with SSRIs), narcotic analgesics, sedating antihistamines and epinephrine cords with antipsychiatric medications.

DEMENTIA

Dementia is a cognitive disorder and it can be associated with the following:

1. Alzheimer's disease
2. HIV disease

3. Parkinson's disease
4. Vascular causes/stroke

Dementia Overview and Facts

Old age, stroke, and Alzheimer's disease are the more common causes of dementia. Aging dementia occurs most commonly in patients 80 years and older and less commonly in patients between the ages of 65 to 70.

Dementia is not a specific disease. Patients with dementia have serious problems with two or more brain functions, such as memory and language. Memory loss is a common symptom of dementia.

A progressive deterioration of intellectual functioning, behavioral and mood changes, and with impairment of occupational and social functions occurs with dementia.

Initially, a clinician will observe subtle changes such as social withdrawal, apathy, and lack of spontaneity. As the dementia progresses, the patient is unable to learn or recall new information, is unable to identify family members, has impaired judgment, gets disoriented often, is unable to clothe or feed independently, and often has impairment of sleep pattern.

The patient becomes agitated, confused, and delusional. The patient loses the ability to think and ultimately is not able to remember and recognize things or people. There is a definite change in, and worsening of, the patient's personality.

Dementia Classification

Depending on the severity, Dementia can be subdivided into the following:

1. **Mild Dementia:** At this stage of dementia, the patient's work or social activities are impaired, but the patient's capacity for independent living remains.
2. **Moderate Dementia:** During this stage of dementia, independent living becomes hazardous.
3. **Severe Dementia:** During this stage of dementia, cognition and function are so impaired that continuous supervision is required.

ALZHEIMER'S DISEASE

Alzheimer's disease is the most common cause of dementia. It often affects the elderly, but in some rare cases, Alzheimer's can affect patients aged 40s through 50s. The exact etiology of Alzheimer's disease is not known, but the disease is familial and associated with old age.

Alzheimer's Disease Pathophysiology

Patients with Alzheimer's disease lose functioning neurons in the brain that deal with cognitive function and memory. There is a buildup of abnormal proteins amyloid beta 42peptide (AB42) and Tau in some of the brain cells.

Alzheimer's Disease Clinical Features

Alzheimer's disease is associated with a characteristic dementia syndrome that has an insidious onset. The dementia is usually slow but has a progressively deteriorating course, terminating in death.

Symptoms often begin with the individuals' gradual withdrawal from active engagement with life.

There is a narrowing of social and other interests, a lessening of mental alertness and adaptability and a lowering of tolerance to new ideas and changes in the routine. The thoughts and activities become self-centered and childlike. There is a preoccupation with the bodily functions of excretion, eating, or digestion.

Progressively, those constantly around the patient will also perceive impairment of memory for recent events, agitation, periods of confusion, impaired judgment, and messiness. In the terminal stages, the patient is reduced to a vegetative state.

An occasional Alzheimer's disease patient may develop a paranoid orientation towards people and/or places; depression or rapid progression of the disease with ultimate delirium.

Alzheimer's Disease Diagnosis

Alzheimer's disease diagnosis can be established with the following:

1. **Medical assessment:** Thorough neurological examination could demonstrate deficits.
2. **Alzheimer's biomarkers:** AB42 and Tau are biomarkers that can assist in the diagnosis of Alzheimer's disease. Low levels of AB42 and high levels of Tau are associated with Alzheimer's disease. Absence of this pattern rules out Alzheimer's disease as being the cause of dementia.
3. **Apolipoprotein E (ApoE) genotyping test:** The presence of two copies of ApoE e4 on the ApoE genotyping test predicts an increased risk of developing Alzheimer's disease after age 65.
   A single copy of ApoE e4 predicts some risk for the disease but the patient may never go on to develop the disease. Be aware that some patients test negative for ApoE e4 and *have* Alzheimer's disease.
4. **Brain MRI:** The MRI shows enlarged ventricles or widening in the folds (sulci) of the cerebral cortex. This indicates brain atrophy.

Alzheimer's Disease Medications and Therapies

Medications available today cannot reverse the changes associated with Alzheimer's disease, but they can slow down the process of dementia. Medications prescribed can only deal with the anxiety, depression, hallucinations, delusions, and insomnia associated with the disease. Family support and involvement in care are crucial adjuncts to the care in these patients.

Acetylcholinesterase Inhibitors

Acetylcholinesterase inhibitors are the treatment of choice for patients with mild to moderate Alzheimer's disease. The drugs in this category work by increasing the concentration of acetylcholine.

Acetylcholine is important in memory, cognitive skills, and thinking. These drugs delay the worsening of some of the Alzheimer's disease–associated symptoms. Common acetylcholinesterase inhibitors used are:

1. **Donepezil (Aricept):** acetylcholinesterase inhibitor
2. **Galantamine (Reminyl):** acetylcholinesterase inhibitor

3. **Rivastigmine (Exelon):** acetylcholinesterase and butyrylcholinesterase inhibitor
4. **Tacrine (Cognex):** acetylcholinesterase inhibitor

Acetylcholinesterase Inhibitor Side Effects

Common side effects are nausea, vomiting, diarrhea, and weight loss.

Vitamin E

Vitamin E is an antioxidant and it is thought to be brain-protective for Alzheimer's patients.

N-methyl d-aspartate (NMDA) Receptor Antagonist: Memantine (Namenda)

Namenda treats moderate to severe Alzheimer's disease by regulating the levels of glutamate. Glutamate helps process, store, and retrieve information in the brain. Namenda is often combined with a cholinesterase inhibitor for the management of moderate to severe Alzheimer's disease.

Adjunctive Drug Therapies

The following are Alzheimer's disease adjunctive drug therapies:

1. **Risperidone and Haloperidol:** These drugs are used when the patient has persistent agitation, delusions, or hallucinations.
2. **Antidepressants:** These drugs are indicated for the management of depression, which occurs more frequently in patients with DAT than in the general population.

Memory Aids

Make "to-do" lists and provide notes to the patient. This helps the patient remember things better, experience less anxiety, and have a calmer living situation.

Treatment for Forgetfulness

Treatment can be counseling or medication, or both.

Upcoming Alzheimer's Drugs

Most of the newer drugs in the process of manufacture for the treatment or prevention of Alzheimer's disease target the amyloid beta 42peptide (AB42) proteins discussed earlier, which accumulate in the brain and are suspected to be the cause of the devastating dementia.

The newer Tau-based medications being tested in animal models reduce the levels of the Tau protein, also discussed earlier. Tau is an essential protein that allows the propagation of nerve impulses. Tau has often been found in the brains of Alzheimer's patients, but its role in the disease and connection to AB42 plaques is unclear.

It has been noted that AB42 seems to be destructive only in the presence of Tau. The rat experimentations have shown memory loss reversal and gene modification, slowing the manufacture of Tau.

ALZHEIMER'S DISEASE SUGGESTED DENTAL GUIDELINES

The following are dental guidelines for Alzheimer's disease:

1. Never leave a dementia or Alzheimer's patient alone in the chair; the patient could unknowingly walk away because of confusion or anxiety.
2. In the initial stages of the disease, written reminders can help Alzheimer's disease patients lead a relatively normal life. This is because in the early stages of the disease, they can remember how to do things, once they are reminded to do them. It is only later that they lose the ability to perform simple tasks.
3. Oral injuries can frequently occur in these patients involving the cheeks, tongue, and alveolar mucosa due to injuries sustained with forks or spoons or during mastication.
4. Poor oral hygiene, increased incidence of caries, and periodontal disease are common findings.
5. Xerostomia often occurs because of the common use of antipsychotic drugs in these patients.
6. **Anesthetics:** Avoid epinephrine in the presence of antipsychotic drugs.
7. **Stress management and analgesics:** Avoid sedatives, hypnotics, narcotic analgesics, and antihistamines in patients with Alzheimer's disease and with all other CNS disorders.
8. Alzheimer's patients do best seeing the same dentist, to maintain consistency and decrease anxiety. Explain all the action and activities that are to occur during a dental appointment. Use short, simple sentences while communicating with the patient.
9. Be aggressive with their dental care. Frequent hygiene recalls (3–4-month intervals), fluoride gel applications, and adjustments of prosthesis are some of the heightened dental needs of these patients.

SCHIZOPHRENIA

Schizophrenia is a chronic, disabling mental illness that can often be severe. Men and women are equally affected.

Schizophrenia is usually diagnosed around the ages of 17–35 years. The illness appears earlier in men than in women and many of the patients are disabled with the disease. Some, however, recover enough with treatment to live a relatively independent life.

Schizophrenia is a disturbance in thinking and perception and a splitting away from reality. These patients are often confused, withdrawn, depressed, and anxious. Hallucinations and/or delusions are common. They do not show any emotions and speak in monotones. Prior to the start of the treatment the patient may be hyperactive, pacing, stationary, or catatonic.

Genes, infections, stresses, and the neurotransmitters dopamine, serotonin, and glutamate have been implicated as causative factors for schizophrenia.

Schizophrenia Symptoms

Schizophrenia is usually associated with the following symptoms:

1. **Delusions:** Delusions are false beliefs held by the patient. These delusions seem very real to the patient.

2. **Hallucinations**: The patient experiences visual, auditory, taste, or smell sensory perceptions or hallucinations. These hallucinations occur in the absence of actual external stimuli.
3. **Disorganized thoughts and behaviors**: These thoughts and behaviors are out of context with reality.
4. **Disorganized speech**: Due to the loss of contact with reality, the patient's speech is in response to hallucinations experienced.
5. **Catatonic behavior**: The patient may be rigid and unresponsive for hours during the catatonic phase.

Schizophrenia Diagnosis

Schizophrenia diagnosis is made when the active symptoms of schizophrenia have been present untreated for at least 6 months or with treatment for only 1 month.

Schizophrenia Treatment

Schizophrenia management is done with neuroleptics and atypical psychotics.

Neuroleptics

These are the older class of drugs that control acute symptoms well but are not that effective in correcting lack of emotional expression and decreased motivation. Drugs that belong to this class include chlorpromazine (Thorazine), fluphenazine (Prolixin), haloperidol (Haldol), molindone (Moban), mesoridazine (Serentil), perphenazine (Trilafon), thioridazine (Mellaril), thiothixene (Navane), and trifluoperazine (Stelazine).

Neuroleptics Side Effects

Hypotension, xerostomia, tachycardia, arrythmia, thrombocytopenia, and leukopenia are side effects of neuroleptics.

Atypical Antipsychotics

The atypical antipsychotics are newer drugs that have minimal or no neurological side effects. These medications have successfully rehabilitated affected patients to become active members of society. Drugs in this category include aripiprazole (Abilify), clozapine (Clozaril), olanzapine (Zyprexa), quetiapine (Seroquel), risperidone (Risperdal), and Ziprasidone (Geodon).

Atypical Antipsychotics Side Effects

These drugs cause **severe** agranulocytosis. The **CBC** must be monitored weekly during the first 6 months of treatment and then every 2 weeks to detect the agranulocytosis.

SCHIZOPHRENIA SUGGESTED DENTAL GUIDELINES

Follow these guidelines:

1. **Anesthetics:** Do not use topical epinephrine or epinephrine-containing local anesthetics with any of the drugs used to treat schizophrenia.
2. **Stress management and analgesics:** Sedative hypnotics, epinephrine, atropine, antihistamines, and narcotics are all contraindicated with antipsychiatric drugs or

CNS-acting drugs. Sedating antihistamines are contraindicated because they enhance sedation.

3. Monitor the CBC and calculate the ANC count in patients on neuroleptics and atypical antipsychotics. Follow the ANC guidelines in patients with leucopenia.

4. Oral side effects and management of the oral lesions are the same as those discussed in the earlier section "Depression and Suggested Dental Alerts."

EATING DISORDERS

Eating disorders are associated with serious disturbances in eating behavior. There is an extreme distorted concern and anxiety about the body shape or size, triggering a severe unhealthy undereating or overeating pattern that is hard to break.

Eating disorders are true medical illnesses that commonly affect adolescent or young adults, and females outnumber males in being affected with the disease.

Anxiety, depression, suicide attempts, low self-esteem, and alcohol and/or substance abuse often coexist with the eating disorders.

Eating disorders, particularly anorexia nervosa, can adversely affect the heart causing renal failure, cardiac arrhythmia, and sudden death in the process.

Eating Disorder Classification

The three most common eating disorders are anorexia nervosa, bulimia, and binge-eating.

Anorexia Nervosa

The patient is very afraid of gaining weight in spite of being extremely thin and grossly underweight. There is true opposition to maintaining ideal body weight. There is a distorted perception of one's own body shape or size and denial that a weight problem exists. This type of patient obsessively goes to extremes to lose even more weight.

The patient picks at food, often eating only select food items and eating infrequently or in small portions. Purging and laxative and diuretic abuse are the additional ways in which the weight is decreased. Serious weight loss results in loss of menstruation in affected females.

Some patients can recover with proper medical intervention, some can go on to suffer chronically with the disease, and still others may develop serious complications and succumb to the disease because of medical complications or suicide. Severe electrolyte loss and hypokalemia (decreased potassium) caused by the purging and undereating precipitates cardiac arrhythmia, kidney failure, and death.

Bulimia

The bulimia patient reacts differently to food when compared with the anorexia nervosa patient. The emphasis is on eating uncontrollably (binge-eating) over a finite time and then eliminating it immediately from the body by forced vomiting.

The patient has no control over the eating, eats fast, and excessively to the point of hurting. The patient is secretive about these practices and is ashamed of the behavior but gets a sense of relief with food elimination by purging.

It is not uncommon for this type of patient to abuse diuretics, laxatives, rigorous exercise, and tools to promote the gag reflex (fingers, throat sticks, spoon, etc.) to assist with vomiting. The patient is usually close to normal body weight but has a distorted perception of her/his own weight.

Bulimia Diagnosis

The patient has to have had at least two food-abuse episodes/week for 3 months to be diagnosed with bulimia.

Binge-Eating

Binge-eating is a variant of bulimia. In binge-eating there is an abnormal compulsion to eat large volumes of food in the shortest possible time, till it hurts and no more can be eaten.

The patient eats in the presence of others and there is tremendous guilt experienced after eating. These patients do not really resort to purging or laxative/diuretic abuse. Consequently, many of these patients are overweight rather than underweight. The etiology and treatment protocols for binge-eating are the same as with bulimia.

Binge-Eating Diagnosis

Binge-eating is considered a true disorder when it happens twice/week for 6 months.

Eating Disorders Treatment

The patient needs to be ready to want to get better because patient participation and commitment is very important. Treatment for anorexia consists of a number of disciplines coming together to help the patient. It is a true team effort to target and address every factor causing the disease. The team includes the physician, psychologist, therapist, nutritionist, family support, and medications when needed.

A patient with associated life-threatening conditions is invariably hospitalized while the others are treated in the outpatient setting. The hospitalized patient's feeds are monitored closely and provided by intravenous therapy.

The anorexia patient needs to gain weight, deal with the psychological conditions promoting the disorder, and learn to maintain the weight.

SSRIs are sometimes used after weight improvement to alleviate anxiety, continue with weight maintenance, and help the patient feel good and maintain a positive attitude.

The same kind of team approach mentioned above is also utilized for the bulimia patient. The patient is encouraged to decrease the meal volume, deal with the underlying psychiatric conditions promoting the eating disorder, develop a healthy attitude toward body shape and size, and take SSRIs to help cope with the recovery process.

EATING DISORDERS SUGGESTED DENTAL GUIDELINES

Follow these guidelines to deal with patients with eating disorders:

1. Always confirm that a patient with an eating disorder is aware of the association of the patient's disease state with enamel erosion, increased incidence of dental caries, and xerostomia. The patient has to "partner" with the dentist in wanting to improve the mouth, reverse the erosion and decay, and maintain the repair.
   Be aware that continuation of the eating disorder will negatively impact on the expensive dentistry. The patient should be coaxed to follow through with the eating disorder recovery process.

2. Confirm that the patient has ongoing psychotherapy support to prevent reverting back to the disorder.
3. Thorough history-taking should include assessment of laxative and diuretic use/abuse.
4. Always check for symptoms and signs of hypokalemia in eating disorder patients: muscle cramps, muscle weakness, tingling numbness in the hands and feet, fatigue, and irregular pulse. Delay dental treatment and refer a patient who is symptomatic for hypokalemia to the medical side.
5. Teach the patient to rinse the mouth with water as soon as the acid is felt in the mouth.
6. Treat the xerostomia and candidiasis, when present, according to the protocol discussed in Chapter 48, "Therapeutic Management of Oral Lesions in the Immune-Competent and Immune-Compromised Patient in the Dental Setting."
7. **Anesthetics:** Avoid epinephrine use in a patient complaining of palpitations or irregular pulse. Epinephrine in the local anesthetic is not contraindicated with the SSRIs.
8. **Stress management, anesthetics, and analgesics:** Epinephrine, sedatives, hypnotics, narcotics and sedating antihistamines are contraindicated with all other psychiatric medications if being used by the patient (Table 52.1).

Table 52.1. Psychiatric medications side effects and epinephrine use in LAs

Psychiatric Drugs Category	Side Effects
Antianxiety Drugs	
Benzodiazepines: Epinephrine can be used.	Xerostomia
Beta Blockers: Limit epinephrine to 2 carpules.	Postural hypotension
Antidepressants with antianxiety effects:	
Monoamine oxidase inhibitors (MAOIs): Avoid epinephrine.	
Selective Serotonin Reuptake Inhibitors (SSRIs): Epinephrine can be used.	
Tricyclic antidepressants: Avoid epinephrine.	
Antidepressant Drugs	
Tricyclic antidepressants (TCAs):	Postural hypotension
Amytriptyline (Elavil)	Tachycardia
Imipramine (Tofranil/Norpramine)	Arrythmia
Nortriptyline (Aventyl)	Xerostomia
Doxepin (Sinequan)	
Avoid Epinephrine.	
Mono Amine Oxidase Inhibitors (MAO-I):	Postural hypotension
Phenelzine (Nardil)	Xerostomia
Isocarboxazid (Marplan)	
Tranylcypromine (Parnate)	
Avoid Epinephrine.	

Table 52.1. *Continued*

Psychiatric Drugs Category	Side Effects
Selective serotonin reuptake inhibitors (SSRIs): Paroxetin (Paxil) Fluoxetin (Prozac) Sertraline (Zoloft) Citalopram (Celexa) **Epinephrine can be used.**	Postural hypotension Xerostomia
Lithium: Avoid epinephrine.	Tremors Anxiety Memory impairment Skin rash Impairment of the renal function Excessive loss of potassium Xerostomia Stomatitis
Treatment for bipolar or manic-depressive psychosis: Lithium Carbonate (Lithane or Lithobid or Lithonate or Eskalith) Carbemazepine (Tegretol) Valproic Acid (Depakote) **Avoid epinephrine with all drugs listed.**	Tremors Anxiety Memory impairment Skin rash Impairment of the renal function Excessive loss of potassium Xerostomia Stomatitis Leukopenia and thrombocytopenia with Valproic acid
Antischizophrenic Drugs **Neuroleptics:** Chlorpromazine (Thorazine) Fluphenazine (Prolixin) Haloperidol (Haldol) Molindone (Moban) Mesoridazine (Serentil) Perphenazine (Trilafon) Thioridazine (Mellaril) Thiothixene (Navane) Trifluoperazine (Stelazine) **Avoid epinephrine with above drugs.**	Hypotension Xerostomia Tachycardia Arrythmia Thrombocytopenia Leukopenia
Atypical antipsychotics: Aripiprazole (Abilify) Clozapine (Clozaril) Olanzapine (Zyprexa) Quetiapine (Seroquel) Risperidone (Risperdal) Ziprasidone (Geodon) **Avoid epinephrine with all drugs listed.**	They cause severe agranulocytosis. Monitor CBC weekly in the first 6 months of care, and then every 2 weeks to detect agranulocytosis.
Alzheimer's Drugs **Acetylcholinesterase inhibitors:** Donepezil (Aricept): Acetylcholinesterase inhibitor Galantamine (Reminyl): Acetylcholinesterase inhibitor Rivastigmine (Exelon): Acetylcholinesterase and Butyrylcholinesterase inhibitor Tacrine (Cognex): Acetylcholinesterase inhibitor **Avoid epinephrine with all drugs listed.**	Nausea Vomiting Diarrhea Weight loss

XX Transplants

53

Organ Transplants, Immunosuppressive Drugs, and Associated Dental Management Guidelines

ORGAN TRANSPLANTS OVERVIEW AND FACTS

Organ transplantation has come a long way from the time the first transplant was done in the early 1950s. Most organ transplants initially had been allografts or tissues from genetically nonidentical donors. This accounted for the less-than-satisfactory outcomes with organ transplants.

Now with newer trends the live-related donor rates have gone up, accounting for an improved outcome and greater hope for organ transplantations.

The success rates for organ transplants have also increased tremendously with the discovery of immunosuppressants cyclosporine and tacrolimus (Prograf). These drugs have improved the survival rates in transplanted patients.

Post–organ transplant care also has seen some changes in the way the patients are managed. The trend now is to keep the patient's immunity at a specific optimal level, such that the need for immunosuppression drugs is decreased. This improves the recipient's immune system response in helping to ward off infections or deal with infections.

Some transplant centers are now providing the patient with steroid-free and calcineurin-inhibitor–free immunosuppressions. The short-term results with these new strategies have been promising so far, but the long-term outcome data needs to show whether this process is really a move in the right direction.

The physician now can utilize **ImmuKnow**®, an assay to assess immune system function from a single blood drop. The test measures the vitality of the patient's immune system, thus allowing the physician to better manage the patient's response to infection and personalize the care to prevent organ rejection.

These newer methods of care will definitely lower the cost of medications in the future and in turn prolong the organ recipient's life.

The major organs transplanted today are bone marrow, heart, lungs, pancreas, liver, and kidneys.

Kidney Transplant Facts

Dialysis is a very expensive option in the long run for renal failure patients. A kidney transplant is also expensive at first, but all in all it has a lower yearly maintenance cost, compared to dialysis.

467

With kidney transplant, the quality of life improves for the patient and there is also an improvement of uremia, anemia, peripheral neuropathy, and autonomic neuropathy.

A kidney transplant can double the life span of kidney failure patients.

The transplanted kidney can be obtained from a cadaver—50% of transplants utilize this source—a live related donor, or a live distant/unrelated donor.

Kidneys obtained from a live donor are much better than those obtained from a nonliving or cadaveric donor.

Liver Transplant Facts

A liver transplant is much more complicated than a kidney transplant because of the complexity of the surgical procedure. To prioritize a patient on the liver transplant list, the severity of a liver failure patient's status is assessed using the model of end-stage liver disease (MELD) criteria. The MELD criteria evaluate the following tests: bilirubin; PT/INR, and serum creatinine. The serum creatinine is the most sensitive mortality risk indicator of liver failure.

Cells Responsible for Prevention of Organ Rejection

The following cells constitute the cell-mediated defenses for the prevention of organ rejection:

1. T-cells: The most important cells
2. Antigen-presenting cells
3. Natural killer cells
4. Monocytes

IMMUNOSUPPRESSANT DRUGS

Immunosuppressants currently available are azathioprine, basiliximab, cyclosporine, daclizumab, muromonab-CD3, mycophenolic acid, mycophenolate mofetil, prednisone, sirolimus, and tacrolimus.

Of these drugs, the ones most commonly used are:

1. Azathioprine (Imuran)
2. The calcineurin inhibitors: Prograf/FK506, cyclosporine (Sandimmune), or tacrolimus
3. Prednisone
4. Mycophenolate mofetil (Cellcept)

AZATHIOPRINE (IMURAN)

Azathioprine (Imuran) Mechanism of Action (MOA)

Azathioprine is an antimetabolite that decreases inflammation and interferes with the growth of rapidly dividing cells. It has a generalized effect on bone marrow, inhibiting production of blood-forming cells, thus preventing rejection.

Azathioprine inhibits the white blood cells causing leucopenia and thrombocytopenia. Always **assess** the **CBC prior** to instituting dental treatment in patients on Imuran.

Azathioprine Side Effects

Common side effects experienced by the patient are cold hands and feet; loss of appetite, upset stomach, diarrhea, and vomiting; fever; mouth sores; sore throat; and unusual bleeding or bruising.

CYCLOSPORINE (SANDIMMUNE)

Cyclosporine is used for the management of organ transplants, severe psoriasis, and rheumatoid arthritis.

Cyclosporine Mechanism of Action (MOA)

Cyclosporine decreases the production of interleukins, resulting in decreased replication of helper and killer T cells.

Cyclosporine (Sandimmune) Facts

Cyclosporine is extensively metabolized by the CytochromeP450 enzyme system in the liver. It is not unusual for the BUN and serum creatinine levels to be elevated during therapy if the cyclosporine levels are not kept in check.

   Cyclosporine can therefore cause hypertension if not regulated well. Nephrotoxicity has occurred in patients receiving high doses of cyclosporine. Cyclosporine levels are monitored regularly every 4–6 weeks. Avoid nephrotoxic drugs in patients on cyclosporine. Cyclosporine is known to cause gingival hyperplasia.

Antibiotics Alert

Macrolides increase cyclosporine toxicity by increasing the intestinal absorption and inhibiting the biliary absorption of cyclosporine.

Antifungal Alert

Fluconazole (Diflucan) also increases cyclosporine toxicity and the mechanism is unknown.

Analgesics Alert

Avoid the use of NSAIDS with cyclosporine because NSAIDS promote nephrotoxicity.

   Avoid the use of trimethoprim-sulphamethoxazole (Bactrim) with cyclosporine because it also promotes nephrotoxicity.

   Note: Bactrim is ineffective in treating oral infections.

Cyclosporine Side Effects

Side effects associated with cyclosporine are diarrhea; increased hair growth; loss of appetite; sinusitis; upset stomach; vomiting; tender, swollen, bleeding gums and gingival hyperplasia; unusual bleeding or bruising; and sore throat, fever, and/or chills.

Cyclosporine Drug Interactions

Avoid the following medications in the dental setting in the presence of cyclosporine: cimetidine (Tagamet), clarithromycin (Biaxin), corticosteroids, erythromycin, Fluconazole (Diflucan), Itraconazole (Sporanox), and Ketoconazole (Nizoral).

TACROLIMUS/PROGRAF/FK506

Tacrolimus is an immunosuppressant that reduces the body's natural immunity in recipients of organ transplants. Prograf is used as an alternate to cyclosporine when cyclosporine cannot be used.

Tacrolimus Mechanism of Action (MOA)

Tacrolimus inhibits cytokine production, including IL-2. It inhibits the expression of IL-2 receptors and blocks cell division.

Tacrolimus Side Effects

Side effects associated with Tacrolimus are diarrhea; vomiting; difficulty breathing and/or wheezing; itching, skin rash, and/or hives; seizures; sore throat, fever, and/or chills; unusual bleeding or bruising.

Tacrolimus Drug Interactions

Avoid the following drugs in the dental setting in the presence of Tacrolimus: antacids, cimetidine (Tagamet), clarithromycin (Biaxin), clotrimazole (Mycelex/Lotrimin), drythromycin, fluconazole (Diflucan), itraconazole (Sporanox), ketoconazole (Nizoral), and methylprednisolone (Medrol).

Prograf/FK506/Tacrolimus Suggested Dental Alert

Prograf can cause anemia. Avoid nephrotoxic drugs in patients on Prograf.

PREDNISONE

Prednisone is an immunosuppressant drug that prevents the body from rejecting a transplanted organ. It is also used to treat certain forms of arthritis, severe allergies, and asthmas, as well as skin, blood, kidney, eye, thyroid, and intestinal disorders.

Prednisone Mechanism of Action (MOA)

Prednisone inhibits interluekin-1 secretions, resulting in decreased replication of cytotoxic T cells. It also has a nonspecific antiinflammatory effect and inhibits the granulocyte function, thus limiting damage to an organ in which the rejection process has already begun.

Prednisone Side Effects

Side effects associated with prednisone are dizziness; easy bruising; upset stomach; skin rash; swollen face, lower legs, or ankles; and vision problems.

Prednisone Suggested Dental Facts and Alerts

Be alert to the following:

1. Always determine the current dose of prednisone and the duration for which the patient has been on corticosteroids.
2. Follow "the rule of twos" in patients who are to undergo major dental surgery, by consulting with the patient's M.D.

3. Check the oral cavity for candidiasis and treat appropriately, when candidiasis is found.

MYCOPHENOLATE MOFETIL (CELLCEPT)

Cellcept is often combined with cyclosporine, Prograf, or Rapamycin to prevent rejection in organ transplant recipients.

Cellcept Mechanism of Action (MOA)

Cellcept lowers the body's immune system by killing the lymphocytes, thus preventing organ rejection.

Cellcept Side Effects

Common side effects are: Fever, chills, or flu symptoms; easy bruising or bleeding; bloody, black, or tarry stools; painful or difficulty urinating; and numbness or tingly feeling.

SUGGESTED DENTAL GUIDELINES FOR ORGAN TRANSPLANT PATIENTS

Follow these guidelines:

1. Prior to the start of routine dental treatment always obtain laboratory tests to confirm that the transplanted organ is optimally functioning. Never just presume that the transplanted organ works well!
2. Obtain a good dental history and perform a thorough dental examination, including full-mouth radiographs.
3. Prioritize the patient's dental problems. Those that are most likely to cause pain, infection, and/or bacteremia in the next 12 months should be taken care of immediately.
4. When treating a **prerenal transplant** patient, follow the **premedication protocol** for shunts and renal failure anesthetic, analgesic, antibiotic (AAAs) suggested guidelines during dentistry.
5. When treating a **preliver transplant** patient, follow the liver failure anesthetic, analgesic, antibiotic (AAAs) suggested guidelines during dentistry.
6. Obtain the CBC and calculate the ANC count in any pretransplant patient. Provide AHA recommended antibiotic premedication if the patient has low ANC counts.
7. Premedication should also be provided in the presence of **ascites** in the preliver transplant patient.
8. In the patient awaiting a liver transplant, evaluate the PT/INR: fresh frozen plasma (FFP) transfusion will be needed if the PT/INR is prolonged.
   Also evaluate the platelet count in the patient awaiting a liver transplant. Platelet replacement will be required if the platelet count is <50 K/mm^3.
9. Pretransplant preparation of the oral cavity is the same as for patients who are to undergo chemotherapy or radiotherapy.
10. Routine dentistry should be **deferred for 6 months**, post–organ transplant.
11. If emergency dental treatment is needed within the first 6 months of the organ transplant, use the AAA guidelines specified for the specific organ during failure (renal failure/cirrhosis).

12. The anesthetics, analgesics, antibiotics (AAAs) used during dentistry will be deter-mined by the current status of the transplanted organ. Obtain appropriate tests to evaluate the status of the transplanted organ and **then** proceed with dentistry.
13. Avoid cimetidine (Tagamet), clarithromycin (Biaxin), corticosteroids, erythromy-cin, fluconazole (Diflucan), itraconazole (Sporanox), and ketoconazole (Nizoral) in the presence of cyclosporine.
14. Avoid the following drugs in the dental setting in the presence of tacrolimus/Prograf/FK506: antacids, cimetidine (Tagamet), clarithromycin (Biaxin), clotrima-zole (Mycelex), erythromycin, fluconazole (Diflucan), itraconazole (Sporanox), ketoconazole (Nizoral), and methylprednisolone (Medrol).
15. If macrolides are the only antibiotics that can be used in the first 6 months of the transplant because of allergy to penicillin, communicate with the patient's M.D. The M.D. can assist with temporarily lowering the cyclosporine dose so the mac-rolide can be safely used.
16. Bone marrow suppression is a genuine concern posttransplant, and these patients have an increased incidence of infections plus increased susceptibility to infections. Determine the ANC and provide appropriate antibiotics when needed. Treat all infections aggressively.
17. If the patient is on steroids, there could be a need for steroid boost prior to major surgery. Always confirm with the patient's physician.
18. Herpangina occurs commonly posttransplant and is very aggressive when it occurs. Treat immediately with valacyclovir (Valtrex) or acyclovir (Zovirax).
19. **Gingival hyperplasia:** Cyclosporine is the leading cause for gingival hyperplasia, posttransplant. The patient can be switched to an alternate medication by the M.D. if the hypertrophy becomes a genuine issue.
20. Potential hypertension can occur with cyclosporine use, so always monitor the BP during dentistry.
21. Consider **premedication** for renal transplant patients that **were** on hemodialysis and still continue to have the shunt even if the ANC is normal.
22. Consider premedication for any organ transplant patient with decreased immunity as indicated by assessment of the total WBC and the ANC counts. Follow the ANC guidelines if the WBC count is below normal.
23. Always look for oral sores and treat accordingly in patients on Imuran.
24. Prograf/FK506 can cause anemia. Follow the anemia AAA suggested guidelines when the CBC indicates anemia.
25. Avoid nephrotoxic drugs in patients on cyclosporine and Prograf.

XXI

Common Laboratory Tests

Comprehensive Metabolic Panel (CMP) and Common Hematological Tests

The Comprehensive Metabolic Panel (CMP) is a series of 14 tests done by a medical laboratory using a fasting blood draw from the patient. The CMP is also called the *Chem 12 Panel*. It is often ordered by the physician to assess the patient's kidney and liver status, electrolytes, proteins, and blood sugar. Once the CMP shows any abnormality, the physician typically orders specific tests to further evaluate the identified disease state.

THE COMPREHENSIVE METABOLIC PANEL (CMP) COMPONENTS

The Comprehensive Metabolic Panel (CMP) includes glucose, calcium, albumin, total protein, sodium, potassium, bicarbonate, chloride, blood urea nitrogen (BUN), creatinine, alkaline phosphatase (ALP), alanine amino transferase (ALT/SGPT), aspartate amino transferase (AST/SGOT), and bilirubin.

COMMON HEMATOLOGICAL TESTS AND DENTISTRY

Common hematological tests reviewed prior to dentistry are:

1. **Complete Blood Count (CBC):** CBC with platelets and WBC differential and erythrocyte sedimentation rate (ESR) are discussed in Chapter 11.
2. **Coagulation Tests:** Prothrombin time (PT)/international normalized ratio (INR), partial thromboplastin time (PTT), and bleeding time (BT) are discussed in Chapter 15.
3. **Renal Assessment Tests:** Serum creatinine (S. Cr.) and blood urea nitrogen (BUN) are discussed in Chapter 28.
4. **Diabetes Assessment Tests:** Fasting blood sugar (FBS), postprandial/postmeal blood sugar (PPBS), and hemoglobin A_1C (HbA_1C) are discussed in Chapter 38.
5. **Liver Assessment Tests:** Hepatic serology and liver function tests (LFTs) are discussed in Chapter 45.
6. **Bone Assessment Tests:** Serum calcium (Ca^{2+}), serum phosphorus (PO_4), and alkaline phosphates (AlkP) are discussed in Chapter 41.

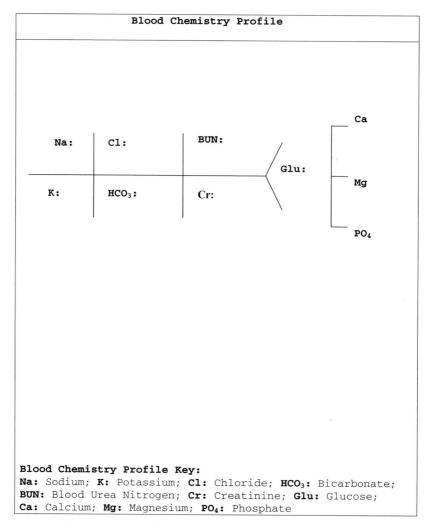

Blood Chemistry Profile

Blood Chemistry Profile Key:
Na: Sodium; **K:** Potassium; **Cl:** Chloride; **HCO₃:** Bicarbonate;
BUN: Blood Urea Nitrogen; **Cr:** Creatinine; **Glu:** Glucose;
Ca: Calcium; **Mg:** Magnesium; **PO₄:** Phosphate

Figure 54.1.   Blood chemistry profile lattice recording.

7. **HIV/AIDS Status Assessment Tests:** The HIV-specific tests CD_4 count, HIV viral load (HIV RNA), CBC w/platelets, WBC differential, LFTs, PT/INR, and serum creatinine are discussed in Chapter 47.

THE COMPREHENSIVE METABOLIC PANEL (CMP) AND DENTISTRY

The CMP ordered by a physician to monitor a medically compromised patient should also be requested and assessed by the treating dentist, using a Medical Consultation Form signed by the patient, who consents release of the information.

The goal is for the dentist to assess the patient's current medical status and modify the dental management with the appropriate use of anesthetics, analgesics, and antibiotics (AAAs) for a successful outcome. The CBC and the CMP, when requested, may occasionally be sent in the standardized lattice format on the Medical Consultation Form itself or in the patient's medical records.

Lattice Pattern Recordings: CBC; PT/INR, and CMP

Figure 54.1 illustrates the blood chemistry profile lattice pattern recording.

Review also Figures 12.1, 45.1, and 45.2 for the standardized lattice pattern recordings.

Appendix
Suggested Reading

HISTORY-TAKING AND PHYSICAL EXAMINATION RESOURCES

Bates B, Bickley LS, Hoekelman RA. A Guide to Physical Examination and History Taking; 6th ed. Philadelphia: J.B Lippincott; 1995.

DeGowin EL, DeGowin RL. Bedside Diagnostic Examination; 3rd ed. New York: Macmillan; 1976.

LOCAL ANESTHETICS RESOURCES

Haas DA. An update on local anesthetics in dentistry. J Can Dent Assoc 2002;68(9):546–551.

Malamed SF. Handbook of Local Anesthesia. 4th ed. St. Louis: Mosby; 1997.

Malamed SF, Gagnon S, Leblanc D. Efficacy of articaine: a new amide local anesthetic. J Am Dent Assoc 2000;131(5):635–642.

USP DI. USP Dispensing Information, 17th ed. The United States Pharmacopeial Convention, Inc., Rockville, MD, 1997,139.

Yang WH, Purchase ECR. Adverse reactions to sulfites. J Can Med Assoc 1985;133:865–880.

ANALGESICS RESOURCES

Physicians Desk Reference, 2007.

Dart RC, Erdman AR, Olson KR, et al. Acetaminophen poisoning: an evidence-based consensus guideline for out-of-hospital management. Clin Toxicol (Phila) 2006;44(1):1–18. [Medline].

Farrell SE. Toxicity, Acetaminophen [serial online]. eMedicine Journal. January 3, 2006. Available at http://www.emedicine.com/emerg/topic819.htm [Full Text]

FDA. Questions and Answers: FDA Regulatory Actions for the COX-2 Selective (includes Bextra, Celebrex, and Vioxx) and Non-Selective Non-Steroidal Antiinflammatory Drugs (NSAIDs). www.fda.gov/cder/drug/infopage/cox2/

Larson AM, Polson J, Fontana RJ, et al. Acetaminophen-induced acute liver failure: results of a United States multicenter, prospective study. Hepatology 2005 Dec;42(6):1364–72. [Medline]

Portenoy RK, Payne R, Coluzzi P, Raschko JW, Lyss A, Busch MA, Frigerio V, Ingham J, Loseth DB, Nordbrock E, Rhiner M. Oral transmucosal fentanyl citrate (OTFC) for the treatment of breakthrough pain in cancer patients: a controlled dose titration study. Pain 1999;79:303–312.

Smilkstein MJ, Knapp GL, Kulig KW, Rumack BH. Efficacy of oral N-acetylcysteine in the treatment of acetaminophen overdose. Analysis of the national multicenter study (1976 to 1985). 1988;319(#24):1557–1562.

Zed and Krenzelok. Treatment of acetaminophen overdose. Am J Health Syst Pharm 1999;56:1081–1091.

www.uptodate.com

ANTIBIOTICS RESOURCES

Alliance for the Prudent Use of Antibiotics. Consumer Information. http://www.tufts.edu/med/apua/Patients/patient.html

American Cancer Society. Infections in Individuals with Cancer. Cancer Resource Center. September 30, 1999. [cited May 27, 2001].

American Cancer Society. Cancer Drugs. Cancer Resource Center. 2000. [cited May 27, 2001].

American Dental Association Council on Scientific Affairs. Antibiotic use in dentistry. JADA 1997;128(5):648. [Medline]

American Dental Association; American Academy of Orthopedic Surgeons. Antibiotic prophylaxis for dental patients with total joint replacements. J Am Dent Assoc 2003;Jul;134(7):895–899. PMID 12892448. [PubMed—indexed for MEDLINE]

CDC. Clostridium difficile infection: Centers for Disease Control and Prevention, 2008.

Dajani AS, Taubert KA, Wildon W, et al. Prevention of bacterial endocarditis: recommendations by the American Heart Association. JADA 1997;128:1142–1151. [Medline]

Dancer SJ. How antibiotics can make us sick: the less obvious adverse effects of antimicrobial chemotherapy. Lancet Infect Dis 2004;4,10:611–619.

Epstein JB, Chong S. A survey of antibiotic use in dentistry. J Am Dent Assoc 2000;131(11):1600–1609.

Goldmann DA, Weinstein RA, Wenzel RP, et al. Strategies to prevent and control the emergence and spread of antimicrobial-resistant microorganisms in hospitals: a challenge to hospital leadership. JAMA 1996;275:234–240.

Guntheroth WG. How important are dental procedures as a cause of infective endocarditis? Am J Cardiol 1984;54:797–801. [Medline]

MEDLINEplus Drug Information. U.S. National Library of Medicine. 24 Jan 2001. [cited May 22, 2001].

Moellering RC, Jr. Linezolid. Summaries for Patients. Annals of Internal Medicine 138 (January 21, 2003):I-44.

Monitoring and management of bacterial resistance to antimicrobial agents: A World Health Organization symposium. Clin Infect Dis 1997;24(suppl 1):S1–S176. [Medline]

Portnof JE, Israel HA, Brause BD, Behrman DA. Dental premedication protocols for patients with knee and hip prostheses. N Y State Dent J 2006 Apr–May;72(3):20–25. PMID 16774168. [PubMed—indexed for MEDLINE]

Simoes JA, et al. Antibiotic resistance patterns of group B streptococcal clinical isolates. Infect Dis Obstet Gynecol 2004;12,1:1–8.

Slavkin HC. Benefit-to-risk ratio: the challenge of antibiotic drug resistance. JADA 1997;128:1447–1451. [Medline]

Strom BL, Abrutyn E, Berlin JA, et al. Dental and cardiac risk factors for infective endocarditis: a population-based case-control study. Ann Intern Med 1998;129:761–769.

Tenover FC, Hughes JM. The challenges of emerging infectious diseases: the development and spread of multiple-resistant bacterial pathogens. JAMA 1996;275(4):300–304.

Wynn RL, Bergman SA, Meiller TF, et al. Antibiotics in treating oral-facial infections of odontogenic origins: An Update. Gen Dent 2001;49(3):238–240,242,244 passim. http://www.medscape.com/viewarticle/569858

ANTIFUNGALS RESOURCE

http://www.nlm.nih.gov/medlineplus/druginformation

ANTIVIRAL RESOURCES

MedLine Plus Drug information: Acyclovir; Valacyclovir. www.nlm.nih.gov/medlineplus/druginfo/medmaster/a681045.html

www.drugs.com/acyclovir.html

www.drugs.com/valacyclovir.html

PRESCRIPTION-WRITING RESOURCES

Materia Medica, Pharmacology, Therapeutics and Prescription Writing. Full text. www.pubmedcentral.nih.gov/articlerender.fcgi?artid=1640934

www.americanpregnancy.org/pregnancyhealth/fdadrugratings.html

www.mrm.uci.edu/DEADrugSchedules.doc

www.perinatology.com/exposures/Drugs/FDACategories.htm

www.usdoj.gov/dea/pubs/csa.html

MEDICAL EMERGENCIES RESOURCES

ADA Council on Dental Therapeutics. Office emergencies and emergency kits. JADA 1980;101:305. [Medline]

Atkin, PA. Management of medical emergencies: For the dental team. British Dent J 2006;200,9:532.

Bochner BS, Lichenstein LM. Anaphylaxis. N Eng J Med 1991; 324:1785–1790.

Brackenridge A, Wallbank H, Lawrenson RA, Russell-Jones D. Emergency management of diabetes and hypoglycaemia. Emerg Med J 2006;23:183–185. doi:10.1136/emj.2005.026252

DeShazo RD, et al. Allergic reactions to drugs and biological agents. JAMA 1997;278:1895–1906.

Fenton AM, et al. Vasovagal syncope. Ann Intern Med November 7, 2000;133:714–725.

Goldstein DS, Spanarkel M, Pitterman A, Toltzis R, Gratz E, Epstein S, et al. Circulatory control mechanisms in vasodepressor syncope. Am Heart J 1982;104:1071–1075. [Medline]

Hass, DA. Management of medical emergencies in the dental office: conditions in each country, the extent of treatment by the dentist. Anesth Prog 2006 Spring;53(1):20–24.

Joint Committee on Allergy, Asthma and Immunology. Practice parameters: The investigation and management of anaphylaxis. J Allerg Clin Immunol 1998;101(6):S465–S528.

Kapoor WN. Syncope. N Engl J Med December 21, 2000;343:1856–1862.

Lott C, Hennes HJ, Dick W. Stroke, A medical emergency. J Accid Emerg Med 1999;16(1):2–7.

Low PA, Opfer-Geheking TL, McPhee BR, et al. Prospective evaluation of clinical characteristics of orthostatic hypotension. Mayo Clin Proc 1995;70(7):617–622.

Mackenzie R, Sutcliff RC. Immediate assessment and management of acute medical emergencies. J Royal Army Med Corps 2004;150,3(SUPP/2):107–118.

Malamed, SF. Managing medical emergencies. J Am Dent Assoc 124(8):40–53.

Manolis AS, Linzer M, Salem D, Estes NA III. Syncope: current diagnostic evaluation and management. Ann Intern Med 1990;112:850–863. [Medline]

Sclater A, Alagiakrishnan K. Orthostatic hypotension. A primary care primer for assessment and treatment. Geriatrics 2004;59(Aug):22–27.

Toback SL. Medical emergency preparedness in office practice. Am Fam Phys 2007;75:1679–1684, 1686.

CONSCIOUS SEDATION RESOURCES

ADA.org. The Use of Sedation and General Anesthesia by Dentists. ADA Statement on The Use of Conscious Sedation, Deep Sedation and General Anesthesia in Dentistry. www.**ada**.org/prof/resources/positions/statements/**use**of.asp J Am Dent Assoc 2002;133;364–365.

ADA Council on Scientific Affairs: The American Dental Association's Guidelines for the Use of Conscious Sedation, Deep Sedation. and General Anesthesia for Dentists. jada.ada.org/cgi/reprint/133/3/364.pdf

Aldrete JA. The post-anesthesia recovery score revisited. J Clin Anesth 1995;7:89–91.

Dental Sedation Teachers Group. Sedation in dentistry. The competent graduate. 2000.

Department of Health. Conscious Sedation in the Provision of Dental Care. Report of an Expert Group on Sedation for Dentistry. Commissioned by the Department of Health. 2003. www.dh.gov.uk

Society for the Advancement of Anaesthesia in Dentistry. Standards for conscious sedation. Report of an Expert Working Group Convened by the Society for the Advancement of Anaesthesia in Dentistry. October 2000.

Society for the Advancement of Anaesthesia in Dentistry and Dental Sedation Teachers Group. Conscious sedation. A referral guide for dental practitioners. September 2001.

White PF, Song D. New criteria for fast-tracking after outpatient anesthesia: A comparison with the modified Aldrete's Scoring System. Anesth Analg 1999;88:1069–1072.

http://www.med.unc.edu/radiology/Sedation/sedstudy.htm

TOP 150 DRUGS RESOURCES

ADA/PDR Guide to Dental Therapeutics, Fourth Edition. American Dental Association, 2006.

http://www.rxlist.com

http://www.drugs.com

ANEMIA RESOURCES

Benjamin LJ, Swinson GI, Nagel RL. Sickle cell anemia day hospital: an approach for the management of uncomplicated painful crises. Blood 2000;95:1130–1136.

Breymann C. Iron deficiency and anemia in pregnancy: modern aspects of diagnosis and therapy. Blood Cells, Molecules, and Diseases. Nov/Dec: 2002.

Conrad ME. Iron deficiency anemia. E Medicine 8 December 2004.

Raymond T. Anemia: diagnosis, treatment and prevention. Midwifery Today. 31 May 1999.

Schier SL. Approach to the adult patient with anemia. Up-to-Date, accessed in Jan 2006, last changed June 2005.

Scrimshaw N. Iron deficiency. Sci Amer 1991;Oct:46–52.

WHO Scientific Group on Nutritional Anaemias. Nutritional anaemias. Report of a WHO Scientific Group (meeting held in Geneva from March 13–17 1967). World Health Organization. Geneva, 1968.

www.nlm.nih.gov/medlineplus/sicklecellanemia.html

www.nlm.nih.gov/medlineplus/thalassemia.html

POLYCYTHEMIA RESOURCES

Anía B, Suman V, Sobell J, Codd M, Silverstein M, Melton L. Trends in the incidence of polycythemia vera among Olmsted County, Minnesota residents, 1935–1989. Am J Hematol 1994;47(2):89–93. PMID 8092146.

Berlin NI. Diagnosis and classification of polycythemias. Semin Hematol 1975;12:339.

Fjellner B, Hägermark O. Pruritus in polycythemia vera: treatment with aspirin and possibility of platelet involvement. Acta Derm Venereol 1979;59(6):505–512. PMID 94209.

Passamonti F, Malabarba L, Orlandi E, Baratè C, Canevari A, Brusamolino E, Bonfichi M, Arcaini L, Caberlon S, Pascutto C, Lazzarino M. Polycythemia vera in young patients: a study on the long-term risk of thrombosis, myelofibrosis and leukemia. Haematologica 2003;88(1):13–8. PMID 12551821.

Torgano G, Mandelli C, Massaro P, Abbiati C, Ponzetto A, Bertinieri G, Bogetto S, Terruzzi E, de Franchis R. Gastroduodenal lesions in polycythaemia vera: frequency and role of Helicobacter pylori. Br J Haematol 2002;117(1):198–202. PMID 11918555.

HEMOCHROMATOSIS RESOURCES

Alexander J, Kowdley KV. Hereditary hemochromatosis: genetics, pathogenesis, and clinical management. Ann Hepatol 2005;Oct–Dec;4(4):240–247.

Beutler E. Hemochromatosis: genetics and pathophysiology. Annu Rev Med 2006;57:331–347.

Kumar V, Abbas AK, Fausto N. Robbins and Cotran Pathologic Basis of Disease. 7th ed. St. Louis: W.B. Saunders; 2005:908–910.915–917.

Olynyk JK, et al. A population-based study of the clinical expression of the hemochromatosis gene. N Engl J Med 1999;Sep 2:341(10):75. PMID 10471457.

BLEEDING DISORDERS RESOURCES

Ball JH. Management of the anticoagulated dental patient. Compend Contin Educ Dent 1996;17:1100–1102,1104,1106 passim.

Blinder D, Manor Y, Martinowitz U, Taicher S, Hashomer T. Dental extractions in patients maintained on continued oral anticoagulant: comparision of local hemostatic modalities. Oral Surg Oral Med Oral Pathol Oral Radiol Endod 1999;88:137–140.

Crowther MA, Donovan D, Harrison L, McGinnis J, Ginsberg J. Low dose oral vitamin K reverses over-anticoagulation due to warfarin. Thromb Haemost 1998;79:1116–1118.

Devani P, Lavery KM, Howell CJ. Dental extractions in patients on warfarin: is alteration of anticoagulant regime necessary? Br J Oral Maxillofac Surg 1998;36:107–111.

Forbes CD, Barr RD, Reid G, et al. Tranexamic acid in control of haemorrhage after dental extraction in haemophilia and Christmas disease. BMJ 1972;2:311–313.

Gasper R, Brenner B, Ardekian L, Peled M, Laufer D. Use of tranexamic acid mouthwash to prevent postoperative bleeding in oral surgery patients on anticoagulant medication. Quintessence Int 1997;28:375–379.

Hirsh J, Dalen J, Anderson DR, et al. Oral anticoagulants: mechanism of action, clinical effectiveness, and optimal therapeutic range. Chest 2001;119(suppl 1):85–215.

Hylek EM, Heiman H, Skates SJ, Sheehan MA, Singer DE. Acetaminophen and other risk factors for excessive warfarin anticoagulation. JAMA 1998;279:657–662.

Jaffer A, Brotman D, Chukwumerije N. When patients on warfarin need surgery. Cleveland Clinic J of Med 2003;70(# 11):973–984.

Johnson-Leong C, Rada RE. The use of low-molecular-weight-heparins in outpatient oral surgery for patients receiving anticoagulation therapy. JADA 2002;1083–1087.

Koopman MM, Prandoni P, Piovella F, et al. Treatment of venous thrombosis with intravenous unfractioated heparin administered in the hospital as compared with subcutaneous low-molecular-weight heparin administered at home. The Tasman study group. N Engl J Med 1996;334:682–687.

Lack of a scientific basis for routine discontinuation of oral anticoagulation therapy before dental treatment. JADA 134:Nov 2003. www.dental.ufl.edu:1180/Offices/Endo/S04_07.doc

Martinowitz U, Sponitz WD. Fibrin tissue adhesives. Thromb Haemost 1997;78:661–666.

Parfitt K, ed. Martindale. The complete drug reference, 32nd ed. London: Pharmaceutical Press; 1999.

Scully C, Cawson RA. Medical Problems in Dentistry. 4th ed. Oxford, London, and Boston: Wright; Butterworth-Heinemann; 1997.

Scully C, Wolff A. Oral surgery in patients on anticoagulant therapy. Oral Surg Oral Med Oral Pathol Oral Radiol Endod 2002;94:57–64.

Silingardi M, Ghirarduzzi A, Tincani E, Iorio A, Iori I. Miconazole oral gel potentiates warfarin anticoagulant activity. Thromb Haemost 2000;83:794–795.

Sindet-Pedersen S, Stenbjerg S. Effect of local antifibrinolytic treatment with tranexamic acid in hemophiliacs undergoing oral surgery. J Oral Maxillofac Surg 1986;44:703–707.

Sindet-Pedersen S. Distribution of tranexamic acid to plasma and saliva after oral administration and mouth rinsing: a pharmacokinetic study. J Clin Pharmacol 1987;27:1005–1008.

Sindet-Pedersen S, Ramstrom G, Bernvil S, Blomback M. Hemostatic effect of tranexamic acid mouthwash in anticoagulant-treated patients undergoing oral surgery. N Engl J Med 1989;320:840–843.

Wahl MJ. Dental surgery in anticoagulated patients. Arch Intern Med 1998;158:1610–1616.

Wahl MJ. Myths of dental surgery in patients receiving anticoagulant therapy. J Am Dent Assoc 2000;131:77–81.

Walsh PN, Rizza CR, Matthews JM, et al. Epsilon-aminocaproic acid therapy for dental extractions in haemophilia and Christmas disease: a double blind controlled trial. Br J Haematol 1971;20:463–475.

Warketin TE, Levine MN, Hirsh J, et al. Heparin-induced thrombocytopenia in patients treated with low-molecular-weight heparin or unfractionated heparin. N Engl J Med 1995;332:1330–1335.

Weibert RT, Le DT, Kayser SR, Rapaport SI. Correction of excessive anticoagulation with low dose oral vitamin K1. Ann Intern Med 1997;126:959–962.

Wells PS, Holbrook AM, Crowther NR, Hirsh J. Interactions of warfarin with drugs and food. Ann Intern Med 1994;121:676–683.

White RH, McKittrick T, Hutchinson R, Twitchell J. Temporary discontinuation of warfarin therapy: changes in the international normalized ratio. Ann Intern Med 1995;122:40–42.

RHEUMATIC FEVER, BACTERIAL ENDOCARDITIS, AND PREMEDICATION RESOURCES

ADA, American Academy of Orthopaedic Surgeons. Advisory statement. Antibiotic prophylaxis for dental patients with total joint replacements. J Am Dent Assoc 1997;Jul;128(7):1004–1008.

ADA, American Academy of Orthopaedic Surgeons. Advisory statement. Antibiotic prophylaxis for dental patients with total joint replacement. J Am Dent Assoc 2003;Jul;134(7):895–859.

AHA. Prevention of Infective endocarditis. Guidelines from the American Heart Association. A Guideline from the American Heart Association Rheumatic Fever, Endocarditis, and Kaasaki Disease Committee, Council on Cardiovascular Disease in the Young, and the council on Clinical Cardiology, Council on Cardiovascular Surgery and Anesthesia, and the Quality of Care and Outcomes Research Interdisciplinary Working Group. Circulation 2007;DOI:10.1161/CIRCULATIONAHA.106.183095.

Dental premedication protocols for patients with knee and hip prostheses. N Y State Dent J. 2006 Apr–May;72(3):20–25. PMID 16774168. [PubMed—indexed for MEDLINE] ime.healthpartners.com/IME/Menu/0,1637,6267,00.html

Ferrieri P. Proceedings of the Jones criteria workshop. Circulation 2002;106:2521–2523.

Jones TD. The diagnosis of rheumatic fever. JAMA 1944;126:481–484.

HYPERTENSION/TIA/CVA/ANGINA/MI/KIDNEY DISEASE RESOURCES

AHA. Clinical Investigation and Reports: Is pulse pressure useful in predicting risk for coronary heart disease? Circulation 1999;100:354–360. © 1999 American Heart Association, Inc.

Albers GW. A review of published TIA treatment recommendations. Albers Neurol 2004;62: S26–S28.

Bertges DJ, Muluk V, Whittle J, Kelley M, MacPherson DS, Muluk SC. Relevance of carotid stenosis progression as a predictor of ischemic neurological outcomes. Arch Intern Med 2003;163:2285–2289.

Chobanian AV, Bakris GL, Black HR, et al., and the National High Blood Pressure Education Program Coordinating Committee. The Seventh Report of the Joint National Committee on Prevention, Detection, Evaluation, and Treatment of High Blood Pressure (JNC7). The JNC 7 Report. JAMA 2003;289:(doi:10.1001/jama.289.19.2560).

Josephson SA, Bryant SO, Mak HK, et al. Clinical practice. Transient ischemic attack. N Engl J Med. 2002 Nov 21;347(21):1687–1692. www.postgradmed.com/issues/2005/01_05/comm_gladstone.shtml

Neal B, MacMahon S, Chapman N. Effects of ACE inhibitors, calcium antagonists, and other blood-pressure-lowering drugs: results of prospectively designed overviews of randomised trials. Blood Pressure Lowering Treatment Trialists' Collaboration. Lancet 2000;356:1955–1964. [CrossRef][ISI][Medline]

Cushman WC, Ford CE, Cutler JA, Margolis KL, Davis BR, Grimm RH, et al. Success and predictors of blood pressure control in diverse North American settings: the antihypertensive and lipid-lowering treatment to prevent heart attack trial (ALLHAT). J Clin Hypertens (Greenwich) 2002;4:393–405. [Medline]

Ezzati M, Lopez AD, Rodgers A, Vander Hoom S, Murray CJ. Selected major risk factors and global and regional burden of disease. Lancet 2002;360:1347–1360. [CrossRef][ISI][Medline]

Janket SJ, Baird AE, Chuang SK, Jones JA. Meta-analysis of periodontal disease and risk of coronary heart disease and stroke. Oral Surg Oral Med Oral Pathol Oral Radiol Endod 2003;95(5):559–569. PMID 12738947.

Levey AS, Bosch JP, Lewis JB, et al. A more accurate method to estimate glomerular filtration rate from serum creatinine: A new prediction equation, Ann Int Med 1999;130:461–470.

Mosca L, Banka CL, Benjamin EJ, et al. Evidence-Based Guidelines for Cardiovascular Disease Prevention in Women: 2007 Update. Circulation.

Pearson TA, Mensah GA, Alexander RW, Anderson JL, Cannon RO III, Criqui M, Fadl YY, Fortmann SP, Hong Y, Myers GL, Rifai N, Smith SC, Jr, Taubert K, Tracy RP, Vinicor F. Markers of inflammation and cardiovascular disease: application to clinical and public health practice: A statement for healthcare professionals from the Centers for Disease Control and Prevention and the American Heart Association. Circulation 2003;107(3):499–511. PMID 12551878.

Pihlstrom BL, Michalowicz BS, Johnson NW. Periodontal diseases. Lancet 2005;366(9499):1809–1820. PMID 16298220.

Scannapieco FA, Bush RB, Paju S. Associations between periodontal disease and risk for atherosclerosis, cardiovascular disease, and stroke. A systematic review. Ann Periodontol 2003;8(1):38–53. PMID 14971247.

Spahr A, Klein E, Khuseyinova N, Boeckh C, Muche R, Kunze M, Rothenbacher D, Pezeshki G, Hoffmeister A, Koenig W. Periodontal infections and coronary heart disease: role of periodontal bacteria and importance of total pathogen burden in the coronary event and periodontal disease (CORODONT) study. Arch Intern Med 2006;166(5):554–559. PMID 16534043.

Transient ischemic attack: review for the emergency physician. Ann Emerg Med 2004 May;43(5):592–604. www.tripdatabase.com/spider.html?itemid=418471

Ulaki SD, Topinka MA, Frasser WR. The Accuracy of the Emergency Physician at Diagnosing CVA/TIA in the Acute Care Setting. Academic Emergency Medicine Volume 7, Number 10 1165, © 2000 Society for Academic Emergency Medicine.

Wilson AM, Ryan MC, Boyle AJ. The novel role of C-reactive protein in cardiovascular disease: risk marker or pathogen. Int J Cardiol 2006;106(3):291–297. PMID 16337036.

Zawada E. (1982). Renal consequences of nonsteroidal antiinflammatory drugs. Postgrad Med 71(5):223–230.

http://www.nhlbi.nih.gov/guidelines/hypertension/jnc7full.pdf

ATRIAL FIBRILLATION RESOURCES

ACC/AHA/ESC. Guidelines for the Management of Patients With Atrial Fibrillation. www.americanheart.org/downloadable/heart/222_ja20017993p_1.pdf

Levy S. Epidemiology and classification of atrial fibrillation. J Cardiovasc Electrophysiol 1998;9(8 Suppl):S78–S82. PMID 9727680.

Levy S. Classification system of atrial fibrillation. Curr Opin Cardiol 2000;15(1):54–57. PMID 10666661.

Prystowsky EN. Management of atrial fibrillation: therapeutic options and clinical decisions. Am J Cardiol 2000;85(10A):3D–11D.

ASTHMA RESOURCES

Jenkins C, Costello J, Hodge L. Systematic review of the prevalence of aspirin-induced asthma and its implications for clinical practice. BMJ 2004;328:434.

Leggett JJ, Johnson BT, Mills M, Gamble J, Heaney LG. Prevalence of gastroesophageal reflux in difficult asthma. Chest 2005;127(4):1227–1231.

Maddox L, Schwartz DA. The pathophysiology of asthma. Annu Rev Med 2002;53:477–498.

National Asthma Education and Prevention Program. Expert Panel Report: Guidelines for the Diagnosis and Management of Asthma. National Institute of Health, Bethesda, MD 1997;97–4051. (http://www.nih.gov/guidelines/asthma/asthgdln.pdf)

National Heart, Lung and Blood Institute. Diseases and Conditions Index. (http://www.nhlbi.nih.gov/health/dci/Diseases/Asthma/Asthma_Treatments.html)

Rodrigo GJ, Rodrigo C, Hall JB. Acute asthma in adults: a review. Chest 2004;125(3):1081–1102.

http://www.webmd.com/asthma/guide/lung-function-tests

COPD RESOURCES

http://www.nhlbi.nih.gov/health/dci/Copd/Copd_Treatments.html
http://www.nhlbi.nih.gov/health/dci/Diseases/Copd/Copd_KeyPoints.html

TUBERCULOSIS RESOURCES

American Thoracic Society/CDC. Targeted tuberculin testing and treatment of latent tuberculosis infection. Am J Respir Crit Care Med 2000;161:S221–S247. Available at http://www.cdc.gov/nchstp/tb/

CDC. Core curriculum on tuberculosis: what the clinician should know, 4th ed. Atlanta, GA: US Department of Health and Human Services, CDC. 2000. Available at http://www.cdc.gov/nchstp/tb/.

CDC. Update: Fatal and severe liver injuries associated with rifampin and pyrazinamide for latent tuberculosis infection, and revisions in American Thoracic Society/CDC recommendations—United States, 2001. MMWR 2001;50:733–735.

CDC. Centers for Disease Control and Prevention, Division of Tuberculosis Elimination. Core Curriculum on Tuberculosis: What the Clinician Should Know. 4th ed. (2000). Updated Aug 2003.

CDC. Treatment of Tuberculosis American Thoracic Society, CDC, and Infectious Diseases Society of America. MMWR 2003;52(RR11);1–77.

CDC. CDC Issues Guidelines on Use of QuantiFERON TB Gold Test MMWR Morb Mortal Wkly Rep. 2005;54(RR-15):49–55.

Food and Drug Administration, Center for Devices and Radiological Health. QuantiFERON®-TB—P010033 [Letter]. Rockville, MD: Food and Drug Administration, 2002. Available at http://www.fda.gov/cdrh/pdf/P010033b.pdf

Geiter LJ, ed. Ending neglect: the elimination of tuberculosis in the United States. Institute of Medicine, Committee on Elimination of Tuberculosis in the United States. Washington, DC: National Academy Press; 2000. Available at http://www.nap.edu/catalog/9837.html

Gostin LO. Controlling the resurgent tuberculosis epidemic: a 50 state survey of TB statutes and proposals for reform. JAMA 1993;269:255—261.

Horsburgh CR, Jr, Feldman S, Ridzon R. Practice guidelines for the treatment of tuberculosis. Clin Infect Dis 2000;31:633–639.

Jasmer RM, Saukkonen JJ, Blumberg HM, Daley CL, Bernardo J, Vittinghoff E, King MD, Kawamura LM, Hopewell PC. Short-course rifampin and pyrazinamide compared with isoniazid for latent tuberculosis infection: a multicenter clinical trial. Short-Course Rifampin and Pyrazinamide for Tuberculosis Infection (SCRIPT) Study Investigators. Ann Intern Med 2002;137:640–647.

Mazurek GH, LoBue PA, Daley CL, et al. Comparison of a whole-blood interferon gamma assay with tuberculin skin testing for detecting latent *Mycobacterium tuberculosis* infection. JAMA 2001;286:1740–1747.

Walley JD, Khan MR, Newell JN, Khan MH. Effectiveness of the direct observation component of DOTS for tuberculosis: a randomised controlled trial in Pakistan. Lancet 2001;357:664–669.

World Health Organization (WHO). Tuberculosis Fact sheet N°104—Global and regional incidence. March 2006, Retrieved on 6 October 2006.

World Health Organization (WHO). What is DOTS? A guide to understanding the WHO-recommended TB control strategy known as DOTS. WHO/CDS/CPC/TB/99.270. Geneva, Switzerland: World Health Organization; 1999. Available at http://www.who.int/gtb/dots

HERBAL RESOURCES

28 ADA Division of Communication. For the dental patient. How medications can affect your oral health. J Am Dent Assoc 2005;136;6:831. [Medline Link] [Context Link] www.co-pulmonarymedicine.com/pt/re/copulmonary/fulltext.00063198-200705000-00006.htm;jsessionid=GL1D2Z0fZ

Complementary & Alternative Medicine: Herbals, surgery, and anesthesia don't always mix. www.newsrx.com/newsletters/Pain-and-Central-Nervous-System-Week/2004-10-04.html

1698 JADA, Vol. 130, December 1999. Herbals May Interact With Anesthesia. jada.ada.org/cgi/reprint/130/12/1700.pdf

ENDOCRINOLOGY RESOURCES

Arlt W, Allolio B. Adrenal insufficiency. Lancet 2003;361:1881–1893.

Howlett TA. An assessment of optimal hydrocortisone replacement therapy. Clin Endocrinol 1997;46:263–268.

Lenart, BA. Atypical fractures of the femoral diaphysis in postmenopausal women taking alendronate. N Engl J Med 2008;358:1304–1306.

Lovas K, Loge JH, Husebye ES. Subjective health status in Norwegian patients with Addison's disease. Clin Endocrinol 2002;56:581–588.

Marx RE, Cillo JE, Ulloa JJ. Oral bisphosphonate-induced osteonecrosis: risk factors, prediction of risk using serum CTX testing, prevention, and treatment. J Oral Maxillofac Surg 2007;65;12:2397–2410.

Monson JP. The assessment of glucocorticoid replacement therapy. Clin Endocrinol 1997;46:269–270.

Peacey SR, Guo CY, Robinson AM, et al. Glucocorticoid replacement therapy: are patients over treated and does it matter? Clin Endocrinol 1997;46:255–261.

Ten S, New M, Maclaren N. Clinical review 130: Addison's disease 2001. J Clin Endocrinol Metab 2001;86:2909–2922.

http://www.endocrinology.org/education/resource/summerschool/2004/ss04/ss04_arl.htm

http://www.ada.org/prof/resourses/topics/osteonecrosis.asp

SEIZURES RESOURCES

www.mayoclinic.com/health/grand-mal-seizure/DS00222

www.mayoclinic.com/health/petit-mal-seizure/DS00216

GASTROINTESTINAL DISEASES RESOURCES

www.digestive.niddk.nih.gov/ddiseases/pubs/colitis/—30k

www.digestive.niddk.nih.gov/ddiseases/pubs/crohns/index

www.digestive.niddk.nih.gov/ddiseases/pubs/ibs/—34k

Geller JL, Adams JS. Proton pump inhibitor therapy and hip fracture risk. JAMA 2007;297:1429.

MedlinePlus. Riboflavin deficiency (ariboflavinosis). National Institute of Health. 2005.

Scully C. Apthous ulceration. NEJM 2006;355:165–172.

Scully C, Gorsky M, Lozada-Nur F. The diagnosis and management of recurrent aphthous stomatitis: a consensus approach. J Am Dent Assoc 2003;134:200–207.

Yang YX, Lewis JD, Epstein S, Metz DC. Long-term Proton Pump Inhibitor Therapy and Risk of Hip Fracture. *JAMA.* 2006;296:2947–2953.

http:// www.digestive.niddk.nih.gov/ddiseases/pubs/gerd/

http://www.cancer.gov/cancertopics/pdq/treatment/colon/patient

http://www.nlm.nih.gov/medlineplus/ulcerativecolitis

www.mayoclinic.com/health/peptic-ulcer/DS00242 2007

www.nlm.nih.gov/medlineplus/celiacdisease.html

HEPATITIS-CIRRHOSIS RESOURCES

AIDS Treatment Data Network. Liver Function Tests: A Simple Fact Sheet. Network www.atdn.org/simple/liverfun.html

Cohen JA, Kaplan MM. The SGOT/SGPT ratio—an indicator of alcoholic liver disease. Dig Dis Sci 1979;24:835–838.

Department of Health and Human Services. Center for Disease Control and Prevention. National Immunization Program.

Diehl AM, Potter J, Boitnott J, Van Duyn MA, Herlong HF, Mezey E. Relationship between pyridoxal 5'-phosphate deficiency and aminotransferase levels in alcoholic hepatitis. Gastroenterol 1984;86:632–636.

Goddard CJ, Warnes TW. Raised liver enzymes in asymptomatic patients: investigation and outcome. Dig Dis 1992;10:218–226.

Haber MM, West AB, Haber AD, Reuben A. Relationship of aminotranferases to liver histological status in chronic hepatitis C. Am J Gastroenterol 1995;90:1250.

Healey CJ, Chapman RW, Fleming KA. Liver histology in hepatitis C infection: a comparison between patients with persistently normal or abnormal transaminases. Gut 1995;37:274–278.

Kamath PS. Clinical approach to the patient with abnormal liver function test results. Mayo Clin Proc 1996;71:1089–1094.

Keeffe EB, Sunderland MC, Gabourel JD. Serum gamma-glutamyl transpeptidase activity in patients receiving chronic phenytoin therapy. Dig Dis Sci 1986;31:1056–1061.

Lieberman D, Phillips D. "Isolated" elevation of alkaline phosphatase: significance in hospitalized patients. J Clin Gastroenterol 1990;12:415–419.

Mendis GP, Gibberd FB, Hunt HA. Plasma activities of hepatic enzymes in patients on anticonvulsant therapy. Seizure 1993;2:319–323.

MMWR. Hepatitis A Vaccination Coverage Among Children Aged 24–35 Months—United States, 2003. MMWR 2005; 54(RR06);141–144.

MMWR. Prevention of Hepatitis A Through Active or Passive Immunization: Recommendations of the Advisory Committee on Immunization Practices (ACIP). MMWR 2006;55(No. RR-07).

Rothschild MA, Oratz M, Schreiber SS. Serum albumin. Hepatol 1988;8:385–401.

Sherman KE. Alanine aminotransferase in clinical practice. Arch Intern Med 1991;151:260–265.

Theal RM, Scott K. Evaluating asymptomatic patients with abnormal liver function test results. Am Fam Physician 1996;53:2111–2119.

Westwood A. The analysis of bilirubin in serum. Ann Clin Biochem 1991;28:119–130.

Whitfield JB, Pounder RE, Neale G, Moss DW. Serum gamma-glutamyl transpeptidase activity in liver disease. Gut 1972;13:702–708.

www.fda.gov/fdac/features/2001/401_hepc.

OCCUPATIONAL POSTEXPOSURE PROPHYLAXIS (PEP) RESOURCES

PEPline: http://www.ucsf.edu/hivcntr/Hotlines/PEPline
HIV/AIDS Treatment Information Service: http://aidsinfo.nih.gov
http://www.hopkins-aids.org

STD RESOURCES

CDC. CDC Guidelines for the Treatment of Sexually Transmitted Diseases: http://www.cdc.gov/nchstp/dstd.html

CDC. Update to CDC's Sexually Transmitted Diseases Treatment Guidelines, 2006: Fluoroquinolones No Longer Recommended for Treatment of Gonococcal Infections. MMWR April 13, 2007.

http://www.cdc.gov/std/healthcomm/fact_sheets.htm

HIV RESOURCES

Aguirre JM, Echebarria MA, Ocina E, Ribacoba L, Montejo M. Reduction of HIV-associated oral lesions after highly active antiretroviral therapy. Oral Surg Oral Med Oral Pathol Oral Radiol Endod 1999;88:114–115.

AHRQ. Management of Dental Patients Who Are HIV Positive. Rockville, Md: Agency for Healthcare Research and Quality; 2001. AHRQ publication 01–E041.

Ball SC, Sepkowitz KA, Jacobs JL. Thalidomide for treatment of oral aphthous ulcers in patients with human immunodeficiency virus: case report and review. Am J Gastroenterol 1997;92:169–170.

Bartlett JG. Serologic tests for the diagnosis of HIV infection, in UpToDate.

Bell DM. Occupational risk of human immunodeficiency virus infection in healthcare workers: an overview. Am J Med 1997;102(5B):9–15. PMID 9845490.

Benson C, Kaplan J, Masur H. Treating opportunistic infections among HIV-infected adults and adolescents: recommendations from CDC, the National Institutes of Health, and the HIV Medicine Association/Infectious Diseases Society of America. Clin Infect Dis 2005;40: S131.

Burgess JA, Johnson BD, Sommers E. Pharmacological management of recurrent oral mucosal ulceration. Drugs 1990;39(1):54–65.

Cassolato, SF, Turnbull RS. Xerostomia: Original Articles: Clinical Aspects and Treatment, Volume 20, No. 2. London: Blackwell Synergy-Geodontology.

Centers for Disease Control and Prevention (CDC). HIV/AIDS Surveillance Report. Atlanta: CDC; 2005.

Centers for Disease Control and Prevention: Guidelines for Preventing Opportunistic infections among HIV-infected persons—2002 Recommendations of the U.S. Public Health Service and the Infectious Disease Society of America. MMWR 2005;51RR-8:1–52.

Chen RY, Accortt NA, Westfall AO, et al. Distribution of health care expenditures for HIV-infected patients. Clin Infect Dis 2006;42L1003–10010.

Chou et al. Screening for HIV: A Review of the Evidence for the U.S. Preventive Services Task Force, Annals of Internal Medicine, Volume 143 Issue 1:55–73.

Farzadegan H, Vlahov D, Solomon L, Muñoz A, Astemborski J, Taylor E, Burnley A, Nelson K. Detection of human immunodeficiency virus type 1 infection by polymerase chain reaction in a cohort of seronegative intravenous drug users. J Infect Dis 1993;168(2):327–331. PMID 8335969.

Grimes RM, Lynch DP. Frequently asked questions about the oral manifestations of HIV/AIDS. JAMA HIV/AIDS Information Center. Accessed April 2000. http://www.ama-assn.org/special/hiv/treatmnt/updates/oral.htm#q2

Hare CB, Pappalardo BL, Busch MP, Phelps B, Alexander SS, Ramstead C, Levy JA, Hecht FM. Negative HIV antibody test results among individuals treated with antiretroviral therapy (ART) during acute/early infection. 2004. The XV International AIDS Conference: Abstract no. MoPeB3107.

HIVdent. Dental Treatment Considerations. Available at www.hivdent.org/DTC/dtctreat-men.htm

Jacobsen JM, Greenspan JS, Spritzler J, Ketter N, Fahey JL, Jackson JB, et al. Thalidomide for the treatment of oral aphthous ulcers in patients with human immunodeficiency virus infection. National Institute of Allergy and Infectious Diseases AIDS Clinical Trials Group. N Engl J Med 1997;336:1487–1493.

Joint United Nations Programme on HIV/AIDS. 2006. Overview of the global AIDS epidemic 2006 Report on the global AIDS epidemic (PDF format).

Joint United Nations Programme on HIV/AIDS. AIDS epidemic update, 2005 (PDF format).

Levine AM, Karim R, Mack W, et al. Neutropenia in human immunodeficiency virus infection: data from the women's interagency HIV study. Arch Intern Med 2006;166:405–410.

Leynaert B, Downs AM, de Vincenzi I. Heterosexual transmission of human immunodeficiency virus: variability of infectivity throughout the course of infection. European Study

Group on Heterosexual Transmission of HIV. Am J Epidemiol 1998;148(1):88–96. PMID 9663408.

Marks G, Crepaz N, Senterfitt JW, Janssen RS. Meta-Analysis of high risk sexual behavior in persons aware and unaware of their HIV status in the United States: implications for HIV prevention programs. J Acquir Immune Defic Syndr 2005;39:446.

McBride D. Management of aphthous ulcers. Am Fam Physician 2000;62:149–154,160.

Palella FJ, Jr, Delaney KM, Moorman AC, Loveless MO, Fuhrer J, Satten GA, Aschman DJ, Holmberg SD. Declining morbidity and mortality among patients with advanced human immunodeficiency virus infection. HIV Outpatient Study Investigators. N Engl J Med 1998;338(13):853–860. PMID 9516219.

Reeves JD, Doms RW. Human Immunodeficiency Virus Type 2. J Gen Virol 2002;83(Pt 6):1253–1265. PMID 12029140.

Ridzon R, Gallagher K, Ciesielski C, et al. Simultaneous transmission of human immunodeficiency virus and hepatitis C virus from a needle-stick injury. N Engl J Med 1997;336:919–922.

Seattle and King County Public Health Department. Update on the HIV Antibody Test Window Period.

Smith DK, Grohskopf LA, Black RJ, Auerbach JD, Veronese F, Struble KA, Cheever L, Johnson M, Paxton LA, Onorato IA, Greenberg AE. Antiretroviral Postexposure Prophylaxis After Sexual, Injection-Drug Use, or Other Nonoccupational Exposure to HIV in the United States. MMWR 2005;54(RR02):1–20.

Sullivan PS, Lansky A, Drake A. HITS-2000 Investigators. Failure to return for HIV test results among persons at high risk for HIV infection: results from a multistate interview project. J Acquir Immune Defic Syndr 2004;15;35:511–518.

Tappuni AR, Flemming GJ. The effect of antiretroviral therapy on the prevalence of oral manifestations in HIV-infected patients: a UK study. Oral Surg Oral Med Oral Pathol Oral Radiol Endod 2001;92:623–628.

UNAIDS/WHO. Policy Statement on HIV Testing (PDF). Accessed October 5, 2006.

Van de Perre P, Simonon A, Msellati P, Hitimana D, Vaira D, Bazubagira A, Van Goethem C, Stevens A, Karita E, Sondag-Thull D. Postnatal transmission of human immunodeficiency virus type 1 from mother to infant. A prospective cohort study in Kigali, Rwanda. N Engl J Med 1991;325(9):593–598. PMID 1812850.

Verpilleux MP, Bastuji-Garin S, Revuz J. Comparative analysis of severe aphthosis and Behçet's disease: 104 cases. Dermatol 1999;198:247–251.

www.projinf.org/indexS.html

ORAL LESIONS RESOURCES

Ball SC, Sepkowitz KA, Jacobs JL. Thalidomide for treatment of oral aphthous ulcers in patients with human immunodeficiency virus: case report and review. Am J Gastroenterol 1997;92:169–170.

Burgess JA, Johnson BD, Sommers E. Pharmacological management of recurrent oral mucosal ulceration. Drugs 1990;39(1):54–65.

Grimes RM, Lynch DP. Frequently asked questions about the oral manifestations of HIV/AIDS. JAMA HIV/AIDS Information Center. Accessed April 2000. http://www.ama-assn.org/special/hiv/treatmnt/updates/oral.htm#q2

Jacobsen JM, Greenspan JS, Spritzler J, Ketter N, Fahey JL, Jackson JB, et al. Thalidomide for the treatment of oral aphthous ulcers in patients with human immunodeficiency virus infection. National Institute of Allergy and Infectious Diseases AIDS Clinical Trials Group. N Engl J Med 1997;336:1487–1493.

McBride D. Management of Aphthous Ulcers. Am Fam Physician 2000;62:149–154,160.

Verpilleux MP, Bastuji-Garin S, Revuz J. Comparative analysis of severe aphthosis and Behçet's disease: 104 cases. Dermatol 1999;198:247–251.

PREGNANCY RESOURCES

Academy of General Dentistry. Pregnancy and Gingivitis. http://www.agd.org/consumer/topics/pregnancy/pregnancy_gingivitis.asp

American Academy of Periodontology. Baby Steps to a Healthy Pregnancy and On-Time Delivery. http://www.perio.org/consumer/pregnancy.htm

American Academy of Periodontology. Periodontal (Gum) Disease. http://www.ada.org/public/resources/glossary.asp#d

American Dental Association FAQs: Pregnancy. http://www.ada.org/public/topics/pregnancy_faq.asp

American Dental Association: Treating Periodontal Disease: Scaling and Root Planing. http://www.ada.org/prof/resources/pubs/jada/patient/patient_23.pdf

American Pregnancy Association: Pregnancy and Dental Work. http://www.americanpregnancy.org/pregnancyhealth/dentalwork.html

Cleveland Clinic. Dental Care During Pregnancy. http://www.clevelandclinic.org/health/health-info/docs/3200/3235.asp

Gaffield ML, Gilbert BJ, Malvitz DM, Romaguera R. Oral health during pregnancy: an analysis of information collected by the pregnancy risk assessment monitoring system. JADA 2001;Jul;132(7):1009–1016.

JADA, Feb 2001: An Update on Radiographic Practices: Information and Recommendations. http://www.ada.org/prof/resources/pubs/jada/reports/report_radiography.pdf

JAMA. Dental Radiography Study Bolsters ADA Recommendations. http://www.ada.org/prof/resources/pubs/adanews/adanewsarticle.asp?articleid=853

Jeffcoat MK, Geurs NC, Reddy MS, Cliver SP, Goldenberg RL, Hauth JC. Periodontal infection and preterm birth: results of a prospective study. JADA 2001;Jul;132(7):875–880.

Jeffcoat MK, Hauth JC, Geurs NC, Reddy MS, Cliver SP, Hodgkins PM, Goldenberg RL. Periodontal disease and preterm birth: results of a pilot intervention study. J Periodontol August 2003;(74, 8).

López NJ, Smith PC, Gutierrez. Higher risk of preterm birth and low birth weight in women with periodontal disease. J Dent Res 2002;81(1):58–63. http://jdr.iadrjournals.org/cgi/content/full/81/1/58

March of Dimes. Preterm Birth. http://www.marchofdimes.com/professionals/14332_1157.asp

Sanchez AR, Kupp LI, Sheridan PJ, Sanchez DR. Maternal chronic infection as a risk factor in preterm low birth weight infants: the link with periodontal infection. J Intl Acad Periodontol 2004;Jul;6(3):89–94.

MALIGNANT HYPERTHERMIA RESOURCES

Denborough MA, Ebeling P, King JO, Zapf PW. Myopathy and malignant hyperpyrexia. Lancet 1970;I:1138–1140.

Larach MG, for the North American Malignant Hyperthermia Group. Standardization of the caffeine halothane muscle contracture test. Anesth Analg 1989;69:511–515.

Malignant Hyperthermia Association of United States. www.mhaus.org/

Nelson TE, Flewellen EH. The malignant hyperthermia syndrome. New Eng J Med 1983;309:416–418. PubMed ID www.hkpp.org/physicians/mh_hyper.html

Nelson TE, Flewellen EH. Malignant hyperthermia: A pharmacogenetic disease of Ca^{++} regulating proteins. Curr Mol Med 2002;2:347–369.

PAGET'S DISEASE RESOURCES

Delmas PD, Meunier PJ. The management of Paget's disease of bone. N Engl J Med 1997;336:558.

Mayo Clinic. Paget's Disease of the Bone. Mayoclinic.com www.mayoclinic.com/health/**pagets-disease**-of-bone/DS00485

MedlinePlus. Paget's disease of Bone. www.nlm.nih.gov/medlineplus/**pagetsdisease**of-bone.html

GOUT RESOURCES

www.medicinenet.com/**gout**/article.htm

MedlinePlus: Gout and Pseudogout. www.nlm.nih.gov/medlineplus/**gout**andpseudo**gout**.html

POLYMYOSITIS AND DERMATOMYOSITIS RESOURCES

Amato AA, Barohn RJ. Idiopathic inflammatory myopathies. Neurol Clin 1997;Aug;15(3):615–648. [Medline]

Briani C, Doria A, Dalakas MC. Update on Idiopathic inflammatory myopathies. Autoimmunity May;2006;39(3):161–170. [Medline]

Christopher-Stine L, Plotz PH. Myositis: an update on pathogenesis. Curr Opin Rheumatol 2004;Nov;16(6):700–706. [Medline]

Dalakas MC, Hohlfeld R. Polymyositis and dermatomyositis. Lancet 2003;Sep 20;362(9388):971–982. [Medline]

Dalakas MC, Sivakumar K. The immunopathologic and inflammatory differences between dermatomyositis, polymyositis and sporadic inclusion body myositis. Curr Opin Neurol 1996;Jun;9(3):235–239. [Medline]

Oddis CV. Idiopathic inflammatory myopathies: a treatment update. Curr Rheumatol Rep 2003;Dec;5(6):431–436. [Medline]

Olsen NJ, Park JH. Inflammatory myopathies: issues in diagnosis and management. Arthritis Care Res 1997;Jun;10(3):200–207. [Medline]

Salomonsson S, Lundberg IE. Cytokines in idiopathic inflammatory myopathies. Autoimmunity May;2006;39(3):177–190. [Medline]

Schnabel A, Hellmich B, Gross WL. Interstitial lung disease in polymyositis and dermatomyositis. Curr Rheumatol Rep 2005;Apr;7(2):99–105. [Medline]

PARKINSON'S DISEASE RESOURCES

Nutt JG, Wooten GF. Supplement to: Diagnosis and initial management of Parkinson's disease. N Engl J Med 2005;353:1021–1027. content.nejm.org/cgi/content/full/353/10/1021/DC1

http://www.ninds.nih.gov/patients/disorder/parkinso/pdhtr.htm

MYASTHENIA GRAVIS RESOURCES

Juel VC. Myasthenia gravis: management of myasthenic crisis and perioperative care. Semin Neurol Mar;2004;24(1):75–81. [Medline]

Keesey JC. Clinical evaluation and management of myasthenia gravis. Muscle Nerve Apr;2004;29(4):484–505. [Medline]

Mehta S. Neuromuscular disease causing acute respiratory failure. Respir Care Sep;2006;51(9):1016–1021; discussion 1021–1023. [Medline]

National Institute of Neurological Disorders and Stroke. Myasthenia Gravis Fact Sheet. www.ninds.nih.gov/disorders/myasthenia_gravis/detail_myasthenia_gravis.htm

Palace J, Vincent A, Beeson D. Myasthenia gravis: diagnostic and management dilemmas. Curr Opin Neurol Oct;2001;14(5):583–589. [Medline]

Pascuzzi RM. The edrophonium test. Semin Neurol Mar;2003;23(1):83–88. [Medline]

Saperstein DS, Barohn RJ. Management of myasthenia gravis. Semin Neurol Mar;2004;24(1):41–8. [Medline]

Vincent A, Palace J, Hilton-Jones D. Myasthenia gravis. Lancet Jun;30;2001;357(9274):2122–2128. [Medline]

www.nlm.nih.gov/medlineplus/**myastheniagravis**.html

MULTIPLE SCLEROSIS RESOURCES

Chemaly D, Lefrançois A, Pérusse R. Oral and maxillofacial manifestations of multiple sclerosis. J Can Dent Assoc 2000;66:600–611.

Commins DJ, Chen JM. Multiple sclerosis: a consideration in acute cranial nerve palsies. Amer J Otol 1997;18:590–595.

Confavreux C, Hutchinson M, Hours MM, et al. Rate of pregnancy-related relapse in multiple sclerosis. Pregnancy in Multiple Sclerosis Group. N Engl J Med 1998 Jul;30;339(5):285–291. [Medline]

Dumas M, Pérusse R. Trigeminal sensory neuropathy: a study of 35 cases. Oral Surg Oral Med Oral Pathol Oral Radiol Endod 1999;87:577–582.

Durelli L, Verdun E, Barbero P, et al. Every-other-day interferon beta-1b versus once-weekly interferon beta-1a for multiple sclerosis: results of a 2-year prospective randomised multicentre study (INCOMIN). Lancet 2002;Apr;27;359(9316):1453–1460. [Medline]

Fukazawa T, Moriwaka F, Hamada K, Hamada T, Tashiro K. Facial palsy in multiple sclerosis. J Neurol 1997;244:631–633.

Goodin DS, Frohman EM, Garmany GP, et al. Disease modifying therapies in multiple sclerosis: report of the Therapeutics and Technology Assessment Subcommittee of the American Academy of Neurology and the MS Council for Clinical Practice Guidelines. Neurol 2002;Jan 22;58(2):169–178. [Medline]

Johnson KP, Brooks BR, Cohen JA, et al. Copolymer 1 reduces relapse rate and improves disability in relapsing-remitting multiple sclerosis: results of a phase III multicenter, double-blind placebo-controlled trial. The Copolymer 1 Multiple Sclerosis Study Group. Neurol 1995;Jul;45(7):1268–1276. [Medline]

Lublin FD, Whitaker JN, Eidelman BH, et al. Management of patients receiving interferon beta-1b for multiple sclerosis: report of a consensus conference. Neurol 1996;Jan;46(1):12–18. [Medline]

McDonald WI, Compston A, Edan G, et al. Recommended diagnostic criteria for multiple sclerosis: guidelines from the International Panel on the diagnosis of multiple sclerosis. Ann Neurol 2001;Jul;50(1):121–127. [Medline]

McGrother CW, Dugmore C, Phillips MJ, Raymond NT, Garrick P, Baird WO. Multiple sclerosis, dental caries and fillings: a case-control study. Br Dent J 1999;187:261–264.

Meaney JF, Watt JW, Eldridge PR, Whitehouse GH, Wells JC, Miles JB. Association between trigeminal neuralgia and multiple sclerosis: role of magnetic resonance imaging. J Neurol Neurosurg Psychiatry 1995;59:253–259.

Noseworthy JH, Lucchinetti C, Rodriguez M, Weinshenker BG. Multiple sclerosis. N Engl J Med 2000;Sep 28;343(13):938–952. [Medline]

Penarrocha Diago P, Bagan Sebastian JV, Alfaro Giner AA, Escrig Orenga VE. Mental nerve neuropathy in systemic cancer. Report of three cases. Oral Surg Oral Med Oral Pathol 1990;69:48–51.

PRISMS Study Group: Randomised double-blind placebo-controlled study of interferon beta-1a in relapsing/remitting multiple sclerosis. PRISMS (Prevention of Relapses and Disability by Interferon beta-1a Subcutaneously in Multiple Sclerosis) Study Group. Lancet 1998;Nov 7;352(9139):1498–1504. [Medline]

Sellebjerg F, Frederiksen JL, Nielsen PM, Olesen J. Double-blind, randomized, placebo-controlled study of oral, high-dose methylprednisolone in attacks of MS. Neurol 1998;Aug;51(2):529–534. [Medline]

Thompson AJ, Polman CH, Miller DH, et al. Primary progressive multiple sclerosis. Brain 1997;Jun;120(Pt 6):1085–1096. [Medline]

Vastag B. Not so fast: research on infectious links to MS questioned. JAMA 2001;Jan 17;285(3):279–281. [Medline]

Weiner HL, Hohol MJ, Khoury SJ, et al. Therapy for multiple sclerosis. Neurol Clin 1995;Feb;13(1):173–196. [Medline]

Weinshenker BG. The natural history of multiple sclerosis. Neurol Clin 1995;Feb;13(1):119–146. [Medline]

www.ninds.nih.gov/disorders/multiple_sclerosis/multiple_sclerosis.htm

HEAD AND NECK CANCERS RESOURCES

American Cancer Society. Cancer Facts and Figures 2006. Atlanta, GA: American Cancer Society; 2007.

Armitage JO. Treatment of non-Hodgkin's lymphoma. N Engl J Med 1993;328(14):1023–1030. [PUBMED Abstract]

Bastion Y, Sebban C, Berger F, et al. Incidence, predictive factors, and outcome of lymphoma transformation in follicular lymphoma patients. J Clin Oncol 1997;15(4):1587–1594. [PUBMED Abstract]

Browman GP, Wong G, Hodson I, et al. Influence of cigarette smoking on the efficacy of radiation therapy in head and neck cancer. N Engl J Med 1993;328(3):159–163. [PUBMED Abstract]

Cabanillas F, Velasquez WS, Hagemeister FB, et al. Clinical, biologic, and histologic features of late relapses in diffuse large cell lymphoma. Blood 1992;79(4):1024–1028. [PUBMED Abstract]

Close LG, Brown PM, Vuitch MF, et al. Microvascular invasion and survival in cancer of the oral cavity and oropharynx. Arch Otolaryngol Head Neck Surg 1989;115(11):1304–1309.

Consensus conference. Magnetic resonance imaging. JAMA 1988;259(14):2132–2138. [PUBMED Abstract]

Day GL, Blot WJ. Second primary tumors in patients with oral cancer. Cancer 1992;70(1):14–19. [PUBMED Abstract]

Jones KR, Lodge-Rigal RD, Reddick RL, et al. Prognostic factors in the recurrence of stage I and II squamous cell cancer of the oral cavity. Arch Otolaryngol Head Neck Surg 1992;118(5):483–485. [PUBMED Abstract]

Langendijk JA, de Jong MA, Leemans ChR, et al. Postoperative radiotherapy in squamous cell carcinoma of the oral cavity: the importance of the overall treatment time. Int J Radiat Oncol Biol Phys 2003;57(3):693–700. [PUBMED Abstract]

Lip and oral cavity. In: American Joint Committee on Cancer: The AJCC Cancer Staging Manual and Handbook. 6th ed. New York: Springer; 2002; pp 23–32. www.amazon.com/AJCC-Cancer-Staging-Manual-6th/dp/0387952713

Po Wing Yuen A, Lam KY, Lam LK, et al. Prognostic factors of clinically stage I and II oral tongue carcinoma—A comparative study of stage, thickness, shape, growth pattern, invasive front malignancy grading, Martinez-Gimeno score, and pathologic features. Head Neck 2002;24(6):513–520. [PUBMED Abstract]

Pui CH, Evans WE. Treatment of acute lymphoblastic leukemia. N Engl J Med 2006;354(2):166–178. [PUBMED Abstract]

Van der Tol IG, de Visscher JG, Jovanovic A, et al. Risk of second primary cancer following treatment of squamous cell carcinoma of the lower lip. Oral Oncol 1999;35(6):571–574. [PUBMED Abstract]

Yuen AR, Kamel OW, Halpern J, et al. Long-term survival after histologic transformation of low-grade follicular lymphoma. J Clin Oncol 1995;13(7):1726–1733. [PUBMED Abstract]

www.cancer.gov/cancertopics/types/hodgkins-lymphoma
www.cancer.gov/cancertopics/types/non-hodgkins-lymphoma

MULTIPLE MYELOMA RESOURCES

Alexanian R, Dimopoulos MA, Delasalle K, Barlogie B. Primary dexamethasone treatment of multiple myeloma. Blood 1992;Aug 15;80(4):887–890. [Medline]

Alyea EP, Anderson KC. Allogeneic bone marrow transplantation in the treatment of multiple myeloma. PPO Updates 2000;14:1–10.

Attal M, Harousseau JL, Stoppa AM, et al. A prospective, randomized trial of autologous bone marrow transplantation and chemotherapy in multiple myeloma. Intergroupe Francais du Myelome. N Engl J Med 1996;Jul 11;335(2):91–97. [Medline]

Barlogie B, Shaughnessy J, Munshi N, Epstein J. Plasma cell myeloma. In: Beutler E, Lichtman M, Coller B, Kipps T, Seligsohn U, eds. Williams Hematology (ed 6). New York: McGraw-Hill; 2001:1279–1304.

Billadeau D, Ahmann G, Greipp P, Van Ness B. The bone marrow of multiple myeloma patients contains B cell populations at different stages of differentiation that are clonally related to the malignant plasma cell. J Exp Med 1993;178:1023–1031.[Abstract]

Bloomfield DJ. Should bisphosphonates be part of the standard therapy of patients with multiple myeloma or bone metastases from other cancers? An evidence-based review. J Clin Oncol 1998;Mar;16(3):1218–1225. [Medline]

Cooper MR, Dear K, McIntyre OR, et al. A randomized clinical trial comparing melphalan/prednisone with or without interferon alfa-2b in newly diagnosed patients with multiple myeloma: a Cancer and Leukemia Group B study. J Clin Oncol 1993;Jan;11(1):155–160. [Medline]

Dimopoulos MA, Moulopoulos A, Smith T, et al. Risk of disease progression in asymptomatic multiple myeloma. Am J Med 1993;Jan;94(1):57–61. [Medline]

Gerull S, Goerner M, Benner A, et al. Long-term outcome of nonmyeloablative allogeneic transplantation in patients with high-risk multiple myeloma. Bone Marrow Transplant 2005;Dec;36(11):963–969. [Medline]

Kuehl WM, Bergsagel PL. Multiple myeloma: evolving genetic events and host interactions. Nat Rev Cancer 2002;2:175–187. [CrossRef][Medline]

Kumar A, Loughran T, Alsina M, et al. Management of multiple myeloma: a systematic review and critical appraisal of published studies. Lancet Oncol 2003;May;4(5):293–304. [Medline]

Kyle RA, Greipp PA. Plasma cell dyscrasias: current status. Crit Rev Oncol Hematol 1988;8(2):93–152. [Medline]

Kyle RA, Rajkumar SV. Multiple Myeloma. N Engld J Med 2004;351:1860–1873.

Kyle RA, Therneau TM, Rajkumar SV, et al. A long-term study of prognosis in monoclonal gammopathy of undetermined significance. N Engl J Med 2002;346:564–569. [Abstract]

Lokhorst HM, Sonneveld P, Cornelissen JJ, et al. Induction therapy with vincristine, adria-mycin, dexamethasone (VAD) and intermediate-dose melphalan (IDM) followed by autologous or allogeneic stem cell transplantation in newly diagnosed multiple myeloma. Bone Marrow Transplant 1999;Feb;23(4):317–322. [Medline]

Ludwig H, Fritz E, Kotzmann H, et al. Erythropoietin treatment of anemia associated with multiple myeloma. N Engl J Med 1990;Jun;14;322(24):1693–1699. [Medline]

Ludwig H, Kumpan W, Sinzinger H. Radiography and bone scintigraphy in multiple myeloma: a comparative analysis. Br J Radiol Mar;1982;55(651):173–181. [Medline]

Moreau P, Hullin C, Garban F, et al. Tandem autologous stem cell transplantation in high-risk de novo multiple myeloma: final results of the prospective and randomized IFM 99–04 protocol. Blood 2006;Jan 1;107(1):397–403, Epub 2005 Sep 6. [Medline]

Nordic Myeloma Study Group. Interferon-alpha 2b added to melphalanprednisone for initial and maintenance therapy in multiple myeloma. A randomized, controlled trial. The Nordic Myeloma Study Group. Ann Intern Med 1996;Jan 15;124(2):212–222. [Medline]

Ross ME, Zhou X, Song G, et al. Classification of pediatric acute lymphoblastic leukemia by gene expression profiling. Blood 2003;102:2951–2959. [Abstract/Free Full Text]

Samson D, Gaminara E, Newland A, et al. Infusion of vincristine and doxorubicin with oral dexamethasone as first-line therapy for multiple myeloma. Lancet 1989;Oct 14;2(8668):882–885. [Medline]

Schreiman JS, McLeod RA, Kyle RA, Beabout JW. Multiple myeloma: evaluation by CT. Radiology Feb;1985;154(2):483–486. [Medline]

Singhal S, Mehta J, Desikan R, et al. Antitumor activity of thalidomide in refractory multiple myeloma. N Engl J Med 1999;Nov 18;341(21):1565–1571. [Medline]

Van de Berg BC, Lecouvet FE, Michaux L, et al. Stage I multiple myeloma: value of MR imaging of the bone marrow in the determination of prognosis. Radiol Oct;1996;201(1):243–246. [Medline]

Yeoh EJ, Ross ME, Shurtleff SA, et al. Classification, subtype discovery, and prediction of outcome in pediatric acute lymphoblastic leukemia by gene expression profiling. Cancer Cell 2002;1:133–143. [CrossRef][Medline]

PSYCHIATRIC CONDITIONS RESOURCES

American Psychiatric Association Work Group on Eating Disorders. Practice guideline for the treatment of patients with eating disorders (revision). Amer J Psychiatry 2000;157(1 Suppl):1–39.

Andreasen NC, Arndt S, Alliger R, et al. Symptoms of schizophrenia. Methods, meanings, and mechanisms. Arch Gen Psychiatry 1995;May;52(5):341–351. [Medline]

Becker AE, Grinspoon SK, Klibanski A, Herzog DB. Eating disorders. N Engl J Med 1999;340(14):1092–1098.

Bruce B, Agras WS. Binge eating in females: a population-based investigation. Intl J Eating Disorders 1992;12:365–373.

Cummings JL, Frank JC, Cherry D, Kohatsu ND, Kemp B, Hewett L, et al. Guidelines for managing Alzheimer's disease: part I. Assessment. Am Fam Physician 2002;65:2263–2272.

Cummings JL, Frank JC, Cherry D, Kohatsu ND, Kemp B, Hewett L, et al. Guidelines for managing Alzheimer's disease: Part II. Treatment. Am Fam Physician 2002;2525–2534.

Davidson JR. Trauma: the impact of post-traumatic stress disorder. J Psychopharmacol 2000;14(2Suppl1):S5–S12.

De Deyn PP, Katz IR, Brodaty H, Lyons B, Greenspan A. Management of agitation, aggression, and psychosis associated with dementia: a pooled analysis including three randomized, placebo-controlled double-blind trials in nursing home residents treated with risperidone. Amer J Alzheimer's Dis & Other Dementias® 2006;21;2:101–108. DOI: 10.117 7/153331750602100209.© 2006 SAGE Publications.

Delagarza VW. Pharmacologic treatment of Alzheimer's disease: an update. Am Fam Physician 2003;68:1365–1372.

Frances A, Mack AH, Ross R, First, MB. 2000. The DSM-IV Classification and Psychopharmacology.

Kane JM. Schizophrenia. N Engl J Med 1996;Jan 4;334(1):34–41. [Medline]

Lagomasino I, Daly R, Stoudemire A. Medical assessment of patients presenting with psychiatric symptoms in the emergency setting. Psychiatr Clin North Am 1999;Dec; 22(4):819–850, viii–ix. [Medline]

Mintzer J, Greenspan A, Caers I, Van Hove I, Kushner S, Weiner M, Gharabawi G, Schneider LS, Am J Geriatr Psychiatry. Risperidone in the treatment of psychosis of Alzheimer disease: results from a prospective clinical trial. Amer J Geriatr Psychiatry 2006;Mar;14(3):280–291.

Small GW, Rabins PV, Barry PP, Buckholtz NS, DeKosky ST, Ferris SH, et al. Diagnosis and treatment of Alzheimer disease and related disorders. Consensus statement of the American Association for Geriatric Psychiatry, the Alzheimer's Association, and the American Geriatrics Society. JAMA 1997;278:1363–1371.

Spitzer RL, Yanovski S, Wadden T, Wing R, Marcus MD, Stunkard A, Devlin M, Mitchell J, Hasin D, Horne RL. Binge eating disorder: its further validation in a multisite study. Intl J Eating Disorders 1993;13(2):137–153.

Strober M, Freeman R, Lampert C, Diamond J, Kaye W. Controlled family study of anorexia nervosa and bulimia nervosa: evidence of shared liability and transmission of partial syndromes. Amer J Psychiatry 2000;157(3):393–401.

Sullivan PF. Mortality in anorexia nervosa. Amer J Psychiatry 1995;152(7):1073–1074.

www.nlm.nih.gov/medlineplus/**dementia**.html

ORGAN TRANSPLANT

Aker S, Ivens K, Guo Z, et al. Cardiovascular complications after renal transplantation. Transplant Proc 1998;Aug;30(5):2039–2042. [Medline] al-Asfari R, Fahdi L, Hadidy S, et al. Medical complications of renal transplantation. Transplant Proc 1999;Dec;31(8):3218. [Medline]

al-Aasfari R, Hadidy S, Yagan S. Infectious complications of kidney transplantation. Transplant Proc 1999;Dec; 31(8):3204. [Medline]

Hricik DE, Whalen CC, Lautman J, et al. Withdrawal of steroids after renal transplantation—clinical predictors of outcome. Transplantation 1992;Jan;53(1):41–45. [Medline]

Jordan ML, Shapiro R, Vivas CA, et al. The use of tacrolimus in renal transplantation. World J Urol 1996;14(4):239–242. [Medline]

Kozaki K, Takeuchi H, Hirano T, et al. Withdrawal or reduction of steroids based on pharmacodynamics assessed by antilymphocyte action after renal transplantation. Transplant Proc 1996;Jun;28(3):1300–1301. [Medline]

Kramer BK, Krager B, Mack M, et al. Steroid withdrawal or steroid avoidance in renal transplant recipients: focus on tacrolimus-based immunosuppressive regimens. Transplant Proc 2005;May;37(4):1789–1791. [Medline]

Levitsky J, Cohen SM. The liver transplant recipient: what you need to know for long-term care. J Fam Pract 2006;Feb;55(2):136–144. [Medline]

Mark W, Berger N, Lechleitner M, et al. Impact of steroid withdrawal on metabolic parameters in a series of 112 enteric/systemic-drained pancreatic transplants. Transplant Proc 2005;May;37(4):1821–1825. [Medline]

McCaughan GW, Koorey DJ. Liver transplantation. Aust N Z J Med 1997;Aug;27(4):371–378. [Medline]

Middleton PF, Duffield M, Lynch SV. Living donor liver transplantation—adult donor outcomes: a systematic review. Liver Transpl 2006 Jan;12(1):24–30. [Medline]

Morris, PJ. Transplantation—A medical miracle of the 20th century. N Engl J Med 2004;351:2678–2680. PMID 15616201.

Muñoz SJ. Long-term management of the liver transplant recipient. Med Clin North Am 1996;Sep;80(5):1103–1120. [Medline]

Oberholzer J, John E, Lumpaopong A, et al. Early discontinuation of steroids is safe and effective in pediatric kidney transplant recipients. Pediatr Transplant 2005;Aug;9(4):456–463. [Medline]

Ojo AO, Meier-Kriesche HU, Hanson JA, et al. Mycophenolate mofetil reduces late renal allograft loss independent of acute rejection. Transplantation 2000;Jun 15;69(11):2405–2409. [Medline]

Organ Procurement and Transplantation Network. Waiting list candidates: Liver. Transplants: Liver. Organ Procurement and Transplantation Network [website].

Perry I, Neuberger J. Immunosuppression: towards a logical approach in liver transplantation. Clin Exp Immunol 2005;Jan;139(1):2–10. [Medline]

Ponticelli C, Tarantino A, Montagnino G, Vegeto A. Use of steroids in renal transplantation. Transplant Proc 1999;Sep;31(6):2210–2211. [Medline]

Puig i Mari JM. Induction treatment with mycophenolate mofetil, cyclosporine, and low-dose steroids with subsequent early withdrawal in renal transplant patients: results of the Spanish Group. Spanish Group of the CellCept Study. Transplant Proc 1999;Sep;31(6):2256–2258. [Medline]

Shapiro R, Jordan ML, Scantlebury VP, et al. Tacrolimus in renal transplantation. Transplant Proc 1996;Aug;28(4):2117–2118. [Medline]

Tintinalli, JE. Liver transplantation. In: Emergency Medicine: A Comprehensive Study Guide. 5th ed. 2004:587–588.

Transplantation Proceedings. Tacrolimus in renal transplantation: a comparison of induction vs noninduction therapy (triple therapy): three-month results. Transplant Proc 1999;Feb–Mar;31(1–2):330–331. [Medline]

US Mycophenolate Mofetil Study Group. Mycophenolate mofetil for the prevention of acute rejection of primary cadaveric kidney transplants: status of the MYC 1866 study at 1 year. Transplant Proc 1997;Feb–Mar;29(1–2):348–349. [Medline]

Varon NF, Alangaden GJ. Emerging trends in infections among renal transplant recipients. Expert Rev Anti Infect Ther 2004;Feb;2(1):95–109. [Medline]

Index

Note: Page numbers followed by f indicate figures; page numbers followed by t indicate tables.